P9-APS-418

Skills Performance Checklists

for

Clinical Nursing Skills & Techniques

Skills Performance Checklists
for

Clinical Nursing Skills & Techniques

Perry, Potter, Ostendorf

*9*th
edition

ELSEVIER

ELSEVIER

3251 Riverport Lane
St. Louis, Missouri 63043

SKILLS PERFORMANCE CHECKLISTS FOR CLINICAL NURSING
SKILLS & TECHNIQUES, NINTH EDITION

ISBN: 978-0-323-48238-7

Copyright © 2018 by Elsevier Inc. All rights reserved.
Previous editions copyrighted 2014, 2010, 2006, 2002, 1998, 1994, 1990, 1986.

All rights reserved. No part of this publication may be reproduced or transmitted in any form or by any means, electronic or mechanical, including photocopying, recording, or any information storage and retrieval system, without permission in writing from the publisher, except that, until further notice, instructors requiring their students to purchase Skills Performance Checklists for Clinical Nursing Skills & Techniques by Anne Griffin Perry, Patricia A. Potter, and Wendy Ostendorf may reproduce the contents or parts thereof for instructional purposes, provided each copy contains a proper copyright notice as follows: Copyright © 2018 by Elsevier Inc.

Details on how to seek permission, further information about the Publisher's permissions policies, and our arrangements with organizations such as the Copyright Clearance Center and the Copyright Licensing Agency can be found at our website: www.elsevier.com/permissions.

This book and the individual contributions contained in it are protected under copyright by the Publisher (other than as may be noted herein).

Notices

Knowledge and best practice in this field are constantly changing. As new research and experience broaden our understanding, changes in research methods, professional practices, or medical treatment may become necessary.

Practitioners and researchers must always rely on their own experience and knowledge in evaluating and using any information, methods, compounds, or experiments described herein. In using such information or methods they should be mindful of their own safety and the safety of others, including parties for whom they have a professional responsibility.

With respect to any drug or pharmaceutical products identified, readers are advised to check the most current information provided (i) on procedures featured or (ii) by the manufacturer of each product to be administered, to verify the recommended dose or formula, the method and duration of administration, and contraindications. It is the responsibility of practitioners, relying on their own experience and knowledge of their patients, to make diagnoses, to determine dosages and the best treatment for each individual patient, and to take all appropriate safety precautions.

To the fullest extent of the law, neither the Publisher nor the authors, contributors, or editors assume any liability for any injury and/or damage to persons or property as a matter of products liability, negligence or otherwise, or from any use or operation of any methods, products, instructions, or ideas contained in the material herein.

Content Strategist: Tamara Myers
Content Development Manager: Jean Sims Fornango/Lisa Newton
Content Development Specialist: Melissa Rawe
Publishing Services Manager: Deepthi Unni
Project Manager: Manchu Mohan
Cover Designer: Muthukumaran Thangaraj

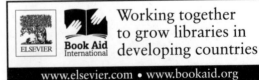

Working together
to grow libraries in
developing countries

www.elsevier.com • www.bookaid.org

Printed in the United States of America

Last digit is the print number: 9 8 7 6 5 4 3 2 1

Contents

Student _____ Date _____

Instructor _____ Date _____

PERFORMANCE CHECKLIST SKILL 2.1 **ADMITTING PATIENTS**

	S	U	NP	Comments

ROOM PREPARATION

1. Performed hand hygiene, prepared room equipment.

2. Ensured equipment is in working order, assembled any special equipment in patient's room.

ASSESSMENT

1. Identified patient using two identifiers.

2. Greeted patient and family by name, introduced self and job title, explained responsibilities in patient's care.

3. Arranged for translation service or speech and language pathologist if necessary.

4. Assessed patient's general appearance, noted signs or symptoms of physical distress.

5. Determined patient's ability to understand and implement health information.

6. Assessed patient's and family's psychological status by noting verbal and nonverbal behaviors and responses.

7. Assessed patient's vital signs, height and weight, and level of discomfort.

8. Assessed for fall risk using scale with grading criteria, considered patient's risk factors.

9. Had family or friends leave room unless patient wishes to have them assist with changing, provided privacy, helped patient undress, assisted patient into comfortable position.

10. Obtained nursing history as soon as possible, applied standards of nursing care adopted by hospital:

    a. Assessed patient's perception of illness and health care needs.

    b. Assessed patient's past medical history.

    c. Assessed presenting signs and symptoms and reason for hospitalization.

    d. Assessed the completed review of health status based on appropriate standards.

Copyright © 2018 by Elsevier Inc. All rights reserved.

	S	U	NP	Comments
e. Assessed risk factors for illness.	——	——	——	————————
f. Assessed history of allergies.	——	——	——	————————
g. Obtained detailed medication history.	——	——	——	————————
h. Assessed patient's knowledge of health problems and expectations of care.	——	——	——	————————
11. Conducted physical assessment of appropriate body systems.	——	——	——	————————
12. Checked health care providers' orders for treatment measures to initiate immediately.	——	——	——	————————
13. Asked patient to identify values regarding health care and expectations of care.	——	——	——	————————
14. Oriented patient to nursing division:				
a. Introduced staff members, introduced patient appropriately.	——	——	——	————————
b. Told patient and family the name of nurse manager, explained that person's role in solving problems.	——	——	——	————————
c. Explained visiting hours and their purpose.	——	——	——	————————
d. Discussed smoking policy, identified smoking areas if available.	——	——	——	————————
e. Demonstrated use of equipment.	——	——	——	————————
f. Showed patient nurse call light, positioned it near patient, had patient demonstrate use and call for assistance if needed.	——	——	——	————————
g. Escorted patient to bathroom if appropriate.	——	——	——	————————
h. Explained hours for mealtime.	——	——	——	————————
i. Described services available.	——	——	——	————————

PLANNING

1. Identified expected outcomes.	——	——	——	————————

IMPLEMENTATION

1. Completed patient medication reconciliation by checking home medication list, updated medication list based on health care provider's orders for treatment.	——	——	——	————————
2. Informed patient about upcoming procedures or treatments.	——	——	——	————————
3. Performed basic comfort measures and administered analgesic, removed and disposed of gloves.	——	——	——	————————
4. Completed learning needs assessment for patient and family.	——	——	——	————————

Copyright © 2018 by Elsevier Inc. All rights reserved.

	S	U	NP	Comments

5. Gave patient and family chance to ask questions about procedures or therapies.
　　___ 　___ 　___ 　_____

6. Collected valuables patient chooses to keep at facility, completed listing sheet, had patient or family sign it, placed values in safe or sent home with family.
　　___ 　___ 　___ 　_____

7. Ensured patient and family have time together alone if desired.
　　___ 　___ 　___ 　_____

8. Ensured call light is within reach and bed is in low position.
　　___ 　___ 　___ 　_____

9. Performed hand hygiene.
　　___ 　___ 　___ 　_____

EVALUATION

1. Had patient explain fall risks, hospital policies, tests, and procedures.
　　___ 　___ 　___ 　_____

2. Asked patient to rate severity of pain.
　　___ 　___ 　___ 　_____

3. Had patient demonstrate use of call light.
　　___ 　___ 　___ 　_____

4. Monitored patient's ability to ambulate independently.
　　___ 　___ 　___ 　_____

5. Checked patient's room setup regularly.
　　___ 　___ 　___ 　_____

6. Identified unexpected outcomes.
　　___ 　___ 　___ 　_____

RECORDING AND REPORTING

1. Recorded history and assessment findings in appropriate log, began to develop nursing plan of care.
　　___ 　___ 　___ 　_____

2. Placed advance directive in medical record if available.
　　___ 　___ 　___ 　_____

3. Notified health care provider of patient's arrival, reported unusual findings, secured admission orders if necessary.
　　___ 　___ 　___ 　_____

Copyright © 2018 by Elsevier Inc. All rights reserved.

Student _____ Date _____

Instructor _____ Date _____

PERFORMANCE CHECKLIST SKILL 2.2   **TRANSFERRING PATIENTS**

	S	U	NP	Comments
ASSESSMENT				
1. Identified patient using two identifiers.	—	—	—	_____
2. Obtained and reviewed transfer order from sending health care provider.	—	—	—	_____
3. Assessed reason for patient's transfer in collaboration with health care provider and appropriate team members.	—	—	—	_____
4. Assessed individuals at high risk for transitional care problems.	—	—	—	_____
5. Explained purpose of transfer, provided time to discuss patient's and family's feelings, obtained written consent if necessary.	—	—	—	_____
6. Assessed patient's current physical condition, determined method for transport.	—	—	—	_____
7. Assessed if patient requires pain relief or other medications.	—	—	—	_____
8. Ensured that staff have notified patient's family of transfer as desired by patient.	—	—	—	_____
PLANNING				
1. Identified expected outcomes.	—	—	—	_____
2. Arranged for patient's transport to an agency by chosen vehicle.	—	—	—	_____
3. Contacted new agency and arranged for bed in appropriate setting if necessary, confirmed willingness of agency to accept patient.	—	—	—	_____
IMPLEMENTATION				
1. Ensured patient's record is complete with individualized care plan.	—	—	—	_____
2. Completed nursing care transfer form appropriately.	—	—	—	_____
3. Completed medication reconciliation appropriately, checked patient's current orders against most recent MAR and original medication list, communicated updated medication list to next provider of care.	—	—	—	_____
4. Had NAP gather and secure patient's personal items, checked entire room and storage areas.	—	—	—	_____

Copyright © 2018 by Elsevier Inc. All rights reserved.

	S	U	NP	Comments

5. Anticipated problems patient may develop before or during transfer, performed necessary therapies.

       —   —   —   _____

6. Assisted in transferring patient safely to stretcher or wheelchair.

       —   —   —   _____

7. Performed and documented final assessment of patient's physical stability.

       —   —   —   _____

8. Accompanied patient to transport vehicle.

       —   —   —   _____

9. Called receiving agency and notified of transfer and patient's status.

       —   —   —   _____

EVALUATION

1. Compared data with previous findings during final assessment.

       —   —   —   _____

2. Inspected patient's alignment and positioning on wheelchair or stretcher.

       —   —   —   _____

3. Ensured equipment for transfer is functioning.

       —   —   —   _____

4. Confirmed patient understands transfer and procedures.

       —   —   —   _____

5. Determined if receiving agency had questions about patient's care.

       —   —   —   _____

6. Identified unexpected outcomes.

       —   —   —   _____

RECORDING AND REPORTING

1. Documented pertinent information if sending patient.

       —   —   —   _____

2. Documented pertinent information if receiving patient.

       —   —   —   _____

Copyright © 2018 by Elsevier Inc. All rights reserved.

Student _____   Date _____

Instructor _____   Date _____

PERFORMANCE CHECKLIST SKILL 2.3   **DISCHARGING PATIENTS**

	S	U	NP	Comments

ASSESSMENT

1. Identified patient using two identifiers.

2. Assessed patient's discharge needs from time of admission, used care plan to focus on ongoing assessments needed.

3. Identified risk factors that may increase risk of patient being readmitted after discharge.

4. Assessed patient's and family's learning needs related to home care, asked patient and family to identify concerns about discharge.

5. Assessed for barriers to learning and patient's health literacy.

6. Assessed for environmental factors within home that interfere with self-care.

7. Assessed patient's anticipated needs after discharge and eligibility for home care reimbursement.

8. Assessed patient's and family's perceptions of health care needs outside the hospital, assessed family caregivers' perceived ability to provide care.

9. Assessed patient's acceptance of health problems.

PLANNING

1. Identified expected outcomes.

IMPLEMENTATION

1. Prepared before day of discharge:

   a. Discussed with patient and family arranging the home to suit patient needs.

   b. Provided patient and family with information about community health care resources.

   c. Conducted teaching lessons with patient and family as soon as possible, reviewed and gave patient discharge materials, referred patient to appropriate Internet resources.

   d. Communicated patient's and family's response to teaching and discharge plans to other team members.

6

Copyright © 2018 by Elsevier Inc. All rights reserved.

	S	U	NP	Comments

2. Performed procedures on day of discharge:

   a. Encouraged patient and family to ask questions and discuss home care.

   b. Checked health care provider's discharge orders for prescriptions, treatment changes, or need for special equipment, arranged for delivery and setup of equipment before patient arrival.

   c. Determined whether patient or family has arranged for transportation.

   d. Provided privacy, assisted as patient dressed and packed personal belongings, checked closets and drawers, obtained copy of valuables list and had items delivered to patient.

   e. Completed medication reconciliation appropriately, checked discharge medication order against MAR and home medication list, provided patient with prescriptions or medications ordered, offered final review of information.

   f. Provided information on follow-up appointments to health care provider's office.

   g. Contacted agency's business office to determine patient need to finalize payment arrangements, arranged for patient or family to visit business office.

   h. Acquired utility cart to move belongings, obtained wheelchair or stretcher for patient.

   i. Assisted patient to wheelchair or stretcher properly, escorted patient to transportation, locked wheelchair wheels, assisted patient and belongings into vehicle.

   j. Returned to divisions, notified appropriate groups of time of discharge, notified housekeeping to clean patient's room.

EVALUATION

1. Asked patient or family member to describe nature of illness, treatment, and symptoms to be reported.

2. Had patient or family members perform any treatments that will continue at home.

3. If a home care nurse, inspected home, identified obstacles, and recommended revisions.

4. Identified unexpected outcomes.

Copyright © 2018 by Elsevier Inc. All rights reserved.

	S	U	NP	Comments

RECORDING AND REPORTING

1. Completed discharge summary form, provided patient with a signed copy. ___ ___ ___ _____

2. Documented unresolved problems and description of arrangements made for resolution in appropriate log. ___ ___ ___ _____

3. Documented patient's vitals and status of health problems at time of discharge in nurses' notes. ___ ___ ___ _____

Copyright © 2018 by Elsevier Inc. All rights reserved.

Student _____ Date _____

Instructor _____ Date _____

PERFORMANCE CHECKLIST SKILL 3.1 **ESTABLISHING THE NURSE-PATIENT RELATIONSHIP**

	S	U	NP	Comments

ASSESSMENT

1. Formulated patient goals and assessment questions.

2. Addressed patient by name, introduced self and role, used clear specific communication.

3. Assessed patient's needs, coping strategies, defenses, and adaptation styles.

4. Assessed patient's need to communicate.

5. Assessed reason patient needs health care.

6. Assessed factors about self and patient that normally influence communication.

7. Assessed personal barriers to communicating with patient.

8. Assessed patient's language and ability to speak.

9. Assessed patient's literacy level.

10. Assessed patient's ability to hear, ensured hearing aid is functional if worn, ensured patient hears and understands words.

11. Observed patient's pattern of communication and verbal or nonverbal behavior.

12. Assessed resources available in selecting communication methods.

13. Assessed patient's readiness to work toward goal attainment.

14. Considered when patient is due to be discharged or transferred.

PLANNING

1. Identified expected outcomes.

2. Prepared patient physically, maintained privacy, and reduced distractions.

3. Planned working phase appropriately.

IMPLEMENTATION

1. Observed patient's nonverbal behaviors, sought clarification where needed.

Copyright © 2018 by Elsevier Inc. All rights reserved.

	S	U	NP	Comments

2. Explained purpose of interaction when information was being shared. ⎯ ⎯ ⎯ _____

3. Continued therapeutic communication skills. ⎯ ⎯ ⎯ _____

4. Identified patient's expectations in seeking health care. ⎯ ⎯ ⎯ _____

5. Encouraged patient to ask for clarification at any time. ⎯ ⎯ ⎯ _____

6. Set mutual goals:

   a. Used therapeutic communication skills. ⎯ ⎯ ⎯ _____

   b. Discussed and prioritized problem areas. ⎯ ⎯ ⎯ _____

   c. Provided information to patient, helped patient express needs and feelings. ⎯ ⎯ ⎯ _____

   d. Used questions carefully and appropriately, asked one question at a time, used direct questions and open-ended statements as much as possible. ⎯ ⎯ ⎯ _____

   e. Avoided communication barriers. ⎯ ⎯ ⎯ _____

7. Communicated with patient during termination phase:

   a. Prepared methods of summarizing information pertinent for patient's aftercare. ⎯ ⎯ ⎯ _____

   b. Used therapeutic communication skills to discuss discharge or termination issues, guided discussion to patient changes in thoughts and behaviors. ⎯ ⎯ ⎯ _____

   c. Summarized with patient what was discussed during the interaction. ⎯ ⎯ ⎯ _____

EVALUATION

1. Observed patient's verbal and nonverbal responses to communication, noted patient's willingness to share information and concerns. ⎯ ⎯ ⎯ _____

2. Noted your response to patient and patient's response to you, reflected on effectiveness of techniques. ⎯ ⎯ ⎯ _____

3. Evaluated patient's ability to work toward identifiable goals, reevaluated and identified barriers if patient goals are not met. ⎯ ⎯ ⎯ _____

4. Summarized and restated goals, reinforced patient strengths, outlined issues requiring work, developed an action plan. ⎯ ⎯ ⎯ _____

5. Identified unexpected outcomes. ⎯ ⎯ ⎯ _____

Copyright © 2018 by Elsevier Inc. All rights reserved.

RECORDING AND REPORTING

	S	U	NP	Comments
1. Recorded pertinent communication, responses to illness or therapies, and responses that demonstrate understanding or lack thereof.	___	___	___	_____
2. Reported relevant information to team members.	___	___	___	_____

Copyright © 2018 by Elsevier Inc. All rights reserved.

Student _____ Date _____

Instructor _____ Date _____

PERFORMANCE CHECKLIST SKILL 3.2 **COMMUNICATING WITH PATIENTS WHO HAVE DIFFICULTY COPING**

	S	U	NP	Comments
ASSESSMENT				
1. Introduced self appropriately, explained purpose of interaction.	___	___	___	_____
2. Assessed factors influencing communication with patient.	___	___	___	_____
3. Assessed for possible factors causing patient anxiety.	___	___	___	_____
4. Discussed with family possible causes of patient's anxiety.	___	___	___	_____
5. Observed for physical, behavioral, and verbal cues that indicate patient is anxious.	___	___	___	_____
6. Observed for physical, behavioral, and verbal cues that indicate patient is depressed.	___	___	___	_____
7. Assessed for possible factors causing patient's depression.	___	___	___	_____
8. Observed for behaviors that indicate the patient is angry.	___	___	___	_____
9. Assessed factors that influence angry patient's communication.	___	___	___	_____
10. Assessed for resources available to help in communicating with potentially violent patient.	___	___	___	_____
11. Assessed for underlying medical condition that may potentially lead to violent behavior.	___	___	___	_____
PLANNING				
1. Identified expected outcomes.	___	___	___	_____
2. Prepared for communication by considering patient goals, time allocation, and resources.	___	___	___	_____
3. Recognized personal level of anxiety, tried to remain calm.	___	___	___	_____
4. Prepared a quiet, calm area; allowed ample personal space.	___	___	___	_____
5. Prepared for de-escalation for an angry patient:				
a. Paused to collect thoughts and feelings.	___	___	___	_____
b. Determined what patient is saying.	___	___	___	_____

Copyright © 2018 by Elsevier Inc. All rights reserved.

	S	U	NP	Comments

c. Prepared environment to de-escalate a potentially violent patient by removing people or factors that provoke anger, maintaining an open exit, and providing privacy.

IMPLEMENTATION

1. Used appropriate nonverbal behaviors and active listening skills, focused on understanding patient's issues.

2. Used appropriate verbal techniques that are clear and concise in responses, acknowledged patient's feelings, provided direction to patient.

3. Helped patient acquire alternative coping strategies.

4. Provided necessary comfort measures.

5. Used open-ended questions.

6. Encouraged and rewarded small decision, made decisions patient is not ready to make.

7. Accepted patient as he or she is, focused on positive feedback, provided positive decision making.

8. Showed honesty and empathy.

9. De-escalated an angry patient appropriately:

   a. Maintained personal space and an open exit, positioned self between patient and exit.

   b. Maintained nonthreatening approach with a calm voice, open body language, and deliberate gestures.

   c. Used therapeutic silence, allowed patient to vent, used active listening.

   d. Responded to anger therapeutically, encouraged verbal expression of anger.

   e. Answered questions calmly and honestly, informed patient of potential consequences and followed through if necessary.

   f. Responded professionally and set limits if patient makes verbal threats to harm others.

   g. Explored alternatives to anger when patient is calm.

EVALUATION

1. Observed for continuing presence of signs and behaviors reflecting anxiety, anger, or depression.

2. Asked patient to describe ways to cope with anxiety, anger, or depression.

Copyright © 2018 by Elsevier Inc. All rights reserved.

	S	U	NP	Comments

3. Evaluated patient's ability to discuss factors causing anxiety, anger, or depression. ⸺ ⸺ ⸺ _____

4. Noted patient's ability to answer questions and problem solve. ⸺ ⸺ ⸺ _____

5. Asked patient to discuss ways to cope in the future and make decisions about own care. ⸺ ⸺ ⸺ _____

6. Identified unexpected outcomes. ⸺ ⸺ ⸺ _____

RECORDING AND REPORTING

1. Recorded cause of patient's anxiety, anger, or depression and any exhibited behaviors. ⸺ ⸺ ⸺ _____

2. Recorded de-escalation techniques used and patient's response. ⸺ ⸺ ⸺ _____

3. Reported methods used to relieve anxiety, anger, and depression and patient's response. ⸺ ⸺ ⸺ _____

Copyright © 2018 by Elsevier Inc. All rights reserved.

Student _____ Date _____

Instructor _____ Date _____

PERFORMANCE CHECKLIST SKILL 3.3 **COMMUNICATING WITH A COGNITIVELY IMPAIRED PATIENT**

	S	U	NP	Comments
ASSESSMENT				
1. Approached patient from the front; assessed physical, behavioral, and verbal cues; assessed orientation status of patient and performed mini-mental examination.	___	___	___	_____
2. Assessed for possible factors causing patient's cognitive impairment.	___	___	___	_____
3. Assessed factors influencing communication with patient.	___	___	___	_____
4. Discussed possible causes of patient's cognitive impairment with family and caregivers.	___	___	___	_____
5. Discussed with family how patient typically communicates with them.	___	___	___	_____
6. Ascertained most effective means of communication with patient.	___	___	___	_____
PLANNING				
1. Identified expected outcomes.	___	___	___	_____
2. Considered type of cognitive impairment, communication impairments, time allocation, and resources.	___	___	___	_____
3. Remained nonjudgmental and aware of own nonverbal cues.	___	___	___	_____
4. Provided a calm environment and reduced distractions.	___	___	___	_____
IMPLEMENTATION				
1. Approached patient from the front.	___	___	___	_____
2. Introduced self, explained purpose of interaction.	___	___	___	_____
3. Used appropriate nonverbal behaviors and active listening skills.	___	___	___	_____
4. Used clear and concise verbal techniques to respond to depressed patient, asked yes-or-no questions.	___	___	___	_____
5. Asked questions one at a time, allowed time for response.	___	___	___	_____
6. Repeated sentences using a steady voice, avoided being too quick to guess patient response.	___	___	___	_____

Copyright © 2018 by Elsevier Inc. All rights reserved.

	S	U	NP	Comments

7. Used assistive and augmentative devices to facilitate communication. ___ ___ ___ _____

8. Provided assistive devices such as eyeglasses or hearing aids. ___ ___ ___ _____

9. Did not argue with or correct patient. ___ ___ ___ _____

10. Maintained meaningful interactions with patient, used creative modes of communication based on patient's comfort and ability. ___ ___ ___ _____

11. Used individualized coping strategies. ___ ___ ___ _____

EVALUATION

1. Observed for clarity and understanding of messages sent and received. ___ ___ ___ _____

2. Observed verbal and nonverbal behaviors. ___ ___ ___ _____

3. Identified unexpected outcomes. ___ ___ ___ _____

RECORDING AND REPORTING

1. Recorded objective and subjective behaviors in nurses' notes. ___ ___ ___ _____

2. Recorded and reported methods used to communicate and patient's response. ___ ___ ___ _____

16

Copyright © 2018 by Elsevier Inc. All rights reserved.

Student _____ Date _____

Instructor _____ Date _____

PERFORMANCE CHECKLIST SKILL 3.4 **COMMUNICATION WITH COLLEAGUES**

	S	U	NP	Comments
ASSESSMENT				
1. Identified purpose of interaction with colleague.	___	___	___	_____
2. Assessed factors influencing communication with others.	___	___	___	_____
3. Considered level of stress in the situation.	___	___	___	_____
PLANNING				
1. Prepared for communication with team members who may have differing needs or concerns.	___	___	___	_____
2. Remained nonjudgmental and aware of own nonverbal cues.	___	___	___	_____
3. Prepared a quiet, calm environment; reduced distractions.	___	___	___	_____
4. Maintained awareness of hierarchical differences as a barrier to communication.	___	___	___	_____
IMPLEMENTATION				
1. Approached colleague from the front, maintained appropriate eye contact.	___	___	___	_____
2. Provided appropriate introduction, explained purpose of interaction.	___	___	___	_____
3. Maintained awareness of body language and tone.	___	___	___	_____
4. Acknowledged and responded to a range of views, allowed equal time for all parties to participate.	___	___	___	_____
5. Used appropriate oral communication skills and active listening, provided feedback and asked for clarification when necessary.	___	___	___	_____
6. Used a range of workplace written communication methods.	___	___	___	_____
7. Encouraged discussion positive and negative feelings.	___	___	___	_____
8. Summarized key themes, helped to develop solutions to the issue.	___	___	___	_____

Copyright © 2018 by Elsevier Inc. All rights reserved.

	S	U	NP	Comments
EVALUATION				
1. Confirmed clarity and understanding of messages.	___	___	___	_____
2. Observed verbal and nonverbal behaviors.	___	___	___	_____
3. Identified unexpected outcomes.	___	___	___	_____
RECORDING AND REPORTING				
1. Recorded successful communication strategies and pertinent changes to patient's plan of care.	___	___	___	_____

Copyright © 2018 by Elsevier Inc. All rights reserved.

Student _____ Date _____

Instructor _____ Date _____

PERFORMANCE CHECKLIST PROCEDURAL GUIDELINE 4.1   **GIVING A HAND-OFF REPORT**

	S	U	NP	Comments
PLANNING				
1. Gathered necessary equipment.	___	___	___	_____
PROCEDURAL STEPS				
1. Implemented an organized format for delivering an appropriate description of patient's needs and problems.	___	___	___	_____
2. Identified electronic patient record using two identifiers.	___	___	___	_____
3. Gathered information from relevant documents.	___	___	___	_____
4. Prioritized information based on patient's needs and problems.	___	___	___	_____
5. Included SBAR documentation in report:				
a. Situation: Patient's name, gender, age, complaints on admission, and current situation.	___	___	___	_____
b. Background information: Allergies, code status, history, special needs, and vaccinations.	___	___	___	_____
c. Assessment data: Objective data from shift with emphasis on changes.	___	___	___	_____
d. Recommendations: Explanation of priorities for oncoming nurse.	___	___	___	_____
6. Asked staff from oncoming shift if they have questions regarding information provided.	___	___	___	_____

Copyright © 2018 by Elsevier Inc. All rights reserved.

Student _____ Date _____

Instructor _____ Date _____

PERFORMANCE CHECKLIST PROCEDURAL GUIDELINE 4.2 **DOCUMENTING NURSES' PROGRESS NOTES**

	S	U	NP	Comments

PLANNING

1. Gathered necessary equipment. ___ ___ ___ _____

PROCEDURAL STEPS

1. Identified patient record using at least two identifiers. ___ ___ ___ _____

2. Reviewed assessment data, problems identified, expected outcomes, nursing interventions, and patient response. ___ ___ ___ _____

3. Documented patient information in the appropriate log, followed charting guidelines. ___ ___ ___ _____

4. Identified information to be documented after patient contact. ___ ___ ___ _____

5. Documented in a timely and orderly fashion, included date and time. ___ ___ ___ _____

6. Documented objective data, select subjective data, nursing actions taken, patient responses, additional plans to be implemented, and to whom information was reported. ___ ___ ___ _____

7. Signed progress note appropriately, indicated level of education and school if you are a student. ___ ___ ___ _____

8. Reviewed previously documented entries with own entries, noted significant changes in patient's status, reported any such changes to patient's health care provider. ___ ___ ___ _____

Copyright © 2018 by Elsevier Inc. All rights reserved.

Student _____ Date _____

Instructor _____ Date _____

PERFORMANCE CHECKLIST PROCEDURAL GUIDELINE 4.3 **ADVERSE EVENT REPORTING**

	S	U	NP	Comments
PLANNING				
1. Gathered necessary equipment.	___	___	___	_____
PROCEDURAL STEPS				
1. Identified the electronic patient record using at least two identifiers.	___	___	___	_____
2. Determined what was involved in the incident and reported exact events appropriately, notified risk management as necessary.	___	___	___	_____
3. Assessed extent of injury to patient or others, included subjective and objective findings.	___	___	___	_____
4. Took steps to restore individual's safety.	___	___	___	_____
5. Called health care provider.	___	___	___	_____
6. Referred injured visitors or staff to emergency department.	___	___	___	_____
7. Completed adverse event report form:				
a. Recorded objective information about the incident, included victim interpretations in quotes.	___	___	___	_____
b. Objectively described patient's or staff member's condition when incident was discovered or observed.	___	___	___	_____
c. Described measures taken by caretakers at the time.	___	___	___	_____
d. Sent completed report to designated department.	___	___	___	_____
8. Documented events in patient's chart when patient is involved:				
a. Entered only objective description.	___	___	___	_____
b. Recorded assessment or intervention activities initiated as result of the event.	___	___	___	_____
c. Did not duplicate all information from report.	___	___	___	_____
d. Did not record that report was completed.	___	___	___	_____
9. Submitted report properly with risk management department or designated persons.	___	___	___	_____

Copyright © 2018 by Elsevier Inc. All rights reserved.

Student _____ Date _____

Instructor _____ Date _____

GUIDELINES FOR MEANINGFUL USE OF AN ELECTRONIC HEALTH RECORDS (EHR)

	S	U	NP	Comments

PLANNING
1. Identified purpose of interaction with colleague. ___ ___ ___ _____

PROCEDURAL STEPS
1. Used organized format for medical reconciliation. ___ ___ ___ _____

2. Identified electronic patient record using two identifiers. ___ ___ ___ _____

3. Gathered information from electronic documentation sources. ___ ___ ___ _____

4. Included two nurses to complete medication reconciliation at time of care transition, assessed current medications, compared to medications on admission if patient is going to be discharged. ___ ___ ___ _____

5. Assessed discrepancies with two nurses. ___ ___ ___ _____

6. Reconciled medication list if patient is to be discharged, provided patient with written reconciled list of medications. ___ ___ ___ _____

7. Taught patient how to keep medication list current. ___ ___ ___ _____

8. Educated patient about medications and importance of sharing current list with health care providers. ___ ___ ___ _____

   Copyright © 2018 by Elsevier Inc. All rights reserved.

Student _____ Date _____

Instructor _____ Date _____

PERFORMANCE CHECKLIST SKILL 5.1 **MEASURING BODY TEMPERATURE**

	S	U	NP	Comments
ASSESSMENT				
1. Identified patient using two identifiers.	___	___	___	_____
2. Determined need to measure patient's body temperature:				
a. Noted patient's risk for temperature alterations.	___	___	___	_____
b. Assessed for other symptoms that accompany temperature alteration.	___	___	___	_____
c. Assessed for factors that normally influence temperature.	___	___	___	_____
3. Determined appropriate measurement site and device for patient.	___	___	___	_____
4. Determined previous baseline temperature and measurement site from patient's record.	___	___	___	_____
5. Assessed patient's knowledge of procedure.	___	___	___	_____
PLANNING				
1. Identified expected outcomes.	___	___	___	_____
2. Explained to patient how you will measure temperature and importance of maintaining proper position.	___	___	___	_____
3. Collected and brought supplies to patient's bedside.	___	___	___	_____
4. Verified patient has had no food, drink, gum, or cigarettes in the past 20 minutes before measuring oral temperature.	___	___	___	_____
IMPLEMENTATION				
1. Performed hand hygiene.	___	___	___	_____
2. Assisted patient to a comfortable position that provides access to temperature site.	___	___	___	_____
3. Obtained temperature reading:				
a. Assessed oral temperature (electronic).				
(1) Applied clean gloves if necessary.	___	___	___	_____
(2) Removed thermometer pack from charger, attached probe stem, grasped top of probe stem appropriately.	___	___	___	_____

Copyright © 2018 by Elsevier Inc. All rights reserved.

	S	U	NP	Comments

(3) Slid disposable probe cover over probe stem until cover locked in place. ___ ___ ___ _____

(4) Asked patient to open mouth, placed thermometer probe under tongue appropriately. ___ ___ ___ _____

(5) Asked patient to hold thermometer probe with lips closed. ___ ___ ___ _____

(6) Left thermometer in place until signal sounded and patient's temperature appeared on display, removed thermometer probe from under patient's tongue. ___ ___ ___ _____

(7) Pushed ejection button to discard probe in the appropriate receptacle. ___ ___ ___ _____

(8) Removed and disposed of gloves if necessary. Performed hand hygiene. ___ ___ ___ _____

(9) Returned thermometer probe stem to storage position. ___ ___ ___ _____

b. Assessed rectal temperature (electronic).

(1) Provided privacy, assisted patient to appropriate position, moved bed linens to expose only anal area. ___ ___ ___ _____

(2) Applied clean gloves, cleansed anal region if necessary, removed soiled gloves, reapplied clean gloves. ___ ___ ___ _____

(3) Removed thermometer pack from charger, attached rectal probe stem to unit, grasped top of probe stem. ___ ___ ___ _____

(4) Slid disposable probe cover over probe stem until cover locked in place. ___ ___ ___ _____

(5) Used single-use package, squeezed lubricant on tissue, dipped probe cover into lubricant and covered appropriately. ___ ___ ___ _____

(6) Exposed patient's anus with nondominant hand, asked patient to breathe and relax. ___ ___ ___ _____

(7) Inserted thermometer appropriately into anus, did not force. ___ ___ ___ _____

(8) Withdrew if resistance was felt. ___ ___ ___ _____

(9) Held probe in position until signal sounded and temperature appeared on display, removed probe from anus. ___ ___ ___ _____

(10) Discarded probe cover appropriately, wiped probe with alcohol swab. ___ ___ ___ _____

Copyright © 2018 by Elsevier Inc. All rights reserved.

	S	U	NP	Comments

(11) Discarded probe cover appropriately, wiped probe with alcohol swab. ___ ___ ___ _____

(12) Wiped patient's anal area with soft tissue, discarded tissue, assisted patient to a comfortable position. ___ ___ ___ _____

(13) Removed and disposed of gloves, performed hand hygiene. ___ ___ ___ _____

c. Assessed axillary temperature (electronic).

(1) Provided privacy, assisted patient to appropriate position, moved clothing or gown away from shoulder and arm. ___ ___ ___ _____

(2) Removed thermometer pack from charger, attached oral thermometer probe stem to unit, grasped top of probe stem. ___ ___ ___ _____

(3) Slid disposable probe cover over stem until cover locked in place. ___ ___ ___ _____

(4) Raised patient's arm away from torso, inspected skin for lesions and perspiration, dried axilla if needed, inserted thermometer into center of axilla, lowered arm properly. ___ ___ ___ _____

(5) Held thermometer in place until signal sounded and temperature appeared on display, removed probe from axilla. ___ ___ ___ _____

(6) Discarded probe cover appropriately. ___ ___ ___ _____

(7) Returned thermometer stem to storage position. ___ ___ ___ _____

(8) Assisted patient to comfortable position, replaced gown. ___ ___ ___ _____

(9) Performed hand hygiene. ___ ___ ___ _____

d. Assessed tympanic membrane temperature.

(1) Assisted patient to appropriate position, obtained temperature from the appropriate ear. ___ ___ ___ _____

(2) Noted presence of earwax. ___ ___ ___ _____

(3) Removed thermometer unit appropriately from charging base. ___ ___ ___ _____

(4) Slid disposable speculum cover over lens tip until it locked in place, did not touch the lens cover. ___ ___ ___ _____

(5) Inserted speculum into ear canal, followed instructions for probe positioning. ___ ___ ___ _____

Copyright © 2018 by Elsevier Inc. All rights reserved.

	S	U	NP	Comments

(6) Once positioned, pressed scan button, left speculum until signal sounded and patient's temperature appeared on display. ___ ___ ___ _____

(7) Removed speculum from auditory meatus, discarded speculum cover appropriately. ___ ___ ___ _____

(8) If second reading was necessary, replaced probe cover and waited 2 minutes before repeating either in same ear or in other ear, considered alternative method. ___ ___ ___ _____

(9) Returned unit to thermometer base. ___ ___ ___ _____

(10) Assisted patient to comfortable position. ___ ___ ___ _____

(11) Performed hand hygiene. ___ ___ ___ _____

e. Assessed temporal artery temperature.

(1) Ensured forehead was dry. ___ ___ ___ _____

(2) Placed sensor firmly on patient's forehead. ___ ___ ___ _____

(3) Pressed red scan button, slowly slid thermometer across forehead, kept sensor flat on skin, lifted sensor after sweeping forehead, touched sensor on neck behind earlobe. Read temperature, released scan button. ___ ___ ___ _____

(4) Cleaned sensor with alcohol swab. ___ ___ ___ _____

4. Informed patient of temperature reading and record measurement. ___ ___ ___ _____

5. Returned thermometer to charger. ___ ___ ___ _____

EVALUATION

1. Established temperature as a baseline if necessary. ___ ___ ___ _____

2. Compared reading with baseline and acceptable range. ___ ___ ___ _____

3. Took temperature 30 minutes after administering antipyretics and every 4 hours until temperature stabilized if patient has a fever. ___ ___ ___ _____

4. Identified unexpected outcomes. ___ ___ ___ _____

RECORDING AND REPORTING

1. Recorded temperature and route in appropriate record. ___ ___ ___ _____

2. Reported abnormal findings to nurse in charge or health care provider. ___ ___ ___ _____

26

Copyright © 2018 by Elsevier Inc. All rights reserved.

Student _____ Date _____

Instructor _____ Date _____

PERFORMANCE CHECKLIST SKILL 5.2 **ASSESSING RADIAL PULSE**

	S	U	NP	Comments
ASSESSMENT				
1. Identified patient using two identifiers.	___	___	___	_____
2. Determined need to assess radial pulse:				
a. Assessed for any risk factors for pulse alterations.	___	___	___	_____
b. Assessed for signs of altered cardiac function.	___	___	___	_____
c. Assessed for signs of peripheral vascular disease.	___	___	___	_____
d. Assessed for factors that influence radial pulse rate and rhythm.	___	___	___	_____
3. Determined patient's previous baseline pulse rate from patient's record.	___	___	___	_____
4. Assessed patient or caregiver knowledge of procedure and rationale for measurement.	___	___	___	_____
PLANNING				
1. Identified expected outcomes.	___	___	___	_____
2. Explained to patient that you will assess HR, encouraged patient to relax, waited before assessing pulse if necessary.	___	___	___	_____
3. Collected appropriate supplies.	___	___	___	_____
IMPLEMENTATION				
1. Performed hand hygiene.	___	___	___	_____
2. Provided privacy if necessary.	___	___	___	_____
3. Assisted patient to appropriate position.	___	___	___	_____
4. Positioned patient's arms appropriately.	___	___	___	_____
5. Compressed pulse against radius, obliterated pulse, relaxed so pulse became palpable.	___	___	___	_____
6. Determined strength of pulse on a scale of 0 to 4+.	___	___	___	_____
7. Used watch to count rate appropriately.	___	___	___	_____
8. Counted rate for 30 seconds if pulse was regular, multiplied total by 2.	___	___	___	_____
9. Counted for 60 seconds if pulse was irregular, assessed frequency and pattern of irregularity.	___	___	___	_____

Copyright © 2018 by Elsevier Inc. All rights reserved.

	S	U	NP	Comments
10. Compared radial pulses bilaterally if pulse was irregular.	___	___	___	_____
11. Assisted patient in returning to a comfortable position.	___	___	___	_____
12. Discussed findings with patient.	___	___	___	_____
13. Performed hand hygiene.	___	___	___	_____

EVALUATION

	S	U	NP	Comments
1. Established radial pulse as baseline if necessary and within acceptable range.	___	___	___	_____
2. Compared pulse rate and character with previous baseline and acceptable range.	___	___	___	_____
3. Identified unexpected outcomes.	___	___	___	_____

RECORDING AND REPORTING

	S	U	NP	Comments
1. Recorded pulse rate and assessment site in appropriate record.	___	___	___	_____
2. Documented measurement of pulse rate after administration of specific therapies in nurses' notes.	___	___	___	_____
3. Reported abnormal findings to nurse in charge or health care provider.	___	___	___	_____

Copyright © 2018 by Elsevier Inc. All rights reserved.

Student _____ Date _____

Instructor _____ Date _____

PERFORMANCE CHECKLIST SKILL 5.3 **ASSESSING APICAL PULSE**

	S	U	NP	Comments
ASSESSMENT				
1. Identified patient using at least two identifiers.	___	___	___	_____
2. Determined need to assess apical pulse:				
a. Assessed for risk factors for apical pulse alteration.	___	___	___	_____
b. Assessed for symptoms of altered cardiac function.	___	___	___	_____
c. Assessed for factors that normally influence apical pulse rate and rhythm.	___	___	___	_____
3. Determined previous baseline if available.	___	___	___	_____
4. Determined any report of latex allergy, ensured stethoscope is latex free if necessary.	___	___	___	_____
5. Assessed patient's knowledge of and skill in taking apical heart rate if necessary.	___	___	___	_____
PLANNING				
1. Identified expected outcomes.	___	___	___	_____
2. Explained to patient that you will assess apical pulse rate, encouraged patient to relax, asked patient not to speak, waited if necessary.	___	___	___	_____
3. Collected appropriate supplies.	___	___	___	_____
IMPLEMENTATION				
1. Performed hand hygiene.	___	___	___	_____
2. Provided privacy if necessary.	___	___	___	_____
3. Assisted patient to appropriate position, moved bed linen and gown to expose sternum and left side of chest.	___	___	___	_____
4. Located anatomic landmarks to identify PMI.	___	___	___	_____
5. Placed diaphragm of stethoscope in palm of hand for 5 to 10 seconds.	___	___	___	_____
6. Placed diaphragm of stethoscope over PMI, auscultated for normal heart sounds.	___	___	___	_____
7. Counted with second hand of watch when heart sounds are heard with regularity.	___	___	___	_____
8. Counted for 30 seconds if pulse is regular, multiplied total by 2.	___	___	___	_____

Copyright © 2018 by Elsevier Inc. All rights reserved.

	S	U	NP	Comments

9. Counted for 60 seconds if pulse is irregular or patient was receiving cardiovascular medication. ___ ___ ___ _____

10. Noted regularity of any dysrhythmia. ___ ___ ___ _____

11. Replaced patient's gown and linen, assisted patient to a comfortable position. ___ ___ ___ _____

12. Discussed findings with patient. ___ ___ ___ _____

13. Performed hand hygiene. ___ ___ ___ _____

14. Cleaned earpieces and diaphragm of stethoscope with alcohol swab. ___ ___ ___ _____

EVALUATION

1. Established apical rate as baseline if necessary and within acceptable range. ___ ___ ___ _____

2. Compared apical rate and character with baseline and acceptable range. ___ ___ ___ _____

3. Identified unexpected outcomes. ___ ___ ___ _____

RECORDING AND REPORTING

1. Recorded apical pulse rate and rhythm on appropriate record, documented location of PMI if pulse not found at fifth ICS and LMCL. ___ ___ ___ _____

2. Documented measurement of apical pulse after administration of specific therapies in nurses' notes. ___ ___ ___ _____

3. Reported abnormal findings to nurse in charge or health care provider. ___ ___ ___ _____

Copyright © 2018 by Elsevier Inc. All rights reserved.

Student _____ Date _____

Instructor _____ Date _____

PERFORMANCE CHECKLIST SKILL 5.4 **ASSESSING RESPIRATIONS**

	S	U	NP	Comments
ASSESSMENT				
1. Identified patient using two identifiers.	___	___	___	_____
2. Determined need to assess patient's respirations:				
a. Assessed for risk factors of respiratory alterations.	___	___	___	_____
b. Assessed for symptoms of respiratory alterations.	___	___	___	_____
c. Assessed for factors that influence the character of respirations.	___	___	___	_____
3. Assessed pertinent laboratory values, including ABGs, pulse oximetry, and CBC.	___	___	___	_____
4. Determined previous baseline respiratory rate.	___	___	___	_____
PLANNING				
1. Identified expected outcomes.	___	___	___	_____
2. Waited before assessing respirations if necessary.	___	___	___	_____
3. Assessed respirations after pulse measurement.	___	___	___	_____
4. Ensured patient was in comfortable position.	___	___	___	_____
IMPLEMENTATION				
1. Performed hand hygiene.	___	___	___	_____
2. Provided privacy.	___	___	___	_____
3. Ensured patient's chest was visible, moved linen or gown.	___	___	___	_____
4. Placed patient's arms in the appropriate position.	___	___	___	_____
5. Observed complete respiratory cycle.	___	___	___	_____
6. Counted rate properly.	___	___	___	_____
7. Counted for 30 seconds if rhythm was regular, multiplied total by 2; counted for 60 seconds if irregular (i.e., too fast or too slow).	___	___	___	_____
8. Noted depth of respirations, assessed depth after counting rate.	___	___	___	_____
9. Noted rhythm of ventilatory cycle.	___	___	___	_____
10. Replaced linen and gown.	___	___	___	_____

Copyright © 2018 by Elsevier Inc. All rights reserved.

	S	U	NP	Comments

11. Performed hand hygiene. ⸺ ⸺ ⸺ _____

12. Discussed findings with patient. ⸺ ⸺ ⸺ _____

EVALUATION

1. Established rate, rhythm, and depth as baseline if necessary. ⸺ ⸺ ⸺ _____

2. Compared respirations with previous baseline. ⸺ ⸺ ⸺ _____

3. Correlated respiratory rate, depth, and rhythm
   with data from pulse oximetry and ABG values. ⸺ ⸺ ⸺ _____

4. Identified unexpected outcomes. ⸺ ⸺ ⸺ _____

RECORDING AND REPORTING

1. Recorded rate, depth, and rhythm in the
   appropriate log. ⸺ ⸺ ⸺ _____

2. Documented measurement after specific therapies in nurses' notes. ⸺ ⸺ ⸺ _____

3. Recorded type and amount of oxygen therapy
   if used. ⸺ ⸺ ⸺ _____

4. Reported abnormal findings to nurse in charge
   or health care provider. ⸺ ⸺ ⸺ _____

Copyright © 2018 by Elsevier Inc. All rights reserved.

Student _____ Date _____

Instructor _____ Date _____

PERFORMANCE CHECKLIST SKILL 5.5 **ASSESSING ARTERIAL BLOOD PRESSURE**

	S	U	NP	Comments
ASSESSMENT				
1. Identified patient using two identifiers.	___	___	___	_____
2. Determined need to assess patient's blood pressure:				
a. Assessed for risk factors of blood pressure alterations.	___	___	___	_____
b. Assessed for symptoms of blood pressure alterations.	___	___	___	_____
c. Assessed for factors that influence blood pressure.	___	___	___	_____
3. Determined appropriate site for blood pressure assessment.	___	___	___	_____
4. Determined previous baseline and assessment site, determined report of latex allergy.	___	___	___	_____
5. Assessed patient's knowledge of procedure and any existing blood pressure alteration.	___	___	___	_____
PLANNING				
1. Identified expected outcomes.	___	___	___	_____
2. Explained to patient that you will assess blood pressure, had patient rest appropriately before measuring, asked patient not to speak.	___	___	___	_____
3. Ensured patient has not exercised, ingested caffeine, or smoked in the past 30 minutes.	___	___	___	_____
4. Selected appropriate cuff size, ensured other necessary equipment is present.	___	___	___	_____
IMPLEMENTATION				
1. Performed hand hygiene.	___	___	___	_____
2. Positioned patient appropriately, ensured room is quiet and relaxing.	___	___	___	_____
3. Assessed BP by auscultation:				
a. Positioned patient appropriately based on which extremity was to be used.	___	___	___	_____
b. Exposed extremity appropriately.	___	___	___	_____
c. Palpated artery, applied bladder of cuff properly above the artery.	___	___	___	_____

Copyright © 2018 by Elsevier Inc. All rights reserved.

	S	U	NP	Comments

d. Positioned manometer gauge vertically at eye level.

e. Measured blood pressure using two-step method.

  (1) Relocated brachial pulse, palpated artery while inflating the cuff to the appropriate pressure, slowly deflated cuff, noted where pulse reappears, deflated cuff, waited 30 seconds.

  (2) Placed stethoscope earpieces in ears, ensured sounds were clear.

  (3) Relocated brachial artery, placed bell or diaphragm of stethoscope over it without touching cuff or clothing.

  (4) Closed valve of pressure bulb, inflated cuff quickly to appropriate pressure.

  (5) Released pressure valve slowly, allowed manometer needle to fall at appropriate rate.

  (6) Noted point on manometer when you heard first clear sound.

  (7) Deflated cuff gradually, noted point at which sound disappeared, listened past the last sound.

f. Measured blood pressure using one-step method.

  (1) Placed stethoscope earpieces in ears, ensured sounds were clear.

  (2) Relocated brachial artery, placed bell or diaphragm of stethoscope over it, did not allow bell or chest piece to touch cuff or clothing.

  (3) Closed valve of pressure bulb, inflated cuff quickly to appropriate pressure.

  (4) Released pressure bulb slowly, allowed manometer to fall at appropriate rate, noted point on manometer when first clear sound was heard.

  (5) Continued to deflate cuff, noted point at which sound disappeared, listened after last sound.

4. Took two measurements at 2 minutes apart, used second as baseline.

5. Removed cuff from patient's arm.

Copyright © 2018 by Elsevier Inc. All rights reserved.

	S	U	NP	Comments

6. Repeated on other limb if necessary.   _____   _____   _____   _____

7. Assessed systolic blood pressure by palpation:

   a. Followed steps 3a–3d of auscultation method.   _____   _____   _____   _____

   b. Located and palpated artery continuously with fingertips, inflated cuff to appropriate pressure.   _____   _____   _____   _____

   c. Slowly released valve, allowed manometer to fall at appropriate rate, noted point at which pulse was palpable again.   _____   _____   _____   _____

   d. Deflated cuff rapidly and completely, removed cuff from patient.   _____   _____   _____   _____

8. Assisted patient to comfortable position, covered extremity if necessary.   _____   _____   _____   _____

9. Discussed findings with patient.   _____   _____   _____   _____

10. Cleaned earpieces and diaphragm of stethoscope with alcohol, wiped cuff with approved disinfectant, performed hand hygiene.   _____   _____   _____   _____

EVALUATION

1. Established baseline if necessary.   _____   _____   _____   _____

2. Compared reading with previous baseline and usual blood pressure for patient's age.   _____   _____   _____   _____

3. Identified unexpected outcomes.   _____   _____   _____   _____

RECORDING AND REPORTING

1. Recorded blood pressure and site assessed in appropriate record.   _____   _____   _____   _____

2. Documented measurement and signs of blood pressure alterations after administration of specific therapies in nurses' notes.   _____   _____   _____   _____

3. Reported abnormal findings to nurse in charge or health care provider.   _____   _____   _____   _____

Copyright © 2018 by Elsevier Inc. All rights reserved.

Student _____ Date _____

Instructor _____ Date _____

PERFORMANCE CHECKLIST PROCEDURAL GUIDELINE 5.1 **NONINVASIVE ELECTRONIC BLOOD PRESSURE MEASUREMENT**

	S	U	NP	Comments
PROCEDURAL STEPS				
1. Identified patient using two identifiers.	——	——	——	_____
2. Assessed need to measure blood pressure, determined patient's baseline blood pressure.	——	——	——	_____
3. Determined appropriateness of using electronic blood pressure measurement.	——	——	——	_____
4. Performed hand hygiene, determined best site for cuff placement, inspected condition of extremities.	——	——	——	_____
5. Collected appropriate equipment at patient's bedside, selected appropriate cuff for patient extremity and machine.	——	——	——	_____
6. Assisted patient to comfortable position, plugged in device, ensured all connections reach.	——	——	——	_____
7. Turned machine on, enabled self-testing of computer systems.	——	——	——	_____
8. Removed constricting clothing.	——	——	——	_____
9. Manually squeezed all air out of cuff and connected it to the connector hose.	——	——	——	_____
10. Wrapped cuff snugly around extremity, verified that one finger fits between cuff and patient's skin, ensured artery arrow was placed correctly.	——	——	——	_____
11. Verified connector hose was not kinked.	——	——	——	_____
12. Set frequency control, pressed start.	——	——	——	_____
13. Set frequency of measurements and upper and lower alarm limits.	——	——	——	_____
14. Obtained additional readings when necessary.	——	——	——	_____
15. Removed cuff at least every 2 hours, removed and cleaned cuff after last use.	——	——	——	_____
16. Discussed findings with patient, performed hand hygiene.	——	——	——	_____

Copyright © 2018 by Elsevier Inc. All rights reserved.

	S	U	NP	Comments

17. Compared electronic blood pressure readings with auscultatory measurements to verify accuracy.

    ____   ____   ____   _____

18. Recorded blood pressure and site assessed in appropriate record, recorded symptoms of blood pressure alterations in nurses' notes, reported abnormal findings to nurse in charge or health care provider.

    ____   ____   ____   _____

Copyright © 2018 by Elsevier Inc. All rights reserved.

Student _____ Date _____

Instructor _____ Date _____

PERFORMANCE CHECKLIST PROCEDURAL GUIDELINE 5.2   **MEASURING OXYGEN SATURATION (PULSE OXIMETRY)**

	S	U	NP	Comments

PROCEDURAL STEPS

1. Identified patient using two identifiers. ___ ___ ___ _____

2. Determined need to measure patient's oxygen saturation, assessed risk factors for decreased oxygen saturation. ___ ___ ___ _____

3. Performed hand hygiene, assessed for symptoms of alterations in oxygen saturation. ___ ___ ___ _____

4. Determined if patient has a latex allergy. ___ ___ ___ _____

5. Assessed for factors that influence measurement of SpO_2. ___ ___ ___ _____

6. Reviewed patient's record for standard of care regarding measurement of SpO_2. ___ ___ ___ _____

7. Determined previous baseline SpO_2 if available. ___ ___ ___ _____

8. Performed hand hygiene, determined most appropriate site for sensor probe placement by measuring capillary refill. ___ ___ ___ _____

9. Arranged equipment at bedside table. ___ ___ ___ _____

10. Positioned patient comfortably, instructed patient to breathe normally. ___ ___ ___ _____

11. Attached sensor to monitoring site, removed nail polish if necessary, instructed patient that probe will not hurt. ___ ___ ___ _____

12. Turned oximeter on, correlated oximeter pulse rate with patient's radial pulse. ___ ___ ___ _____

13. Left sensor in place until readout reached constant value and pulse display reached full strength, informed patient of oximeter alarm, read SpO_2 on display. ___ ___ ___ _____

14. Determined limits for SpO_2, verified that alarms are on, assessed skin integrity under sensor probe every 2 hours, relocated if necessary. ___ ___ ___ _____

15. Removed probe and turned oximeter off if planning to check SpO_2 intermittently, stored sensor appropriately. ___ ___ ___ _____

16. Discussed findings with patient, performed hand hygiene. ___ ___ ___ _____

Copyright © 2018 by Elsevier Inc. All rights reserved.

	S	U	NP	Comments

17. Compared SpO$_2$ readings with baseline and acceptable SpO$_2$.

    — — — _____

18. Recorded SpO$_2$ in appropriate record, recorded symptoms of oxygen saturation alterations in nurses' notes.

    — — — _____

19. Reported abnormal findings to nurse in charge or health care provider.

    — — — _____

Copyright © 2018 by Elsevier Inc. All rights reserved.

Student _____ Date _____

Instructor _____ Date _____

PERFORMANCE CHECKLIST SKILL 6.1 **GENERAL SURVEY**

	S	U	NP	Comments

ASSESSMENT

1. Noted if patient has had any acute distress, deferred general survey if needed.

2. Reviewed graphic sheet for previous vital signs, considered factors that may alter values.

3. Determined patient's primary language, obtained an appropriate interpreter if necessary.

4. Confirmed primary reason patient has sought health care.

5. Identified patient's normal height, weight, and BMI, determined amount of any weight gain or loss, assessed if patient is dieting or exercising.

6. Asked if patient has noticed any changes in condition of skin.

7. Reviewed patient's past I&O records.

8. Reviewed patient's perceptions about personal health.

9. Assessed for evidence of latex allergy, asked if patient has food allergies or must avoid latex products.

PLANNING

1. Identified expected outcomes.

2. Explained to patient that process is routine to check for areas of concern, asked patient to tell if any areas hurt when touched.

3. Performed hand hygiene, assembled necessary equipment, positioned patient appropriately.

IMPLEMENTATION

1. Noted patient's verbal and nonverbal behaviors throughout assessment, determined LOC and orientation.

2. Obtained temperature, pulse, respirations, and BP as necessary; informed patient of vital signs.

3. Noted patient's gender, race, age, and external physical features.

4. Rephrased a question if it is possible patient misunderstands.

40

Copyright © 2018 by Elsevier Inc. All rights reserved.

	S	U	NP	Comments

5. Asked short, to-the-point questions if patient responses are inappropriate. ___ ___ ___ _____

6. Gave simple commands if patient cannot respond to questions about orientation. ___ ___ ___ _____

7. Assessed affect and mood, noted if verbal and nonverbal signals match. ___ ___ ___ _____

8. Watched patient interact with family or caregiver, assessed for signs of abuse. ___ ___ ___ _____

9. Observed for signs of abuse, especially in children, females, and older adults; reported findings if necessary. ___ ___ ___ _____

10. Assessed posture and position. ___ ___ ___ _____

11. Assessed body movements for coordination, tremors, and mobility. ___ ___ ___ _____

12. Assessed speech for intelligibility and association. ___ ___ ___ _____

13. Observed hygiene and grooming for presence or absence of makeup, type of clothing, and cleanliness:

   a. Observed characteristics of hair. ___ ___ ___ _____

   b. Inspected condition of nails. ___ ___ ___ _____

   c. Assessed presence or absence of body hair. ___ ___ ___ _____

14. Inspected exposed areas of skin, asked if patient has noticed changes. ___ ___ ___ _____

15. Inspected skin surfaces, compared symmetry of body parts, looked for skin color variations. ___ ___ ___ _____

16. Inspected color of face, oral mucosa, lips, conjunctiva, sclera, palms, and nail beds. ___ ___ ___ _____

17. Palpated intact skin with ungloved fingertips for texture and moisture:

   a. Noted texture of skin and any localized areas of hardness or lesions. ___ ___ ___ _____

   b. Palpated areas that appear irregular in texture. ___ ___ ___ _____

   c. Palpated temperature using back of hand, compared symmetrical body parts, noted temperature differences. ___ ___ ___ _____

18. Applied clean gloves, inspected character if secretions, removed gloves. ___ ___ ___ _____

19. Assessed skin turgor at sternum, forearm, or abdomen. ___ ___ ___ _____

Copyright © 2018 by Elsevier Inc. All rights reserved.

	S	U	NP	Comments

20. Assessed condition of skin for pressure areas; if found, applied gentle pressure and released, noted skin color. ___ ___ ___ _____

21. Inspected color, location, texture, size, shape, and types of any lesions; noted grouping and distribution:

   a. Applied clean gloves if necessary; palpated lesion to determine mobility, contour, and consistency. ___ ___ ___ _____

   b. Noted if patient feels any tenderness. ___ ___ ___ _____

   c. Measured size of lesion appropriately. ___ ___ ___ _____

22. Removed gloves, discarded used supplies and gloves appropriately, assisted patient to comfortable position, performed hand hygiene. ___ ___ ___ _____

EVALUATION

1. Observed for evidence of physical or emotional distress, which may alter data. ___ ___ ___ _____

2. Compared assessment findings with previous observations. ___ ___ ___ _____

3. Asked patient if there is information that has not been discussed. ___ ___ ___ _____

4. Identified unexpected outcomes. ___ ___ ___ _____

RECORDING AND REPORTING

1. Recorded patient's vital signs in the appropriate log. ___ ___ ___ _____

2. Recorded description of alterations in general appearance in the appropriate log. ___ ___ ___ _____

3. Described patient's behaviors objectively, included patient's self-report. ___ ___ ___ _____

4. Documented evaluation of patient learning. ___ ___ ___ _____

5. Reported abnormalities and acute symptoms to nurse in charge or health care provider. ___ ___ ___ _____

Copyright © 2018 by Elsevier Inc. All rights reserved.

Student _____ Date _____

Instructor _____ Date _____

PERFORMANCE CHECKLIST SKILL 6.2 **HEAD AND NECK ASSESSMENT**

	S	U	NP	Comments
ASSESSMENT				
1. Assessed for history of headache, dizziness, pain, or stiffness.	___	___	___	_____
2. Determined if patient has history of eye disease, diabetes mellitus, or hypertension.	___	___	___	_____
3. Asked if patient has experienced blurred vision, flashing lights, halos around lights, or reduced visual field.	___	___	___	_____
4. Asked if patient has experienced ear pain, itching, discharge, vertigo, tinnitus, or change in hearing.	___	___	___	_____
5. Reviewed patient's occupational history.	___	___	___	_____
6. Asked if patient has a history of allergies, nasal discharge, epistaxis, or postnasal drip.	___	___	___	_____
7. Determined if the patient smokes or chews tobacco.	___	___	___	_____
PLANNING				
1. Identified expected outcomes.	___	___	___	_____
2. Told patient you will be completing a routine examination of the head and neck.	___	___	___	_____
3. Anticipated teaching topics.	___	___	___	_____
4. Performed hand hygiene, assembled necessary equipment.	___	___	___	_____
IMPLEMENTATION				
1. Positioned patient appropriately.	___	___	___	_____
2. Inspected the head; noted position, facial features, and symmetry.	___	___	___	_____
3. Assessed the eyes:				
a. Inspected position of eyes, color, condition of conjunctiva, and movement.	___	___	___	_____
b. Assessed patient's near vision and far vision.	___	___	___	_____
c. Inspected pupils for size, shape, and equality.	___	___	___	_____
d. Tested papillary reflexes properly, tested for accommodation.	___	___	___	_____

Copyright © 2018 by Elsevier Inc. All rights reserved.

	S	U	NP	Comments

4. Assessed hearing, noted patient's response to questions and presence of a hearing aid, asked patient to repeat short words if necessary. ⎯ ⎯ ⎯ _____

5. Inspected nose externally; noted color of mucosa, lesions, discharge, swelling, or bleeding; consulted with health care provider if drainage was infectious. ⎯ ⎯ ⎯ _____

6. Inspected nares in patients with NG, NI, or nasotracheal tube; stabilized tube as needed. ⎯ ⎯ ⎯ _____

7. Inspected sinuses properly. ⎯ ⎯ ⎯ _____

8. Assessed mouth, discussed signs of oral cancer:

   a. Applied clean gloves; inspected lips for color, texture, hydration, and lesions. ⎯ ⎯ ⎯ _____

   b. Inspected teeth; noted position and alignment; noted color, presence of dental caries, tartar, and extraction sites. ⎯ ⎯ ⎯ _____

   c. Inspected mucosa and gums, determined if dentures of retainers are comfortable. ⎯ ⎯ ⎯ _____

   d. Palpated oral lesions if present for tenderness, size, and consistency. ⎯ ⎯ ⎯ _____

9. Inspected and palpated neck:

   a. Asked patient if there is history of pain or difficulty with neck movement. ⎯ ⎯ ⎯ _____

   b. Inspected neck for bilateral symmetry of muscles, asked patient to flex and hyperextend neck and turn head side to side. ⎯ ⎯ ⎯ _____

   c. Positioned patient appropriately; inspected area where lymph nodes are distributed properly; compared both sides; noted if nodes are large, fixed, inflamed, or tender. ⎯ ⎯ ⎯ _____

10. Removed gloves, discarded used supplies and gloves in proper receptacle, helped patient to comfortable position, performed hand hygiene. ⎯ ⎯ ⎯ _____

EVALUATION

1. Compared assessment findings with previous observation. ⎯ ⎯ ⎯ _____

2. Asked patient to describe common symptoms of eye, ear, sinus, or mouth disease. ⎯ ⎯ ⎯ _____

3. Asked patient to list occupational safety precautions. ⎯ ⎯ ⎯ _____

4. Identified unexpected outcomes. ⎯ ⎯ ⎯ _____

Copyright © 2018 by Elsevier Inc. All rights reserved.

	S	U	NP	Comments

RECORDING AND REPORTING

1. Recorded all findings, including abnormal findings, in appropriate record. ___ ___ ___ _____

2. Documented own evaluation of patient learning. ___ ___ ___ _____

3. Reported any unexpected findings to nurse in charge or health care provider. ___ ___ ___ _____

Copyright © 2018 by Elsevier Inc. All rights reserved.

Student _____ Date _____

Instructor _____ Date _____

PERFORMANCE CHECKLIST SKILL 6.3 **THORAX AND LUNG ASSESSMENT**

	S	U	NP	Comments

ASSESSMENT

1. Assessed history of tobacco and marijuana use (i.e., type, duration, and amount in pack-years), determined length of time since smoking if patient quit.   ___ ___ ___ _____

2. Asked if patient experiences respiratory alterations.   ___ ___ ___ _____

3. Determined if patient works in environment containing pollutants, radiation, or second-hand smoke.   ___ ___ ___ _____

4. Reviewed history for risk factors and/or exposure to infectious diseases (e.g., HIV, TB).   ___ ___ ___ _____

5. Asked if patient had history of persistent cough, hemoptysis, unexplained weight loss, fatigue, night sweats, or fever.   ___ ___ ___ _____

6. Asked if patient has history of chronic hoarseness.   ___ ___ ___ _____

7. Assessed for history of allergies.   ___ ___ ___ _____

8. Reviewed family history for cancer, TB, allergies, or COPD.   ___ ___ ___ _____

PLANNING

1. Identified expected outcomes.   ___ ___ ___ _____

2. Anticipated teaching topics, including risk factors for lung disease.   ___ ___ ___ _____

3. Performed hand hygiene, assembled necessary equipment.   ___ ___ ___ _____

IMPLEMENTATION

1. Positioned patient and prepared for examination:

   a. Positioned patient appropriately.   ___ ___ ___ _____

   b. Removed gown from posterior chest, kept front of chest and legs covered, removed the gown from area being examined as you proceed.   ___ ___ ___ _____

2. Inspected posterior thorax:

   a. Removed gown from posterior chest, kept front of chest and legs covered, removed the gown from area being examined as you proceed.   ___ ___ ___ _____

Copyright © 2018 by Elsevier Inc. All rights reserved.

	S	U	NP	Comments

b. Determined rate and rhythm of breathing, had patient relax.

   ____   ____   ____   _____

c. Palpated for masses, pulsations, unusual movement, or areas of localized tenderness; palpated suspicious mass or size, shape, and typical qualities of lesions.

   ____   ____   ____   _____

d. Assessed chest expansion; stood behind patient, placed thumbs properly around spine, noted movement of thumbs as patient breathes.

   ____   ____   ____   _____

e. Auscultated breath sounds; had patient take slow, deep mouth breaths; listened to entire inspiration and expiration at each position; compared breath sounds over both sides; asked patient to breathe deeper if necessary.

   ____   ____   ____   _____

f. Had patient cough if adventitious sounds were heard, listened again to determine if sound was cleared with coughing.

   ____   ____   ____   _____

3. Inspected lateral thorax:

a. Instructed patient to raise arms, inspected chest wall for same characteristics as reviewed for posterior chest.

   ____   ____   ____   _____

b. Extended palpation and auscultation to lateral sides of chest.

   ____   ____   ____   _____

4. Inspected anterior thorax:

a. Inspected accessory muscles of breathing, noted effort to breathe.

   ____   ____   ____   _____

b. Inspected width or spread of angle made by coastal margins and tip of sternum.

   ____   ____   ____   _____

c. Observed patient's breathing pattern, as well as symmetry and degree of chest wall and abdominal movement.

   ____   ____   ____   _____

d. Palpated anterior thoracic muscles and ribs for lumps, masses, tenderness, or unusual movement.

   ____   ____   ____   _____

e. Palpated anterior chest excursion appropriately.

   ____   ____   ____   _____

f. Auscultated anterior thorax properly.

   ____   ____   ____   _____

5. Cleaned and stored stethoscope, performed hand hygiene.

   ____   ____   ____   _____

EVALUATION

1. Compared respiratory findings with assessment characteristics for thorax and lungs.

   ____   ____   ____   _____

2. Had patient identify factors leading to lung diseases.

   ____   ____   ____   _____

3. Identified unexpected outcomes.

   ____   ____   ____   _____

Copyright © 2018 by Elsevier Inc. All rights reserved.

	S	U	NP	Comments

RECORDING AND REPORTING

1. Documented patient's respiratory rate and character and other physical assessments in the appropriate record.   ___ ___ ___ _____

2. Reported abnormalities to nurse in charge or health care provider.   ___ ___ ___ _____

3. Documented evaluation of patient learning.   ___ ___ ___ _____

Copyright © 2018 by Elsevier Inc. All rights reserved.

Student _____ Date _____

Instructor _____ Date _____

PERFORMANCE CHECKLIST SKILL 6.4   **CARDIOVASCULAR ASSESSMENT**

	S	U	NP	Comments
ASSESSMENT				
1. Assessed patient for history of smoking, alcohol intake, caffeine intake, use of "recreational" drugs, exercise habits, and dietary patterns.	___	___	___	_____
2. Determined if patient is taking medications for cardiovascular function and if patient knows their purpose, dosage, and side effects.	___	___	___	_____
3. Asked if patient has experienced the cardinal symptoms of heart disease, asked if symptoms occurred while exercising or at rest.	___	___	___	_____
4. Determined onset, factors, quality, region, severity, and radiation of any reported chest pain.	___	___	___	_____
5. Assessed family history for heart disease, diabetes, high cholesterol or lipids, hypertension, stroke, or rheumatic heart disease.	___	___	___	_____
6. Asked patient about history of preexisting heart conditions, heart surgery, or vascular disease.	___	___	___	_____
7. Determined if patient experiences leg cramps, numbness or tingling in extremities, sensation of cold hands or feet, pain in legs, or swelling or cyanosis of extremities.	___	___	___	_____
8. Asked if any leg pain or cramping was present, asked if it was relieved by walking or standing or if it occurred during sleep.	___	___	___	_____
9. Asked women if they wear tight-fitting underwear or hosiery or sit or lie in bed with legs crossed.	___	___	___	_____
PLANNING				
1. Identified expected outcomes.	___	___	___	_____
2. Anticipated teaching topics, including risk for heart and vascular disease.	___	___	___	_____
3. Performed hand hygiene, prepared necessary supplies.	___	___	___	_____
IMPLEMENTATION				
1. Assisted patient in being as relaxed and comfortable as possible.	___	___	___	_____
2. Had patient assume proper position.	___	___	___	_____

Copyright © 2018 by Elsevier Inc. All rights reserved.

	S	U	NP	Comments

3. Explained procedure, avoided facial gestures reflecting concern. ___ ___ ___ _____

4. Ensured that room was quiet. ___ ___ ___ _____

5. Assessed the heart:

  a. Formed a mental image of the exact location of the heart. ___ ___ ___ _____

  b. Found the angle of Louis, slipped finger down each side to feel adjacent ribs. ___ ___ ___ _____

  c. Found the following anatomic landmarks:

    (1) The aortic area. ___ ___ ___ _____

    (2) The pulmonic area. ___ ___ ___ _____

    (3) The second pulmonic area. ___ ___ ___ _____

    (4) The tricuspid area. ___ ___ ___ _____

    (5) The mitral area. ___ ___ ___ _____

    (6) The epigastric area. ___ ___ ___ _____

  d. Stood to the patient's right, inspected and palpated the precordium, noted visible pulsations and more exaggerated lifts, palpated for pulsations at all landmarks. ___ ___ ___ _____

  e. Located PMI. ___ ___ ___ _____

  f. Turned patient onto left side if necessary. ___ ___ ___ _____

  g. Inspected epigastric area, palpated abdominal aorta, noted a localized strong beat. ___ ___ ___ _____

  h. Auscultated heart sounds properly.

    (1) Positioned patient appropriately. ___ ___ ___ _____

    (2) Asked patient not to speak but to breathe comfortably, began with diaphragm of the stethoscope and alternated with the bell, avoided jumping from one area to another. ___ ___ ___ _____

    (3) Moved systematically around the heart sound locations in the proper order. ___ ___ ___ _____

    (4) Listened for S_2 at each site. ___ ___ ___ _____

    (5) Counted each lub-dub as one heartbeat, counted number of beats for 1 minute. ___ ___ ___ _____

    (6) Assessed heart rhythm by noting time between S_1 and S_2 and time between S_2 and the next S_1, listened to the full cycle at each area, noted regular intervals between each sequence. ___ ___ ___ _____

Copyright © 2018 by Elsevier Inc. All rights reserved.

	S	U	NP	Comments

(7) Compared apical and radial pulses when heart rate is irregular, asked a colleague for assistance if needed.

    i. Auscultated for extra heart sounds at each site, noted pitch, loudness, duration, timing, location on chest wall, and where heard in cardiac cycle.

      (1) Listened for low-pitched extra sounds with the bell of the stethoscope.

      (2) Positioned patient properly, asked patient to hold breath, listened for friction rubs.

    j. Auscultated for heart murmurs over each auscultation site.

      (1) Noted intensity and location where you can best hear any murmur detected.

      (2) Noted pitch of the murmur.

6. Assessed neck vessels:

    a. Positioned patient appropriately.

    b. Inspected both sides of neck for obvious arterial pulsations.

    c. Palpated each carotid artery appropriately; asked patient to raise chin slightly; noted rate, rhythm, strength, and elasticity; noted if pulse changed during breathing.

    d. Auscultated for blowing sound over each carotid artery with bell of stethoscope, asked patient to hold a breath for a few heartbeats so respiratory sounds do not interfere with auscultation.

7. Performed peripheral vascular assessment:

    a. Inspected lower extremities for changes in color and conditions of the skin, compared skin color with patient lying and standing.

    b. Palpated edematous areas, noted mobility, consistency, and tenderness.

    c. Assessed for pitting edema properly.

    d. Measured circumference of extremity with tape measure.

    e. Checked capillary refill properly.

    f. Asked if patient experienced pain or tenderness, checked for signs of phlebitis or DVT.

Copyright © 2018 by Elsevier Inc. All rights reserved.

	S	U	NP	Comments

g. Palpated each peripheral artery for equality and elasticity starting at the distal end of each, noted ease with which it sprang back and strength of pulse.

   (1) Palpated radial pulse properly. ＿＿ ＿＿ ＿＿ ＿＿＿＿＿＿＿＿＿

   (2) Palpated ulnar pulse properly. ＿＿ ＿＿ ＿＿ ＿＿＿＿＿＿＿＿＿

   (3) Palpated brachial pulse properly. ＿＿ ＿＿ ＿＿ ＿＿＿＿＿＿＿＿＿

   (4) Positioned patient appropriately, palpated dorsalis pedis pulse properly. ＿＿ ＿＿ ＿＿ ＿＿＿＿＿＿＿＿＿

   (5) Palpated posterior tibial pulse properly. ＿＿ ＿＿ ＿＿ ＿＿＿＿＿＿＿＿＿

   (6) Palpated popliteal pulse properly, repositioned patient if needed. ＿＿ ＿＿ ＿＿ ＿＿＿＿＿＿＿＿＿

   (7) Applied gloves, positioned patient properly, palpated femoral pulse properly. ＿＿ ＿＿ ＿＿ ＿＿＿＿＿＿＿＿＿

h. Used a Doppler instrument if necessary.

   (1) Applied conducting gel to either patient's skin or transducer tip of probe, turned on Doppler. ＿＿ ＿＿ ＿＿ ＿＿＿＿＿＿＿＿＿

   (2) Applied ultrasound probe to skin, changed Doppler angle until pulsation is audible, wiped gel from patient and Doppler. ＿＿ ＿＿ ＿＿ ＿＿＿＿＿＿＿＿＿

8. Removed gloves, discarded used supplies and glove appropriately, helped patient to comfortable position, performed hand hygiene. ＿＿ ＿＿ ＿＿ ＿＿＿＿＿＿＿＿＿

EVALUATION

1. Compared findings with normal assessment characteristics of heart and vascular system. ＿＿ ＿＿ ＿＿ ＿＿＿＿＿＿＿＿＿

2. Asked another nurse to confirm assessment if heart sounds are not audible or pulses are not palpable. ＿＿ ＿＿ ＿＿ ＿＿＿＿＿＿＿＿＿

3. Asked patient to describe behaviors that increase risk for heart and vascular disease. ＿＿ ＿＿ ＿＿ ＿＿＿＿＿＿＿＿＿

4. Compared pulses and capillary refill bilaterally with previous assessment. ＿＿ ＿＿ ＿＿ ＿＿＿＿＿＿＿＿＿

5. Identified unexpected outcomes. ＿＿ ＿＿ ＿＿ ＿＿＿＿＿＿＿＿＿

RECORDING AND REPORTING

1. Documented quality, intensity, rate, and rhythm of heart sounds and peripheral pulses in appropriate record. ＿＿ ＿＿ ＿＿ ＿＿＿＿＿＿＿＿＿

2. Documented additional cardiac findings, JVP, and condition of extremities in appropriate record. ＿＿ ＿＿ ＿＿ ＿＿＿＿＿＿＿＿＿

Copyright © 2018 by Elsevier Inc. All rights reserved.

	S	U	NP	Comments

3. Documented activity level and subjective data related to fatigue, shortness of breath, and chest pain.

4. Documented evaluation of patient learning.

5. Reported any irregularities in heart function and indications of impaired arterial blood flow immediately to health care provider.

6. Reported changes in peripheral circulation to health care provider.

Copyright © 2018 by Elsevier Inc. All rights reserved.

Student _____ Date _____

Instructor _____ Date _____

PERFORMANCE CHECKLIST SKILL 6.5 **ABDOMINAL ASSESSMENT**

	S	U	NP	Comments

ASSESSMENT

1. Assessed character of any reported abdominal or lower back pain. ____ ____ ____ _____

2. Observed patient's movement and position. ____ ____ ____ _____

3. Assessed patient's normal bowel habits. ____ ____ ____ _____

4. Determined if patient has had abdominal surgery, trauma, or diagnostic tests of the GI tract. ____ ____ ____ _____

5. Assessed if patient has had recent weight changes or intolerance to diet. ____ ____ ____ _____

6. Assessed for indications of GI alterations. ____ ____ ____ _____

7. Determined if patient takes antiinflammatory medications or antibiotic. ____ ____ ____ _____

8. Reviewed family history of cancer, kidney disease, alcoholism, hypertension, or heart disease. ____ ____ ____ _____

9. Reviewed patient's history for risks of HBV exposure. ____ ____ ____ _____

PLANNING

1. Identified expected outcomes. ____ ____ ____ _____

2. Anticipated teaching topics including warning signs of colorectal cancer. ____ ____ ____ _____

3. Performed hand hygiene, gathered necessary supplies. ____ ____ ____ _____

IMPLEMENTATION

1. Prepared patient for abdominal assessment:

   a. Asked if patient needs to empty bladder or defecate. ____ ____ ____ _____

   b. Kept patient's upper chest and legs draped. ____ ____ ____ _____

   c. Ensured that room was warm. ____ ____ ____ _____

   d. Positioned patient properly. ____ ____ ____ _____

   e. Exposed area from just above the xiphoid process down to the symphysis pubis. ____ ____ ____ _____

   f. Maintained conversation during assessment except during auscultation, explained steps calmly and slowly. ____ ____ ____ _____

   g. Asked patient to point to tender areas. ____ ____ ____ _____

54

Copyright © 2018 by Elsevier Inc. All rights reserved.

	S	U	NP	Comments

2. Performed abdominal assessment:

a. Identified landmarks dividing abdominal region into quadrants. ____ ____ ____ _____

b. Inspected skin of abdomen's surface for color, scars, venous patterns, rashes, lesions, stretch marks, and artificial openings; observed lesions for characteristics described in skill 6.1. ____ ____ ____ _____

c. Asked if patient self-administers injections if bruising was noted. ____ ____ ____ _____

d. Inspected contour, symmetry, and surface motion of the abdomen; noted masses, bulging, or distention. ____ ____ ____ _____

e. Noted if any distention was generalized, looked for flanks on each side. ____ ____ ____ _____

f. Measured size of abdominal girth if you suspected distention, used the marking pen to indicate where tape measure was applied. ____ ____ ____ _____

g. Turned off suction connected to an NG or NI tube momentarily. ____ ____ ____ _____

h. Auscultated bowel sounds appropriately, asked patient not to talk, listened at least 5 minutes before describing sounds as absent. ____ ____ ____ _____

i. Auscultated for vascular sounds with bell of stethoscope over the epigastric region and each quadrant. ____ ____ ____ _____

j. Positioned patient appropriately, percussed each of the four quadrants, noted areas of tympany and dullness. ____ ____ ____ _____

k. Asked patient if abdomen feels unusually tight, determined if this was a recent development. ____ ____ ____ _____

l. Positioned patient appropriately, percussed over each CVA along scapular lines, noted if patient experienced pain. ____ ____ ____ _____

m. Lightly palpated over each quadrant, palpated painful areas last.

   (1) Noted muscular resistance, distention, tenderness, and superficial masses; observed patient's face for signs of discomfort. ____ ____ ____ _____

   (2) Noted if abdomen was firm or soft to touch. ____ ____ ____ _____

n. Palpated for a smooth round mass below umbilicus and above symphysis pubis, asked if patient had sensation of needing to void. ____ ____ ____ _____

Copyright © 2018 by Elsevier Inc. All rights reserved.

	S	U	NP	Comments

o. Noted size, location, shape, consistency, tenderness, mobility, and texture of any masses palpated. ___ ___ ___ _____

p. Pressed one hand slowly into tender areas and released quickly, noted if pain was aggravated. ___ ___ ___ _____

EVALUATION

1. Compared assessment findings with previous assessment characteristics to identify changes. ___ ___ ___ _____

2. Asked patient to describe signs and symptoms of colorectal cancer. ___ ___ ___ _____

3. Identified unexpected outcomes. ___ ___ ___ _____

RECORDING AND REPORTING

1. Documented appearance of abdomen, quality of bowel sounds, presence of distention, abdominal circumference, and presence and location of tenderness in appropriate record. ___ ___ ___ _____

2. Documented evaluation of patient learning. ___ ___ ___ _____

3. Recorded patient's ability to void and defecate, included description of output. ___ ___ ___ _____

4. Reported serious abnormal findings to nurse in charge and health care provider. ___ ___ ___ _____

Copyright © 2018 by Elsevier Inc. All rights reserved.

Student _____ Date _____

Instructor _____ Date _____

PERFORMANCE CHECKLIST SKILL 6.6 **GENITALIA AND RECTUM ASSESSMENT**

	S	U	NP	Comments
ASSESSMENT				
1. Assessed female patient:				
a. Determined if patient has symptoms of vaginal discharge, painful or swollen perianal tissue, or genital lesions.	___	___	___	_____
b. Determined if patient has symptoms or history of genitourinary problems.	___	___	___	_____
c. Asked if patient has had signs of bleeding outside of normal menstruation or after menopause or has had unusual vaginal discharge.	___	___	___	_____
d. Determined if patient has received HPV vaccine.	___	___	___	_____
e. Determined if patient has history of HPV, first pregnancy before age 17, smoking, obesity, diet low in fruits and vegetables, or has had multiple full-term pregnancies.	___	___	___	_____
f. Determined if patient is older than 63; is obese; has history of ovarian dysfunction, breast or endometrial cancer, or endometriosis; has family history of reproductive cancer; has history of infertility or nulliparity; or uses estrogen as hormone replacement therapy.	___	___	___	_____
g. Determined if patient is postmenopausal, obese, or infertile; had early menarche or late menopause; has history of hypertension, diabetes, gallbladder disease, or polycystic ovary disease; has family history of endometrial, breast, or colon cancer; or has history of estrogen-related exposure.	___	___	___	_____
h. Determined patient's knowledge of risk factors and signs of gynecological cancers.	___	___	___	_____
2. Assessed male patient:				
a. Reviewed normal elimination pattern.	___	___	___	_____
b. Asked if patient has noted penile pain or swelling, genital lesions, or urethral discharge.	___	___	___	_____
c. Determined if patient has noted heaviness or painless enlargement or irregular lumps of testis.	___	___	___	_____

Copyright © 2018 by Elsevier Inc. All rights reserved.

	S	U	NP	Comments

d. Determined if patient reported any enlargement of inguinal area; assessed if any enlargement was intermittent, associated with straining, and painful; assessed whether coughing, lifting, or straining at stool causes pain. ___ ___ ___ _____

e. Asked if patient has experienced weak or interrupted urine flow, difficulty with urinating, polyuria, nocturia, hematuria, or dysuria; determined if patient has continuing pain in lower back, pelvis, or upper thighs. ___ ___ ___ _____

f. Assessed patient's knowledge of risk factors and signs of prostate and testicular cancer. ___ ___ ___ _____

3. Assessed in all patients:

   a. Determined whether patient has experienced rectal bleeding or pain, black or tarry stools, or change in bowel habits. ___ ___ ___ _____

   b. Determined whether patient has personal or family history of colorectal cancer, polyps, or chronic inflammatory bowel disease, asked if patient is over age 50. ___ ___ ___ _____

   c. Inquired about dietary habits. ___ ___ ___ _____

   d. Determined if patient is obese, is physically inactive, smokes, has type 2 diabetes, or consumes alcohol. ___ ___ ___ _____

   e. Assessed medication history for use of laxatives or cathartic medications. ___ ___ ___ _____

   f. Assessed for use of codeine or iron preparations. ___ ___ ___ _____

   g. Assessed patient's knowledge of risks and signs of colorectal cancer. ___ ___ ___ _____

PLANNING

1. Identified expected outcomes. ___ ___ ___ _____

2. Anticipated teaching topics including warning signs of colorectal cancer. ___ ___ ___ _____

3. Performed hand hygiene, prepared necessary supplies. ___ ___ ___ _____

IMPLEMENTATION

1. Prepared patient for assessment:

   a. Asked if patient needs to empty bladder or defecate. ___ ___ ___ _____

   b. Kept patient's upper chest and legs draped, kept room warm. ___ ___ ___ _____

   c. Positioned patient appropriately. ___ ___ ___ _____

   d. Applied clean gloves. ___ ___ ___ _____

58

Copyright © 2018 by Elsevier Inc. All rights reserved.

	S	U	NP	Comments

2. Performed female genitalia examination:

   a. Exposed perineal area, repositioned sheet as needed. ____ ____ ____ _____

   b. Inspected surface characteristics of perineum; retracted labia majora; observed for inflammation, edema, lesions, or lacerations; noted if there was any discharge. ____ ____ ____ _____

3. Performed male genitalia examination:

   a. Exposed perineal area, observed for rashes, excoriations, or lesions. ____ ____ ____ _____

   b. Inspected and palpated all penile surfaces. ____ ____ ____ _____

   c. Inspected and palpated testicular surfaces. ____ ____ ____ _____

   d. Palpated testes, asked if patient experiences tenderness with palpation. ____ ____ ____ _____

4. Assessed rectum:

   a. Positioned patient appropriately. ____ ____ ____ _____

   b. Viewed perianal and sacrococcygeal areas by retracting buttocks using nondominant hand. ____ ____ ____ _____

   c. Inspected anal tissue for skin characteristics, lesions, external hemorrhoids, ulcers, inflammation, rashes, and excoriation. ____ ____ ____ _____

5. Removed and discarded gloves, discarded disposable supplies, helped patient to comfortable position, performed hand hygiene. ____ ____ ____ _____

EVALUATION

1. Compared assessment findings with previous assessment characteristics to identify changes. ____ ____ ____ _____

2. Asked patient to describe signs and symptoms of appropriate cancers. ____ ____ ____ _____

3. Asked patient to identify guidelines for HPV vaccination. ____ ____ ____ _____

4. Identified unexpected outcomes. ____ ____ ____ _____

RECORDING AND REPORTING

1. Documented results of assessment in appropriate record. ____ ____ ____ _____

2. Recorded patient's ability to void, including description of output. ____ ____ ____ _____

3. Documented evaluation of patient learning. ____ ____ ____ _____

4. Reported abnormalities to nurse in charge and health care provider. ____ ____ ____ _____

Copyright © 2018 by Elsevier Inc. All rights reserved.

Student _____ Date _____

Instructor _____ Date _____

PERFORMANCE CHECKLIST SKILL 6.7 **MUSCULOSKELETAL AND NEUROLOGICAL ASSESSMENT**

	S	U	NP	Comments
ASSESSMENT				
1. Reviewed patient history for alcohol intake of more than two drinks per day; inadequate intake of protein, vitamin D, or calcium; thin and light body frame; family history of osteoporosis; white or Asian ancestry; sedentary lifestyle; long-term use of certain medications; certain medical conditions.	⎯	⎯	⎯	_____
2. Determined if patient has been screened for osteoporosis.	⎯	⎯	⎯	_____
3. Asked patient to describe history of alteration in bone, muscle, or joint function and location of alteration.	⎯	⎯	⎯	_____
4. Assessed nature and extent of patient's musculoskeletal pain, asked if walking affects reported lower extremity pain or cramping, assessed distance walked and pain before, during, and after activity.	⎯	⎯	⎯	_____
5. Assessed for height and weight, noted if there is a decrease in women older than 50.	⎯	⎯	⎯	_____
6. Determined if patient uses analgesics, antipsychotics, antidepressants, nervous system stimulants, or recreational drugs.	⎯	⎯	⎯	_____
7. Determined if patient had recent history of seizures or convulsions; clarified sequence of events; character of any symptoms; and relationship to time of day, fatigue, or stress.	⎯	⎯	⎯	_____
8. Screened patient for headache, tremors, dizziness, vertigo, numbness or tingling, visual changes, weakness, pain, or changes in speech.	⎯	⎯	⎯	_____
9. Discussed with spouse, family member, or friends any recent changes in behavior.	⎯	⎯	⎯	_____
10. Assessed patient for history of change in vision, hearing, smell, taste, or touch.	⎯	⎯	⎯	_____
11. Reviewed history for drug toxicity, serious infection, metabolic disturbances, heart failure, and severe anemia if patient displays sudden acute confusion.	⎯	⎯	⎯	_____

Copyright © 2018 by Elsevier Inc. All rights reserved.

	S	U	NP	Comments

12. Reviewed history for head or spinal cord injury, meningitis, congenital anomalies, neurologic disease, or psychiatric counseling. ___ ___ ___ _____

PLANNING

1. Identified expected outcomes. ___ ___ ___ _____

2. Performed hand hygiene, gathered necessary supplies. ___ ___ ___ _____

IMPLEMENTATION

1. Prepared patient for assessment:

    a. Integrated musculoskeletal and neurologic assessments during other portions of assessment or care. ___ ___ ___ _____

    b. Planned time for short rest periods during assessment. ___ ___ ___ _____

2. Assessed musculoskeletal system:

    a. Observed ability to use arms and hands for grasping objects. ___ ___ ___ _____

    b. Assessed muscle strength of upper extremities by applying gradual increase in pressure to muscle group. ___ ___ ___ _____

    c. Assessed hand grasp strength appropriately. ___ ___ ___ _____

    d. Asked patient to maintain pressure against resistance on arm or leg, compared strength of symmetrical muscle groups, noted weakness. ___ ___ ___ _____

    e. Exposed muscles and joints, observed body alignment in different positions. ___ ___ ___ _____

    f. Inspected gait as patient walked, had patient use assistive devices if appropriate. ___ ___ ___ _____

    g. Performed the Get Up and Go Test. ___ ___ ___ _____

    h. Stood behind patient; observed postural alignment; looked sideways at cervical, thoracic, and lumbar curves. ___ ___ ___ _____

    i. Made a general observation of extremities. ___ ___ ___ _____

    j. Palpated bones, joints, and surrounding tissue in involved areas; noted heat, tenderness, edema, or resistance to pressure. ___ ___ ___ _____

    k. Asked patient to put major joint through its full ROM, observed equality of active and passive motion in same body parts. ___ ___ ___ _____

    l. Palpated joint for swelling, stiffness, tenderness, and heat; noted any redness. ___ ___ ___ _____

    m. Assessed muscle tone in major muscle groups. ___ ___ ___ _____

Copyright © 2018 by Elsevier Inc. All rights reserved.

	S	U	NP	Comments

3. Performed neurologic assessment:

   a. Assessed LOC and orientation. ___ ___ ___ _____

   b. Assessed CNs.

     (1) Assessed EOM for CNs III, IV, and VI. ___ ___ ___ _____

     (2) Applied light sensation with cotton ball to symmetrical areas of the face. ___ ___ ___ _____

     (3) Had patient frown, smile, puff cheeks, and raise eyebrows for CN VII, noted symmetry. ___ ___ ___ _____

     (4) Had patient speak and swallow for CNs IX and X, checked midline uvula and symmetrical rise of uvula and soft palate, elicited gag reflex. ___ ___ ___ _____

   c. Assessed extremities for sensation, performed sensory test with patient's eyes closed.

     (1) Asked patient to indicate when sharp or dull sensation was felt as sharp and blunt ends of tongue blade were alternately applied to symmetrical areas. ___ ___ ___ _____

     (2) Applied light wisp of cotton in symmetrical areas. ___ ___ ___ _____

     (3) Grasped finger or toe, alternated moving up and down, asked patient to state whether digit was up or down. ___ ___ ___ _____

   d. Assessed motor and cerebellar function.

     (1) Had patient walk across the room, turn, and come back, noted use of assistive devices. ___ ___ ___ _____

     (2) Had patient stand straight first with eyes open and then closed, observed for swaying. ___ ___ ___ _____

   e. Assessed DTRs.

     (1) Determined necessity to monitor DTRs. ___ ___ ___ _____

     (2) Compared sides for each reflex tested and assigned a grade. ___ ___ ___ _____

     (3) Palpated the patellar tendon just below the patella, tapped pointed end of reflex hammer on the tendon. ___ ___ ___ _____

     (4) Stroked lateral aspect of the sole from the heel to the ball of the foot. ___ ___ ___ _____

     (5) Noted presence of Babinski's reflex. ___ ___ ___ _____

4. Disposed of supplies, performed hand hygiene. ___ ___ ___ _____

Copyright © 2018 by Elsevier Inc. All rights reserved.

	S	U	NP	Comments

EVALUATION

1. Compared muscle strength and ROM with previous physical assessment.

2. Compared neurologic status with previous assessment.

3. Evaluated level of patient discomfort on the appropriate pain scale.

4. Identified unexpected outcomes.

RECORDING AND REPORTING

1. Documented posture, gait, muscle strength, and ROM in appropriate record.

2. Documented LOC, orientation, papillary response, sensation, and reflex response in appropriate record.

3. Documented evaluation of patient learning.

4. Reported to nurse in charge or health care provider acute pain, sudden muscle weakness, change in LOC, or change in size or pupillary reaction.

Copyright © 2018 by Elsevier Inc. All rights reserved.

Student _____ Date _____

Instructor _____ Date _____

PERFORMANCE CHECKLIST PROCEDURAL GUIDELINE 6.1   **MONITORING INTAKE AND OUTPUT**

	S	U	NP	Comments
PROCEDURAL STEPS				
1. Identified patients with conditions that increase fluid loss.	——	——	——	_____
2. Identified patients with impaired swallowing, unconscious patients, and patients with impaired mobility.	——	——	——	_____
3. Identified patients on medication that influences fluid balance.	——	——	——	_____
4. Assessed signs and symptoms of dehydration and fluid overload.	——	——	——	_____
5. Weighed patients daily using same scale, same time of day, and comparable clothing.	——	——	——	_____
6. Monitored laboratory reports including urine specific gravity and Hct.	——	——	——	_____
7. Assessed patient's and family's knowledge of purpose and process of I&O measurement.	——	——	——	_____
8. Explained to patient and family the reason I&O are important.	——	——	——	_____
9. Performed hand hygiene.	——	——	——	_____
10. Measured and recorded all intake of fluid appropriately.	——	——	——	_____
11. Instructed patient and family to call you or NAP to empty contents of urinal, urine hat, or commode every time patient uses it; instructed them to monitor incontinence, vomiting, and excessive perspiration and to report it to the nurse.	——	——	——	_____
12. Informed patient and family that drainage bag and tube drainage are closely monitored, measured, and recorded and who is responsible, ensured graduation container was clearly marked.	——	——	——	_____
13. Applied clean gloves; measured drainage as indicated; noted color and characteristics; wore mask, eye protection, or gown if needed.	——	——	——	_____
14. Removed gloves and disposed of them properly, performed hand hygiene.	——	——	——	_____

Copyright © 2018 by Elsevier Inc. All rights reserved.

	S	U	NP	Comments
15. Noted I&O balance or imbalance, reported urine output less than 30 mL/hr or significant changes in daily weight.	____	____	____	_____
16. Documented on I&O form or electronic record.	____	____	____	_____

Copyright © 2018 by Elsevier Inc. All rights reserved.

Student _____ Date _____

Instructor _____ Date _____

PERFORMANCE CHECKLIST SKILL 7.1   **URINE SPECIMEN COLLECTION: MIDSTREAM (CLEAN-VOIDED) URINE; STERILE URINARY CATHETER**

	S	U	NP	Comments
ASSESSMENT				
1. Identified patient using two identifiers.	___	___	___	_____
2. Assessed patient's or family's understanding of purpose of test and method of collection.	___	___	___	_____
3. Assessed patient's ability to assist with urine specimen collection.	___	___	___	_____
4. Assessed for signs of UTI.	___	___	___	_____
5. Referred to agency procedures for collection methods.	___	___	___	_____
PLANNING				
1. Identified expected outcomes.	___	___	___	_____
IMPLEMENTATION				
1. Performed hand hygiene, checked labels and completed laboratory requisition for container.	___	___	___	_____
2. Provided privacy, allowed mobile patient to collect specimen in bathroom.	___	___	___	_____
3. Collected clean-voided urine specimen:				
a. Applied clean gloves, gave patient supplies to clean perineum or assisted patient in cleansing perineum, removed and disposed of gloves.	___	___	___	_____
b. Opened package of commercial specimen kit using aseptic technique.	___	___	___	_____
c. Poured antiseptic solution over cotton balls if necessary.	___	___	___	_____
d. Opened specimen container, maintained sterility of inside of container, placed cap properly.	___	___	___	_____
e. Assisted or allowed patient to cleanse perineum and collect specimen, informed patient antiseptic would feel cold.	___	___	___	_____
(1) For male patient:				
(a) Held penis with one hand, cleansed meatus properly, had patient retract foreskin if necessary, returned foreskin when done.	___	___	___	_____

Copyright © 2018 by Elsevier Inc. All rights reserved.

	S	U	NP	Comments

    (b) Rinsed area and dried if agency procedure indicates.

    (c) Had patient pass container through urine stream after patient initiated stream.

  (2) For female patient:

    (a) Spread labia minora with fingers of nondominant hand or had patient assist.

    (b) Cleansed urethral area appropriately, used fresh swab for each fold.

    (c) Rinsed area and dried with cotton ball if agency procedure indicates.

    (d) Passed specimen container into urine stream after patient initiated stream.

  f. Removed specimen container before flow stopped and before releasing labia or penis, assisted with personal hygiene as appropriate.

  g. Replaced cap on container, touched only outside.

  h. Cleaned urine from exterior surface of container.

4. Collected urine from indwelling urinary catheter:

  a. Explained use of needleless syringe and that patient would not experience discomfort.

  b. Explained need to clamp catheter 10 to 15 minutes before obtaining specimen and that it could not be obtained from drainage bag.

  c. Applied clean gloves, clamped drainage tubing below withdrawal site.

  d. Positioned patient properly, located port, cleansed port with disinfectant and allowed to dry.

  e. Attached needleless Luer-Lok syringe to port appropriately.

  f. Withdrew appropriate amount for culture for routine urinalysis.

  g. Transferred urine from syringe to appropriate container.

  h. Placed lid tightly on container.

  i. Unclamped catheter, ensured urine was flowing freely.

Copyright © 2018 by Elsevier Inc. All rights reserved.

	S	U	NP	Comments

5. Secured label to container, completed label properly.

6. Disposed of soiled supplies, removed and discarded gloves, performed hand hygiene.

7. Sent specimen and requisition to laboratory within 20 minutes, refrigerated specimen if necessary.

EVALUATION

1. Inspected clean-voided specimen for contamination.

2. Evaluated patient's urine C&S report for bacterial growth.

3. Observed urinary drainage system to ensure it was intact and patent.

4. Asked patient to explains steps in procedure.

5. Identified unexpected outcomes.

RECORDING AND REPORTING

1. Recorded collection of specimen in appropriate log.

2. Documented evaluation of patient learning.

3. Reported any abnormal findings to health care provider.

Copyright © 2018 by Elsevier Inc. All rights reserved.

Student _____ Date _____

Instructor _____ Date _____

PERFORMANCE CHECKLIST PROCEDURAL GUIDELINE 7.1 **COLLECTING A TIMED SPECIMEN**

	S	U	NP	Comments

PROCEDURAL STEPS

1. Identified patient using two identifiers, compared identifiers with patient's MAR. ___ ___ ___ _____

2. Explained reason for specimen collection, how patient can help, and that urine must be free of contaminants. ___ ___ ___ _____

3. Placed collection container in bathroom, included can of ice if indicated; posted signs reminding of timed urine collection; ensured personnel in receiving area collected and saved urine if patient left unit. ___ ___ ___ _____

4. Had patient drink two to four glasses of water about 30 minutes before times of collection. ___ ___ ___ _____

5. Performed hand hygiene, applied clean gloves, discarded first specimen as test began, indicated time test began on requisition, ensured patient began test with empty bladder, began collecting all urine for designated time. ___ ___ ___ _____

6. Measured volume of each voiding if I&O was to be recorded, placed all urine in labeled specimen bottles with appropriate additives. ___ ___ ___ _____

7. Kept specimen bottle in refrigerator or ice in bathroom to prevent decomposition of urine unless instructed otherwise. ___ ___ ___ _____

8. Encouraged patient to drink two glasses of water 1 hour before collection ended and empty bladder during last 15 minutes of collection period. ___ ___ ___ _____

9. Performed hand hygiene, applied clean gloves, collected final specimen, labeled specimen appropriately, attached requisition, sent to laboratory, removed gloves, performed hand hygiene. ___ ___ ___ _____

10. Removed signs, informed patient specimen collection period was complete. ___ ___ ___ _____

Copyright © 2018 by Elsevier Inc. All rights reserved.

Student _____ Date _____

Instructor _____ Date _____

PERFORMANCE CHECKLIST PROCEDURAL GUIDELINE 7.2 **URINE SCREENING FOR GLUCOSE, KETONES, PROTEIN, BLOOD, AND PH**

	S	U	NP	Comments

PROCEDURAL STEPS

1. Identified patient using two identifiers, compared identifiers with information on MAR.

2. Determined if double-voided specimen was needed for glucose testing; asked patient to void, discard, and drink water if necessary.

3. Performed hand hygiene, applied clean gloves, asked patient to collect fresh random urine specimen or removed specimen from catheter port.

4. Immersed end of reagent strip into urine container, removed strip immediately and tapped against side of container to remove excess urine.

5. Held strip in horizontal position.

6. Timed number of seconds on container, compared color of strip with color chart.

7. Discussed test results with patient, discarded urine, removed and discarded gloves, performed hand hygiene.

8. Recorded results immediately in appropriate log, reported reading to health care provider.

Copyright © 2018 by Elsevier Inc. All rights reserved.

Student _____ Date _____

Instructor _____ Date _____

PERFORMANCE CHECKLIST SKILL 7.2 **MEASURING OCCULT BLOOD IN STOOL**

	S	U	NP	Comments
ASSESSMENT				
1. Identified patient using two identifiers, compared identifiers with information in MAR.	___	___	___	_____
2. Assessed patient or caregiver for understanding of need for stool test.	___	___	___	_____
3. Assessed patient's ability to cooperate with procedure and collect specimen.	___	___	___	_____
4. Assessed patient's medical history for GI disorders.	___	___	___	_____
5. Reviewed patient's medications for drugs that contribute to GI bleeding.	___	___	___	_____
6. Referred to health care provider's orders for medication or dietary modifications before test.	___	___	___	_____
PLANNING				
1. Identified expected outcomes.	___	___	___	_____
2. Explained procedure to patient or family member, discussed reason for collection and how patient can help, explained that feces must be free of contaminants.	___	___	___	_____
3. Arranged for any needed dietary or medication restrictions.	___	___	___	_____
IMPLEMENTATION				
1. Performed hand hygiene.	___	___	___	_____
2. Applied clean gloves; obtained uncontaminated specimen in clean, dry container.	___	___	___	_____
3. Used tip of wooden applicator to obtain small portion of feces.	___	___	___	_____
4. Measured for occult blood:				
a. Performed Hemoccult slide test.				
(1) Opened flap of slide, applied thin smear of stool on paper in first box.	___	___	___	_____
(2) Obtained a second specimen from a different portion of stool, applied to second box of slide.	___	___	___	_____

Copyright © 2018 by Elsevier Inc. All rights reserved.

	S	U	NP	Comments

(3) Closed slide cover, turned slide over, opened cardboard flap, applied two drops of developing solution on each box of guaiac paper. ___ ___ ___ _____

(4) Read results at the appropriate time, noted color changes. ___ ___ ___ _____

(5) Disposed of test slide in proper receptacle. ___ ___ ___ _____

b. Performed test using Hematest tablets.

(1) Placed stool on guaiac paper and Hematest tablet on top of stool specimen, applied tap water, allowed to flow onto paper. ___ ___ ___ _____

(2) Observed color of paper at appropriate time. ___ ___ ___ _____

(3) Disposed of tablet and paper properly. ___ ___ ___ _____

5. Wrapped wooden applicator in paper towel, grabbed properly, removed gloves over wrapped applicator, disposed in proper receptacle, performed hand hygiene. ___ ___ ___ _____

EVALUATION

1. Noted color changes in guaiac paper. ___ ___ ___ _____

2. Asked patient to explain steps in stool specimen collection. ___ ___ ___ _____

3. Noted character of stool specimen. ___ ___ ___ _____

4. Identified unexpected outcomes. ___ ___ ___ _____

RECORDING AND REPORTING

1. Recorded results of test and stool characteristics in appropriate log. ___ ___ ___ _____

2. Documented evaluation of patient learning. ___ ___ ___ _____

3. Reported positive test results to health care provider. ___ ___ ___ _____

Copyright © 2018 by Elsevier Inc. All rights reserved.

Student _____ Date _____

Instructor _____ Date _____

PERFORMANCE CHECKLIST SKILL 7.3 **MEASURING OCCULT BLOOD IN GASTRIC SECRETIONS (GASTROCCULT)**

	S	U	NP	Comments

ASSESSMENT

1. Identified patient using two identifiers, compared identifiers with information on MAR. ___ ___ ___ _____

2. Assessed patient's or family members' understanding of need for test. ___ ___ ___ _____

3. Assessed patient's medical history for bleeding or GI disorders. ___ ___ ___ _____

4. Assessed patient's medical history for GI disorders. ___ ___ ___ _____

PLANNING

1. Identified expected outcomes. ___ ___ ___ _____

2. Explained procedure to patient or family, discussed why collection was necessary. ___ ___ ___ _____

IMPLEMENTATION

1. Performed hand hygiene. ___ ___ ___ _____

2. Verified NG tube placement. ___ ___ ___ _____

3. Obtained specimen by disconnecting tube from suction or gravity drainage from tube, aspirated fluid properly from the tube. ___ ___ ___ _____

4. Obtained sample of emesis from basin properly. ___ ___ ___ _____

5. Performed Gastroccult test:

   a. Applied one drop of gastric sample to Gastroccult blood test slide properly. ___ ___ ___ _____

   b. Applied two drops of developer solution over sample and one drop between positive and negative performance monitors. ___ ___ ___ _____

   c. Verified that performance monitor turns blue in 30 seconds. ___ ___ ___ _____

   d. Compared color of gastric sample with that of performance monitor at the appropriate time. ___ ___ ___ _____

   e. Disposed of test slide, applicator, and syringe in proper receptacle; reconnected enteral tube to drainage system if needed; removed gloves; performed hand hygiene. ___ ___ ___ _____

Copyright © 2018 by Elsevier Inc. All rights reserved.

	S	U	NP	Comments

EVALUATION

1. Noted character of gastric secretions.

2. Noted changes in guaiac paper.

3. Asked patient to explain the purpose of the procedure.

4. Identified unexpected outcomes.

RECORDING AND REPORTING

1. Recorded results of test and unusual characteristics of gastric contents in appropriate log.

2. Documented evaluation of patient learning.

3. Reported positive test results to health care provider.

Copyright © 2018 by Elsevier Inc. All rights reserved.

Student _____ Date _____

Instructor _____ Date _____

PERFORMANCE CHECKLIST SKILL 7.4 **COLLECTING NOSE AND THROAT SPECIMENS FOR CULTURE**

	S	U	NP	Comments

ASSESSMENT

1. Identified patient using at least two identifiers, compared identifiers with information on MAR. ____ ____ ____ _____

2. Assessed patient's understanding of purpose for procedure and ability to cooperate, obtained assistance if required. ____ ____ ____ _____

3. Inspected condition of nares and drainage from nasal mucosa and sinuses. ____ ____ ____ _____

4. Determined if patient experienced postnasal drip, sinus headache, tenderness, congestion, sore throat, or exposure to others with similar symptoms. ____ ____ ____ _____

5. Applied clean gloves, assessed condition of posterior pharynx. ____ ____ ____ _____

6. Reviewed health care provider's orders to determine if nose, throat, or both cultures were needed. ____ ____ ____ _____

PLANNING

1. Identified expected outcomes. ____ ____ ____ _____

2. Planned to do culture at appropriate time. ____ ____ ____ _____

3. Explained procedure to patient or family, discussed reason for specimen collection and how patient can help. ____ ____ ____ _____

4. Explained sensations patient may feel during procedure. ____ ____ ____ _____

IMPLEMENTATION

1. Asked patient to sit appropriately. ____ ____ ____ _____

2. Performed hand hygiene, had swab ready to use. ____ ____ ____ _____

3. Collected throat culture:

   a. Applied clean gloves. ____ ____ ____ _____

   b. Instructed patient to tilt head properly. ____ ____ ____ _____

   c. Asked patient to open mouth and say "ah," depressed tongue properly, illuminated with penlight as needed. ____ ____ ____ _____

   d. Inserted swab without touching lips, teeth, tongue, cheeks, or uvula. ____ ____ ____ _____

Copyright © 2018 by Elsevier Inc. All rights reserved.

	S	U	NP	Comments

e. Swabbed tonsillar area properly, made contact with inflamed sites. ___ ___ ___ _____

f. Withdrew swab without touching oral structures. ___ ___ ___ _____

4. Collected nasal culture:

a. Applied clean gloves ___ ___ ___ _____

b. Encouraged patient to blow nose, checked nostrils for patency, selected appropriate nostril. ___ ___ ___ _____

c. Had patient tilt head properly. ___ ___ ___ _____

d. Inserted nasal speculum properly. ___ ___ ___ _____

e. Passed swab into nostril until it reached portion of mucosa that was inflamed or contained exudates, rotated swab quickly. ___ ___ ___ _____

f. Removed swab without touching sides of speculum or nasal canal. ___ ___ ___ _____

g. Removed nasal speculum and placed in basin, offered patient facial tissue. ___ ___ ___ _____

5. Inserted swab into culture tube, crushed ampule at bottom of tube with gauze to protect fingers. ___ ___ ___ _____

6. Placed tip of swab into liquid medium, placed top securely on top of tube. ___ ___ ___ _____

7. Attached completed identification label and requisition to culture tube in front of patient, noted if patient was taking antibiotic or if specific organism was suspected. ___ ___ ___ _____

8. Enclosed specimen in plastic biohazard bag, sent to laboratory. ___ ___ ___ _____

9. Returned patient to comfortable position, removed and disposed of gloves, performed hand hygiene. ___ ___ ___ _____

EVALUATION

1. Checked laboratory record for results of culture test. ___ ___ ___ _____

2. Asked patient to explain purpose of culture. ___ ___ ___ _____

3. Identified unexpected outcomes. ___ ___ ___ _____

RECORDING AND REPORTING

1. Described appearance of mucosal structures and recorded specimen collection in appropriate log. ___ ___ ___ _____

2. Documented evaluation of patient learning. ___ ___ ___ _____

3. Reported unusual test results to health care provider. ___ ___ ___ _____

Copyright © 2018 by Elsevier Inc. All rights reserved.

Student _____ Date _____

Instructor _____ Date _____

PERFORMANCE CHECKLIST SKILL 7.5 **OBTAINING VAGINAL OR URETHRAL DISCHARGE SPECIMENS**

	S	U	NP	Comments
ASSESSMENT				
1. Identified patient using two identifiers, compared identifiers with MAR.	—	—	—	_____
2. Assessed patient understanding of need for culture and ability to cooperate with procedure.	—	—	—	_____
3. Performed hand hygiene; applied clean gloves; assessed condition of external genitalia and urethra, meatus, and vaginal orifice; observed for redness, swelling, tenderness, and discharge that was whitish; removed and discarded gloves; performed hand hygiene.	—	—	—	_____
4. Asked patient about dysuria, localized pruritus of genitalia, or lower abdominal pain.	—	—	—	_____
5. Gathered and recorded sexual history of patient if symptoms suggested STI.	—	—	—	_____
6. Referred to health care provider's order to determine if culture was to be vaginal or urethral.	—	—	—	_____
PLANNING				
1. Identified expected outcomes.	—	—	—	_____
2. Explained procedure to patient and/or family, discussed reason for specimen collection and how patient can help. Instructed female patient not to douche 24 hours before obtaining culture, instructed male patient not to urinate for 1 hour before obtaining urethral culture.	—	—	—	_____
IMPLEMENTATION				
1. Performed hand hygiene, applied clean gloves.	—	—	—	_____
2. Provided privacy.	—	—	—	_____
3. Assisted patient to appropriate position, raised gown, draped body parts to be exposed properly.	—	—	—	_____
4. Directed light source onto perineum if needed.	—	—	—	_____
5. Opened culture tube, held swab in dominant hand.	—	—	—	_____
6. Instructed patient to deep breathe slowly.	—	—	—	_____

Copyright © 2018 by Elsevier Inc. All rights reserved.

	S	U	NP	Comments

7. Obtained specimen properly:

   a. For female patient:

      (1) Separated labia with nondominant hand to expose vaginal orifice. ___ ___ ___ _____

      (2) Touched tip of swab into discharge pool or vaginal orifice, did not touch skin or mucosa. ___ ___ ___ _____

      (3) Exposed urethral meatus, pulled labia minora upward and back. ___ ___ ___ _____

      (4) Used clean swab, applied tip to meatus where discharge was visible, avoided touching labia. ___ ___ ___ _____

   b. For male patient:

      (1) Grasped penis appropriately, gently retracted foreskin if necessary. ___ ___ ___ _____

      (2) Held swab appropriately, applied to area of discharge. ___ ___ ___ _____

      (3) Introduced swab into meatus if necessary. ___ ___ ___ _____

      (4) Returned foreskin to natural position. ___ ___ ___ _____

8. Returned each swab to culture tube, secured top. ___ ___ ___ _____

9. Wrapped ampule with gauze if using commercial culture tube, crushed ampule, pushed tip into fluid medium. ___ ___ ___ _____

10. Removed and discarded gloves, performed hand hygiene. ___ ___ ___ _____

11. Labeled each culture tube with ID label, affixed requisition and conformed identifiers in front of patient. ___ ___ ___ _____

12. Sent specimen immediately to laboratory or refrigerator. ___ ___ ___ _____

13. Assisted patient to comfortable position, assisted with personal hygiene as needed, replaced gown, removed and discarded drape. ___ ___ ___ _____

EVALUATION

1. Reviewed laboratory results for evidence of pathogens. ___ ___ ___ _____

2. Continued to monitor whether discharge was present and, if it was, observed color and amount. ___ ___ ___ _____

3. Asked patient to explain steps of procedure. ___ ___ ___ _____

4. Identified unexpected outcomes. ___ ___ ___ _____

Copyright © 2018 by Elsevier Inc. All rights reserved.

	S	U	NP	Comments

RECORDING AND REPORTING

1. Recorded types of cultures and date and time sent to laboratory in the appropriate log. ____ ____ ____ _____

2. Documented evaluation of patient learning. ____ ____ ____ _____

3. Reported laboratory results to nurse in charge or health care provider. ____ ____ ____ _____

Copyright © 2018 by Elsevier Inc. All rights reserved.

Student _____ Date _____

Instructor _____ Date _____

PERFORMANCE CHECKLIST PROCEDURAL GUIDELINE 7.3 **COLLECTING A SPUTUM SPECIMEN BY EXPECTORATION**

	S	U	NP	Comments

PROCEDURAL STEPS

1. Identified patient using two identifiers, compared identifiers with information on MAR. ___ ___ ___ _____

2. Provided opportunity to rinse mouth with water. ___ ___ ___ _____

3. Performed hand hygiene, applied clean gloves, provided sputum cup, instructed patient not to touch inside of container. ___ ___ ___ _____

4. Had patient take deep breaths with full exhalation and then take full inhalation followed by a forceful cough, ensured sputum was expectorated directly into specimen container. ___ ___ ___ _____

5. Repeated until enough sputum had been collected. ___ ___ ___ _____

6. Secured lid on container, wiped outside of container with disinfectant. ___ ___ ___ _____

7. Offered patient tissues and mouth care, disposed of tissues properly. ___ ___ ___ _____

8. Removed and disposed of gloves, performed hand hygiene. ___ ___ ___ _____

9. Attached completed ID label and requisition to side of container, confirmed identifiers in patient's presence. ___ ___ ___ _____

10. Enclosed specimen in biohazard bag. ___ ___ ___ _____

Copyright © 2018 by Elsevier Inc. All rights reserved.

Student _____ Date _____

Instructor _____ Date _____

PERFORMANCE CHECKLIST SKILL 7.6   **COLLECTING A SPUTUM SPECIMEN BY SUCTION**

	S	U	NP	Comments
ASSESSMENT				
1. Identified patient using two identifiers, compared identifiers with MAR.	___	___	___	_____
2. Checked health care provider's orders for type of analysis and specifications.	___	___	___	_____
3. Assessed patient's level of understanding or procedure and purpose.	___	___	___	_____
4. Assessed when patient last ate a meal or had tube feeding.	___	___	___	_____
5. Determined type of assistance needed by patient to obtain specimen.	___	___	___	_____
6. Assessed patient's respiratory status.	___	___	___	_____
PLANNING				
1. Identified expected outcomes.	___	___	___	_____
2. Explained procedure and purpose, instructed patient to breathe normally.	___	___	___	_____
IMPLEMENTATION				
1. Provided privacy.	___	___	___	_____
2. Positioned patient properly.	___	___	___	_____
3. Performed hand hygiene, applied clean glove to nondominant hand, prepared suction device, determined if device was functioning properly.	___	___	___	_____
4. Directed light source onto perineum if needed.	___	___	___	_____
5. Applied sterile glove to dominant hand or used clean glove.	___	___	___	_____
6. Connected sterile suction catheter to rubber tubing on sputum trap.	___	U	NP	_____
7. Lubricated suction catheter tip with sterile water.	___	___	___	_____
8. Inserted suction catheter through appropriate tube without applying suction.	___	___	___	_____
9. Advanced catheter into trachea, warned patient to expect to cough.	___	___	___	_____
10. Applied suction appropriately as patient coughs.	___	___	___	_____

Copyright © 2018 by Elsevier Inc. All rights reserved.

	S	U	NP	Comments

11. Released suction, removed catheter, turned off suction. ___ ___ ___ _____

12. Detached catheter from specimen trap, disposed of catheter in appropriate receptacle. ___ ___ ___ _____

13. Secured top on container, detached suction tubing and connected rubber tubing to plastic adapter. ___ ___ ___ _____

14. Wiped outside of container with disinfectant. ___ ___ ___ _____

15. Offered patient tissues, disposed of tissues in emesis basin or appropriate container. ___ ___ ___ _____

16. Removed and disposed of gloves, performed hand hygiene. ___ ___ ___ _____

17. Labeled with ID label on side of specimen container, confirmed identifiers in front of patient, placed specimen in appropriate container, attached requisition. ___ ___ ___ _____

18. Sent specimen immediately to laboratory or refrigerated. ___ ___ ___ _____

19. Offered patient mouth care if desired. ___ ___ ___ _____

EVALUATION

1. Observed patient's respiratory status throughout procedure, measured oxygen saturation if necessary. ___ ___ ___ _____

2. Noted anxiety or discomfort in patient. ___ ___ ___ _____

3. Observed character of sputum. ___ ___ ___ _____

4. Referred to laboratory reports for test results. ___ ___ ___ _____

5. Asked patient to explain purpose and steps of procedure. ___ ___ ___ _____

6. Identified unexpected outcomes. ___ ___ ___ _____

RECORDING AND REPORTING

1. Recorded all pertinent information in appropriate log. ___ ___ ___ _____

2. Reported unusual sputum characteristics to nurse in charge or health care provider. ___ ___ ___ _____

3. Documented evaluation of patient learning. ___ ___ ___ _____

4. Reported abnormal laboratory findings to health care provider, initiated isolation techniques if necessary. ___ ___ ___ _____

5. Noted on requisition if patient was receiving antibiotics. ___ ___ ___ _____

Copyright © 2018 by Elsevier Inc. All rights reserved.

Student _____ Date _____

Instructor _____ Date _____

PERFORMANCE CHECKLIST SKILL 7.7   **OBTAINING WOUND DRAINAGE SPECIMENS**

	S	U	NP	Comments
ASSESSMENT				
1. Identified patient using two identifiers, compared identifiers with MAR.	___	___	___	_____
2. Assessed patient's understanding of need to culture and ability to cooperate with procedure.	___	___	___	_____
3. Assessed patient for signs of fever, chills, or excessive thirst; noted if WBC count was elevated.	___	___	___	_____
4. Asked patient about extent and type of pain at wound site, gave analgesic before dressing changes if necessary.	___	___	___	_____
5. Determined when dressing change was scheduled, performed wound assessment as part of procedure.	___	___	___	_____
6. Reviewed health care provider's orders for aerobic or anaerobic culture.	___	___	___	_____
7. Performed hand hygiene, applied clean gloves, removed old dressings and disposed properly, removed gloves and performed hand hygiene, applied sterile gloves to palpate wound, observed for signs of infection, discarded gloves, performed hand hygiene.	___	___	___	_____
PLANNING				
1. Identified expected outcomes.	___	___	___	_____
2. Determined and requested analgesic, administered as ordered and if needed.	___	___	___	_____
3. Explained reason for wound culture and how it would be collected.	___	___	___	_____
4. Explained that patient may feel tickling sensation.	___	___	___	_____
IMPLEMENTATION				
1. Provided privacy.	___	___	___	_____
2. Performed hand hygiene, applied clean gloves.	___	___	___	_____
3. Cleansed area around wound edges properly with antiseptic swab, removed old exudate.	___	___	___	_____
4. Discarded swab, removed and disposed of gloves, performed hand hygiene.	___	___	___	_____

Copyright © 2018 by Elsevier Inc. All rights reserved.

	S	U	NP	Comments

5. Opened packages of culture tube and dressing supplies, applied sterile gloves.   ___ ___ ___ _____

6. Obtained cultures:

   a. Aerobic culture.

     (1) Took swab from tube, inserted into wound in area of drainage, rotated swab gently, returned swab to tube, wrapped ampule in gauze, crushed ampule of medium, pushed swab into fluid.   ___ ___ ___ _____

   b. Anaerobic culture.

     (1) Took swab from culture tube, swabbed deeply into draining body cavity, rotated, returned swab to culture tube.   ___ ___ ___ _____

    OR:

     (2) Inserted syringe into wound, aspirated exudates, attached needle, expelled all air, injected drainage into culture tube.   ___ ___ ___ _____

7. Removed and disposed of gloves, performed hand hygiene.   ___ ___ ___ _____

8. Placed specimen label on each culture tube and verified identifiers in front of patient, indicated if patient was receiving antibiotics.   ___ ___ ___ _____

9. Sent specimens to the laboratory immediately.   ___ ___ ___ _____

10. Cleaned wound per order, applied new sterile dressing, secured dressing appropriately.   ___ ___ ___ _____

11. Removed and disposed of gloves and soiled supplies appropriately, performed hand hygiene.   ___ ___ ___ _____

12. Assisted patient to comfortable position.   ___ ___ ___ _____

EVALUATION

1. Obtained laboratory report for results of culture.   ___ ___ ___ _____

2. Observed character of wound drainage.   ___ ___ ___ _____

3. Observed edges of wound for redness and bleeding.   ___ ___ ___ _____

4. Asked patient to explain purpose and steps of procedure.   ___ ___ ___ _____

5. Identified unexpected outcomes.   ___ ___ ___ _____

RECORDING AND REPORTING

1. Recorded all pertinent information about specimens and wound characteristics in appropriate log.   ___ ___ ___ _____

2. Reported evidence of infection to health care provider.   ___ ___ ___ _____

Copyright © 2018 by Elsevier Inc. All rights reserved.

	S	U	NP	Comments
3. Documented evaluation of patient learning.	____	____	____	_____
4. Recorded patient's tolerance of procedure and response to analgesics.	____	____	____	_____

Copyright © 2018 by Elsevier Inc. All rights reserved.

Student _____ Date _____

Instructor _____ Date _____

PERFORMANCE CHECKLIST SKILL 7.8   **COLLECTING BLOOD SPECIMENS AND CULTURE BY VENIPUNCTURE (SYRINGE AND VACUTAINER METHOD)**

	S	U	NP	Comments
ASSESSMENT				
1. Identified patient using two identifiers, compared identifiers with MAR.	___	___	___	_____
2. Determined if patient understands purpose of procedure and ability to cooperate.	___	___	___	_____
3. Determined if special conditions need to be met before specimen collection.	___	___	___	_____
4. Assessed patient for possible risks associated with venipuncture, reviewed medication history.	___	___	___	_____
5. Assessed patient for contraindicated sites for venipuncture.	___	___	___	_____
6. Identified presence of tape sensitivities or latex or povidone-iodine allergies.	___	___	___	_____
7. Assessed for systemic signs of bacteremia.	___	___	___	_____
8. Reviewed health care provider's orders for types of tests.	___	___	___	_____
PLANNING				
1. Identified expected outcomes.	___	___	___	_____
2. Explained procedure to patient, described purpose of tests, explained sensations patient would feel.	___	___	___	_____
IMPLEMENTATION				
1. Brought equipment to bedside and organized.	___	___	___	_____
2. Provided privacy, performed hand hygiene.	___	___	___	_____
3. Raised or lowered bed to comfortable height.	___	___	___	_____
4. Assisted patient to appropriate position.	___	___	___	_____
5. Applied tourniquet properly:				
a. Positioned tourniquet properly above site.	___	___	___	_____
b. Crossed tourniquet over patient's arm, placed over gown sleeve if appropriate.	___	___	___	_____
c. Held tourniquet between fingers, tucked loop between patient's arm and tourniquet.	___	___	___	_____
6. Did not keep tourniquet on patient longer than 1 minute.	___	___	___	_____

86

Copyright © 2018 by Elsevier Inc. All rights reserved.

	S	U	NP	Comments

7. Inspected extremity for best site.   ____ ____ ____ _____

8. Applied clean gloves, palpated selected vein, noted rigidity of vein.   ____ ____ ____ _____

9. Obtained blood specimen:

   a. Syringe method.

     (1) Had syringe with appropriate needle attached.   ____ ____ ____ _____

     (2) Cleansed venipuncture site properly with antiseptic, allowed to dry, used appropriate antiseptic.   ____ ____ ____ _____

     (3) Removed needle cover, informed patient that "stick" lasts a few seconds.   ____ ____ ____ _____

     (4) Placed thumb or forefinger below site, pulled skin taut, stretched until vein was stabilized.   ____ ____ ____ _____

     (5) Held syringe and needle properly above arm bevel up.   ____ ____ ____ _____

     (6) Inserted needle into vein, stopped when "pop" was felt.   ____ ____ ____ _____

     (7) Held syringe, pulled back plunger.   ____ ____ ____ _____

     (8) Observed for blood return.   ____ ____ ____ _____

     (9) Obtained desired amount of blood, kept needle stabilized.   ____ ____ ____ _____

     (10) Released tourniquet.   ____ ____ ____ _____

     (11) Applied gauze without applying pressure, withdrew needle, applied pressure, checked for hematoma.   ____ ____ ____ _____

     (12) Activated safety cover, discarded needle in appropriate container.   ____ ____ ____ _____

     (13) Attached syringe to transfer device, attached tube, allowed vacuum to fill tube appropriately, removed and filled other tubes as appropriate, rotated tubes properly.   ____ ____ ____ _____

   b. Vacutainer system method.

     (1) Attached double-ended needle to Vacutainer tube.   ____ ____ ____ _____

     (2) Had proper tube resting inside Vacutainer device, did not puncture stopper.   ____ ____ ____ _____

     (3) Cleansed venipuncture site properly, allowed to dry.   ____ ____ ____ _____

Copyright © 2018 by Elsevier Inc. All rights reserved.

	S	U	NP	Comments

(4) Removed needle cover, informed patient that "stick" would only last a few seconds. ___ ___ ___ _____

(5) Placed thumb and forefinger below site, pulled skin taut, stretched skin until vein stabilized. ___ ___ ___ _____

(6) Held needle at appropriate angle from arm bevel up. ___ ___ ___ _____

(7) Inserted needle into vein. ___ ___ ___ _____

(8) Grasped Vacutainer securely, advanced specimen tube into needle of holder. ___ ___ ___ _____

(9) Noted flow of blood into tube. ___ ___ ___ _____

(10) Grasped Vacutainer firmly, removed tube, inserted additional tube as needed, rotated each tube properly. ___ ___ ___ _____

(11) Released tourniquet after tubes were filled. ___ ___ ___ _____

(12) Applied gauze pad over site without applying pressure, withdrew needle with Vacutainer. ___ ___ ___ _____

(13) Applied pressure over site with gauze or antiseptic pad until bleeding stops, observed for hematoma, taped dressing securely. ___ ___ ___ _____

(14) Disposed of syringe, needle, gauze and other supplies appropriately. ___ ___ ___ _____

c. Blood culture.

(1) Cleansed site with antiseptic swab, allowed to dry. ___ ___ ___ _____

(2) Cleaned tops of culture bottles properly, allowed to dry. ___ ___ ___ _____

(3) Collected appropriate amount of venous blood from each venipuncture site. ___ ___ ___ _____

(4) Activated safety guard, discarded needle, replaced with new sterile needle before injecting blood sample into culture bottle. ___ ___ ___ _____

(5) Filled anaerobic bottle first if both aerobic and anaerobic cultures were needed. ___ ___ ___ _____

(6) Mixed blood in each culture bottle. ___ ___ ___ _____

Copyright © 2018 by Elsevier Inc. All rights reserved.

	S	U	NP	Comments

d. CVC collection.

(1) Selected appropriate port, turned off IV pumps, clamped lumens.

    ____ ____ ____ _____

(2) Wiped all Luer-Lok caps or removed alcohol-impregnated cap, attached saline syringe to selected port, released clamp, aspirated for blood return, flushed with saline, used appropriate-sized syringe, removed syringe.

    ____ ____ ____ _____

(3) Wiped port with alcohol, attached syringe, aspirated 5 mL of blood and discarded, reclamped catheter, wiped port, attached Luer-Lok syringe, unclamped catheter, aspirated blood. Reclamped catheter, removed syringe, cleansed catheter port, attached Vacutainer with proper attachment, inserted specimen tube, allowed tube to fill.

    ____ ____ ____ _____

(4) For Vacutainer method, clamped catheter, attached needleless connecter to holder, placed blood tube into holder, disinfected cap, inserted needleless connection in cap, unclamped catheter, advanced blood tube into holder, allowed blood to fill tube, clamped catheter, discarded first tube in biohazard container, attached specimen tubes to Vacutainer with Luer-Lok adapted, unclamped catheter, obtained blood specimens.

    ____ ____ ____ _____

(5) Clamped catheter, removed Vacutainer holder and needleless connection from cap, disinfected with alcohol.

    ____ ____ ____ _____

(6) Attached prefilled NS syringe; flushed using push, pause method; ensured positive pressure for lumen; removed and locked lumen syringe properly; if positive pressure is not verified, held syringe plunger steady; locked off lumen with slide cap, removed syringe; reattached alcohol-impregnated cap.

    ____ ____ ____ _____

(7) Rotate tubes appropriately.

    ____ ____ ____ _____

10. Checked tubes for sign of external contamination with blood, decontaminated if necessary.

    ____ ____ ____ _____

11. Removed gloves after specimen was obtained and spillage was cleaned.

    ____ ____ ____ _____

12. Assisted patient to comfortable position.

    ____ ____ ____ _____

Copyright © 2018 by Elsevier Inc. All rights reserved.

	S	U	NP	Comments

13. Attached properly completed labels to each tube, affixed requisition and verified identifiers in front of patient.   ____ ____ ____ _____

14. Placed specimens in biohazard bag, sent to laboratory within 30 minutes.   ____ ____ ____ _____

15. Performed hand hygiene.   ____ ____ ____ _____

EVALUATION

1. Inspected venipuncture site for homeostasis.   ____ ____ ____ _____

2. Determined if patient remained anxious or fearful.   ____ ____ ____ _____

3. Checked laboratory report for test results.   ____ ____ ____ _____

4. Asked patient to explain purpose and steps of procedure.   ____ ____ ____ _____

5. Identified unexpected outcomes.   ____ ____ ____ _____

RECORDING AND REPORTING

1. Recorded all pertinent information in appropriate log.   ____ ____ ____ _____

2. Documented evaluation of patient learning.   ____ ____ ____ _____

3. Reported any STAT or abnormal test results of health care provider.   ____ ____ ____ _____

Copyright © 2018 by Elsevier Inc. All rights reserved.

Student _____ Date _____

Instructor _____ Date _____

PERFORMANCE CHECKLIST SKILL 7.9 **BLOOD GLUCOSE MONITORING**

	S	U	NP	Comments

ASSESSMENT

1. Identified patient using two identifiers, compared identifiers with MAR.   ___ ___ ___ _____

2. Assessed patient's understanding of procedure and purpose of blood glucose monitoring, determined if patient understood how to perform test and its importance in glucose control.   ___ ___ ___ _____

3. Determined if specific conditions needed to be met before or after sample collection.   ___ ___ ___ _____

4. Determined if risks exist for performing skin puncture.   ___ ___ ___ _____

5. Assessed area of skin to be used as puncture site; inspected fingers and forearms for edema, inflammations, cuts, and sores; avoided areas of bruising and open lesions; avoided hand on side of mastectomy.   ___ ___ ___ _____

6. Reviewed health care provider's orders for time or frequency of measurement.   ___ ___ ___ _____

7. Assessed ability of patient to perform testing at home and to handle skin-puncturing device if necessary.   ___ ___ ___ _____

PLANNING

1. Identified expected outcomes.   ___ ___ ___ _____

2. Explained procedure and purpose to patient and family, offered opportunity to practice testing procedures, provided resources and teaching aids.   ___ ___ ___ _____

IMPLEMENTATION

1. Performed hand hygiene, instructed adult to perform hand hygiene, rinsed and dried.   ___ ___ ___ _____

2. Positioned patient appropriately.   ___ ___ ___ _____

3. Removed reagent strip from vial and cap, checked code on test strip vial, used proper test strips.   ___ ___ ___ _____

4. Inserted strip into meter, did not bend strip.   ___ ___ ___ _____

5. Removed unused reagent strip from meter; placed on clean, dry surface with test pad facing up.   ___ ___ ___ _____

Copyright © 2018 by Elsevier Inc. All rights reserved.

	S	U	NP	Comments

6. Matched code on screen with code from test strip vial, confirmed codes.

| | ___ | ___ | ___ | _____ |

7. Performed hand hygiene, applied clean gloves, prepared lancet device properly.

| | ___ | ___ | ___ | _____ |

8. Obtained blood sample:

   a. Wiped finger or forearm with antiseptic, chose appropriate area for puncture site.

| | ___ | ___ | ___ | _____ |

   b. Held area to be punctured in dependent position, did not massage finger site.

| | ___ | ___ | ___ | _____ |

   c. Held tip of lancet against area of skin chosen for test site, pressed release button, removed device.

| | ___ | ___ | ___ | _____ |

   d. Squeezed fingertip until round blood drop forms.

| | ___ | ___ | ___ | _____ |

9. Obtained test results:

   a. Ensured meter was still on, brought test strip to drop of blood, ensured adequate sample was obtained.

| | ___ | ___ | ___ | _____ |

   b. Read glucose test result on the screen.

| | ___ | ___ | ___ | _____ |

10. Turned meter off; disposed of test strip, lancet, and gloves in proper receptacle.

| | ___ | ___ | ___ | _____ |

11. Performed hand hygiene.

| | ___ | ___ | ___ | _____ |

12. Discussed test results with patient, encouraged questions and participation.

| | ___ | ___ | ___ | _____ |

EVALUATION

1. Inspected puncture site for bleeding and tissue injury.

| | ___ | ___ | ___ | _____ |

2. Compared glucose meter reading with normal levels and previous results.

| | ___ | ___ | ___ | _____ |

3. Asked patient to explain how to obtain blood glucose reading.

| | ___ | ___ | ___ | _____ |

4. Identified unexpected outcomes.

| | ___ | ___ | ___ | _____ |

RECORDING AND REPORTING

1. Recorded procedure and glucose level in appropriate log, took action for abnormal range.

| | ___ | ___ | ___ | _____ |

2. Described patient response in notes.

| | ___ | ___ | ___ | _____ |

3. Described explanations or teaching provided in notes.

| | ___ | ___ | ___ | _____ |

4. Described evaluation of patient learning.

| | ___ | ___ | ___ | _____ |

5. Recorded and reported abnormal blood glucose levels.

| | ___ | ___ | ___ | _____ |

Copyright © 2018 by Elsevier Inc. All rights reserved.

Student _____   Date _____

Instructor _____   Date _____

PERFORMANCE CHECKLIST SKILL 7.10 **OBTAINING AN ARTERIAL SPECIMEN FOR BLOOD GAS MEASUREMENT**

	S	U	NP	Comments
ASSESSMENT				
1. Identified patient using two identifiers, compared identifiers with MAR.	___	___	___	_____
2. Assessed factors that influence ABG measurements, including hyperventilation or hypoventilation and body temperature.	___	___	___	_____
3. Identified medications that may influence ABG measurement.	___	___	___	_____
4. Assessed respiratory status.	___	___	___	_____
5. Reviewed criteria for choosing site for ABG sample:				
a. Assessed collateral blood flow with Allen test.	___	___	___	_____
b. Assessed accessibility of vessel.	___	___	___	_____
c. Assessed tissue surrounding artery.	___	___	___	_____
d. Assessed that arteries were not directly adjacent to veins.	___	___	___	_____
6. Assessed arterial sites (radial, brachial, and femoral arteries) for use in obtaining specimen.	___	___	___	_____
7. Reviewed baseline ABG values for patient.	___	___	___	_____
8. Determined patient's knowledge about ABG procedure.	___	___	___	_____
PLANNING				
1. Identified expected outcomes.	___	___	___	_____
2. Prepared heparinized syringe properly.	___	___	___	_____
3. Explained steps and purpose of procedure to patient.	___	___	___	_____

Copyright © 2018 by Elsevier Inc. All rights reserved.

	S	U	NP	Comments

IMPLEMENTATION

1. Performed hand hygiene. _____ _____ _____ _____

2. Palpated selected site with fingertips. _____ _____ _____ _____

3. Elevated patient's wrist with small pillow, asked patient to extend fingers downward, stabilized artery with hyperextension of wrist. _____ _____ _____ _____

4. Applied clean gloves, cleaned area of maximal impulse with alcohol or antiseptic, allowed to dry. _____ _____ _____ _____

5. Held gauze pad with same fingers used to palpate artery. _____ _____ _____ _____

6. Used corner of gauze pad to point to site. _____ _____ _____ _____

7. Held needle bevel up, inserted at appropriate angle, prepared patient for painful stick. _____ _____ _____ _____

8. Stopped advancing needle at appropriate time. _____ _____ _____ _____

9. Allowed arterial pulsations to pump appropriate amount of blood into syringe. _____ _____ _____ _____

10. Held gauze pad over puncture site, withdrew syringe and needle, activated safety guard over needle. _____ _____ _____ _____

11. Applied pressure over and proximal to puncture site with pad. _____ _____ _____ _____

12. Maintained continuous pressure for appropriate time, had another nurse remove safety needle and attach filter cap if needed. _____ _____ _____ _____

13. Inspected site visually for signs of bleeding or hematoma formation. _____ _____ _____ _____

14. Palpated artery below or distal to puncture site. _____ _____ _____ _____

15. Took syringe, removed safety needle, discarded in biohazard container, attached filter cap to syringe or covered tip with gauze to dispel air. _____ _____ _____ _____

16. Placed ID label on syringe in front of patient, confirmed identifiers, placed syringe in cup of crushed ice, attached requisition to sample. _____ _____ _____ _____

17. Placed sample in biohazard bag, sent to laboratory immediately. _____ _____ _____ _____

18. Removed gloves, performed hand hygiene. _____ _____ _____ _____

Copyright © 2018 by Elsevier Inc. All rights reserved.

	S	U	NP	Comments

EVALUATION

1. Inspected puncture site and area distal for complications. ____ ____ ____ _____

2. Reviewed results of sample as soon as possible. ____ ____ ____ _____

3. Asked patient to explain how to obtain arterial blood gas specimen. ____ ____ ____ _____

4. Identified unexpected outcomes. ____ ____ ____ _____

RECORDING AND REPORTING

1. Recorded all pertinent information in the appropriate log. ____ ____ ____ _____

2. Reported ABG results to health care provider. ____ ____ ____ _____

3. Reported patient's FiO_2 and any ventilator settings. ____ ____ ____ _____

4. Described evaluation of patient learning. ____ ____ ____ _____

5. Recorded results of test in nurses' notes. ____ ____ ____ _____

Copyright © 2018 by Elsevier Inc. All rights reserved.

Student _____ Date _____

Instructor _____ Date _____

PERFORMANCE CHECKLIST SKILL 8.1 **INTRAVENOUS MODERATE SEDATION**

	S	U	NP	Comments

ASSESSMENT

1. Identified patient using two identifiers, compared identifiers with information in MAR.

2. Verified type of procedure scheduled and procedure site with patient.

3. Verified that a preprocedure medication reconciliation and H&P examination were completed.

4. Verified that informed consent was obtained at an appropriate time.

5. Assessed patient's past history if adverse reaction to IV sedation.

6. Verified patient's ASA Physical Status Classification.

7. Assessed patient for risk factors increasing likelihood of adverse event.

8. Assessed patient's history for substance abuse or liver/kidney disease.

9. Verified patient has not ingested food or fluids for at least 4 hours.

10. Determined if patient was allergic to latex, antiseptic, tape, or anesthetic solutions.

11. Assessed patient's level of understanding of procedure, including any concerns.

12. Assessed baseline vital signs.

13. Determined patient's height and weight.

14. Assessed patient's baseline status via agency's scoring system.

PLANNING

1. Identify expected outcomes.

2. Explained to patient that sedation would cause relaxation and amnesia but he or she would be awake during the procedure, taught patient nonverbal signals if necessary.

3. Explained that close monitoring does not indicate a problem.

96

Copyright © 2018 by Elsevier Inc. All rights reserved.

	S	U	NP	Comments

4. Explained to patient major steps of procedure. ___ ___ ___ _____

5. Positioned patient as needed for procedure. ___ ___ ___ _____

IMPLEMENTATION

1. Established peripheral IV access. ___ ___ ___ _____

2. Implemented Universal Precautions protocol properly in presence of appropriate health care team members. ___ ___ ___ _____

3. Monitored heart rate and SpO_2 continuously during diagnostic procedure; monitored airway patency, respiratory rate and depth, blood pressure, and LOC and responsiveness; kept oxygen and suction equipment nearby. ___ ___ ___ _____

4. Observed for verbal and nonverbal evidence of pain, grimacing, or eye opening. ___ ___ ___ _____

5. Assessed level of sedation using appropriate scale. ___ ___ ___ _____

6. Repositioned patient as needed without interrupting. ___ ___ ___ _____

EVALUATION

1. Monitored patient throughout the procedure using the Modified Ramsay Sedation Scale. ___ ___ ___ _____

2. Used Aldrete score after procedure; monitored LOC, respiratory rate, oxygen saturation, blood pressure, heart rate and rhythm, and pain score. ___ ___ ___ _____

3. Asked patient to repeat back what he or she understands regarding procedure or any postprocedure patient instructions. ___ ___ ___ _____

4. Had patient's driver explain postprocedure education and sign appropriate documents. ___ ___ ___ _____

5. Asked patient to describe the medications he or she will take home. ___ ___ ___ _____

6. Identified unexpected outcomes. ___ ___ ___ _____

RECORDING AND REPORTING

1. Documented vital signs, SpO_2, end-tidal CO_2, and sedation level at the appropriate times. ___ ___ ___ _____

2. Recorded all information related to drugs and fluids given during and after procedure. ___ ___ ___ _____

3. Reported any respiratory distress, cardiac compromise, or unexpected altered mental status to health care provider immediately. ___ ___ ___ _____

4. Documented discharge teaching, medication reconciliation, discontinuation of IV access, final/discharge assessment, and to whom/how discharged. ___ ___ ___ _____

5. Documented evaluation of patient learning. ___ ___ ___ _____

Copyright © 2018 by Elsevier Inc. All rights reserved.

Student _____ Date _____

Instructor _____ Date _____

PERFORMANCE CHECKLIST SKILL 8.2 **CONTRAST MEDIA STUDIES: ARTERIOGRAM (ANGIOGRAM), CARDIAC CATHETERIZATION, AND INTRAVENOUS PYELOGRAM**

	S	U	NP	Comments
ASSESSMENT				
1. Identified patient using two identifiers, compared identifiers with information in MAR.	___	___	___	_____
2. Verified type of procedure scheduled and procedure site with patient.	___	___	___	_____
3. Verified that informed consent was obtained at appropriate time.	___	___	___	_____
4. Determined if patient was taking anticoagulants, aspirin, or nonsteroidal medication.	___	___	___	_____
5. Assessed patient for history of allergies and previous reaction to contrast agent, notified cardiologist or radiologist if necessary.	___	___	___	_____
6. Reviewed medical record for contraindications.	___	___	___	_____
7. Assessed patient's bleeding and coagulation status.	___	___	___	_____
8. Obtained vital signs and peripheral pulses, auscultated heart and lungs, obtained weight if needed.	___	___	___	_____
9. Assessed patient's hydration status.	___	___	___	_____
10. Assessed patient's level of understanding of procedures, including any concerns.	___	___	___	_____
11. Determined type of arteriogram scheduled, verified details if necessary.	___	___	___	_____
12. Determined and documented last time of ingested food, drink, or medications.	___	___	___	_____
13. Reviewed health care provider's order for preprocedure medications, hydration, antihistamines, and IV sedation.	___	___	___	_____
PLANNING				
1. Identified expected outcomes.	___	___	___	_____
2. Explained to patient purpose of procedure and what would happen.	___	___	___	_____
3. Removed all of patient's jewelry and metal objects.	___	___	___	_____
4. Completed appropriate preprocedure preparation for IVP or cardiac catheterization.	___	___	___	_____

Copyright © 2018 by Elsevier Inc. All rights reserved.

	S	U	NP	Comments

5. Verified availability of emergent cardiac surgery if necessary and patient's ASA classification. ___ ___ ___ _____

IMPLEMENTATION

1. Had patient empty bladder or bowels before procedure. ___ ___ ___ _____

2. Prepared cardiac monitor, pulse oximeter, and/or end-tidal CO_2 monitor. ___ ___ ___ _____

3. Performed hand hygiene, applied appropriate PPE. ___ ___ ___ _____

4. Provided IV access using large-bore cannula, removed gloves. ___ ___ ___ _____

5. Helped patient to a comfortable position on x-ray table, immobilized extremity, padded any bony prominences. ___ ___ ___ _____

6. Took time-out to verify patient's name, type of procedure, and site. ___ ___ ___ _____

7. Monitored vital signs, SpO_2, end-tidal CO_2; palpated peripheral pulses for arterial procedures. ___ ___ ___ _____

8. Told patient that he or she may experience chest pain and severe hot flash for a few seconds during injection of dye. ___ ___ ___ _____

9. Applied necessary PPE; draped patient, leaving puncture site exposed. ___ ___ ___ _____

10. Observed patient while physician worked for signs of anaphylaxis if iodinated dye was used. ___ ___ ___ _____

11. Assisted with measuring cardiac volumes and pressure for cardiac catheterization. ___ ___ ___ _____

12. Monitored levels of sedation and LOC if appropriate. ___ ___ ___ _____

13. Removed and discarded gloves, performed hand hygiene. ___ ___ ___ _____

14. Kept extremity immobilized for 2 to 6 hours, used orthopedic bedpan if necessary. ___ ___ ___ _____

15. Emphasized need to lie flat for 6 to 12 hours. ___ ___ ___ _____

16. Encouraged patient to drink fluids. ___ ___ ___ _____

EVALUATION

1. Evaluated patient's body position and comfort during procedure. ___ ___ ___ _____

2. Monitored vital signs and oxygen saturation, assessed for signs of cardiac complications at appropriate intervals. ___ ___ ___ _____

Copyright © 2018 by Elsevier Inc. All rights reserved.

	S	U	NP	Comments

3. Monitored for complications:

   a. Performed neurovascular checks properly, used a Doppler ultrasonic stethoscope if necessary. ___ ___ ___ _____

   b. Assessed vascular access site for bleeding and hematoma. ___ ___ ___ _____

   c. Auscultated heart and lungs, compared with preprocedure findings. ___ ___ ___ _____

   d. Observed patient for possible delayed reaction to iodine. ___ ___ ___ _____

4. Evaluated level of sedation, LOC, and SpO_2; used Aldrete Scale. ___ ___ ___ _____

5. Assessed postprocedure laboratory values. ___ ___ ___ _____

6. Had patient rate discomfort on pain scale. ___ ___ ___ _____

7. Asked patient to describe signs of an allergic reaction. ___ ___ ___ _____

8. Identified unexpected outcomes. ___ ___ ___ _____

RECORDING AND REPORTING

1. Recorded patient's status; recorded any drainage from puncture site, appearance of dressing, and condition of puncture site. ___ ___ ___ _____

2. Reported problems to health care provider if necessary. ___ ___ ___ _____

3. Documented evaluation of patient learning. ___ ___ ___ _____

Copyright © 2018 by Elsevier Inc. All rights reserved.

Student _____ Date _____

Instructor _____ Date _____

PERFORMANCE CHECKLIST SKILL 8.3 **ASSISTING WITH ASPIRATIONS: BONE MARROW ASPIRATION/ BIOPSY, LUMBAR PUNCTURE, PARACENTESIS, AND THORACENTESIS**

	S	U	NP	Comments
ASSESSMENT				
1. Identified patient using two identifiers, compared identifiers with information on MAR.	___	___	___	_____
2. Verified type of procedure scheduled, purpose, and procedure site with patient and medical record.	___	___	___	_____
3. Verified that informed consent was obtained at an appropriate time.	___	___	___	_____
4. Determined patient's ability to assume position and stay still, discussed need for premedication with health care provider.	___	___	___	_____
5. Obtained vital signs, SpO_2/end-tidal CO_2 value, and weight; obtained abdominal girth measurement if necessary; assessed lower extremity movement, sensation, and muscle strength.	___	___	___	_____
6. Instructed patient to empty bladder.	___	___	___	_____
7. Assessed patient's coagulation status.	___	___	___	_____
8. Determined whether patient was allergic to antiseptic, latex, or anesthetic solutions.	___	___	___	_____
9. Assessed patient's level of understanding of procedure, including any concerns.	___	___	___	_____
10. Assessed baseline pain level.	___	___	___	_____
PLANNING				
1. Identified expected outcomes.	___	___	___	_____
2. Explained steps of skin preparation, anesthetic injection, needle insertion, and position required.	___	___	___	_____
3. Premedicated for pain or anxiety if ordered.	___	___	___	_____
4. Verified recent chest x-ray examination.	___	___	___	_____
IMPLEMENTATION				
1. Performed hand hygiene.	___	___	___	_____
2. Set up sterile tray or opened supplies.	___	___	___	_____
3. Took time-out to verify patient's name, type of procedure, and procedure site with patient and team.	___	___	___	_____

Copyright © 2018 by Elsevier Inc. All rights reserved.

	S	U	NP	Comments

4. Assisted patient in maintaining correct position, reassured patient while explaining procedure.

5. Explained to patient that pain might occur when lidocaine was injected and that pressure might occur when tissue or fluid was aspirated.

6. Assessed patient's condition during procedure, including respiratory status, vital signs, and complaints of pain.

7. Noted character of aspirate.

8. Properly labeled specimen in presence of patient, transported to laboratory in proper container, labeled specimens in order of collection.

9. Assisted with pressure over insertion site and application of gauze after needle was removed.

10. Removed PPE, discarded appropriately, performed hand hygiene.

EVALUATION

1. Monitored LOC, vital signs, and SpO_2/end-tidal CO_2 at appropriate intervals.

2. Inspected dressing over puncture site for signs of infection, inspected area under patient for bleeding, avoided disrupting healing clot at site.

3. Evaluated pain score.

4. Measured abdominal girth and respirations following paracentesis, compared with preprocedure assessments.

5. Asked patient to describe expectations after the procedure.

6. Identified unexpected outcomes.

RECORDING AND REPORTING

1. Recorded all pertinent information in the appropriate log.

2. Reported changes in vital signs, unexpected pain, or excessive drainage to health care provider immediately.

Copyright © 2018 by Elsevier Inc. All rights reserved.

Student _____ Date _____

Instructor _____ Date _____

PERFORMANCE CHECKLIST SKILL 8.4 **CARE OF PATIENT UNDERGOING BRONCHOSCOPY**

	S	U	NP	Comments

ASSESSMENT

1. Identified patient using at least two identifiers, compared identifiers with information on MAR. ___ ___ ___ _____

2. Verified type of procedure scheduled and procedure site with patient. ___ ___ ___ _____

3. Verified that informed consent was obtained at the appropriate time. ___ ___ ___ _____

4. Assessed patient's history for inability to tolerate interruption of high-flow oxygen if necessary. ___ ___ ___ _____

5. Obtained baseline vital signs, SpO_2, and end-tidal CO_2 values. ___ ___ ___ _____

6. Assessed type of cough, sputum produced, and heart and lung sounds. ___ ___ ___ _____

7. Determined purpose of procedure. ___ ___ ___ _____

8. Determined whether patient was allergic to local anesthetic. ___ ___ ___ _____

9. Assessed need for preprocedure medication. ___ ___ ___ _____

10. Assessed time patient last ingested food, fluids, or medications. ___ ___ ___ _____

11. Assessed patient's level of understanding of procedure, including any concerns. ___ ___ ___ _____

PLANNING

1. Identified expected outcomes. ___ ___ ___ _____

2. Administered atropine, opioid, or antianxiety agent 30 minutes before procedure. ___ ___ ___ _____

3. Explained procedure to patient. ___ ___ ___ _____

4. Removed and safely stored patient's dentures/eyeglasses. ___ ___ ___ _____

IMPLEMENTATION

1. Assessed current IV access or established new access. ___ ___ ___ _____

2. Assisted patient to assume appropriate position. ___ ___ ___ _____

3. Took time-out to verify patient's name, type of procedure, and procedure site with patient and team. ___ ___ ___ _____

Copyright © 2018 by Elsevier Inc. All rights reserved.

	S	U	NP	Comments

4. Performed hand hygiene, applied PPE, positioned tip of suction catheter for easy access to patient's mouth.

5. Instructed patient not to swallow the local anesthetic, provided emesis basin.

6. Assisted patient throughout procedure with explanations, verbal reassurance, and support.

7. Assessed patient's pulse, BP, respirations, SpO_2, end-tidal CO_2, and breathing capacity; observed degree of restlessness, capillary refill, and color of nail beds.

8. Noted characteristics of suctioned material.

9. Wiped patient's mouth and nose to remove lubricant with gloved hand after bronchoscope was removed.

10. Instructed patient not to eat or drink until gag reflex had returned, tested for presence of gag reflex properly.

11. Removed protective equipment, discarded it, and performed hand hygiene.

EVALUATION

1. Monitored vital signs, SpO_2, and end-tidal CO_2.

2. Observed character and amount of sputum.

3. Observed respiratory status closely, palpated for facial or neck crepitus.

4. Assessed for return of gag reflex.

5. Asked patient to describe postprocedure normal and abnormal symptoms.

6. Identified unexpected outcomes.

RECORDING AND REPORTING

1. Recorded all pertinent information in the appropriate log, documented time of gag reflex return.

2. Reported bleeding, respiratory distress, or changes in vital signs to health care provider immediately, reported results of procedure to appropriate health care personnel.

3. Documented evaluation of patient learning.

Copyright © 2018 by Elsevier Inc. All rights reserved.

Student _____ Date _____

Instructor _____ Date _____

PERFORMANCE CHECKLIST SKILL 8.5 **CARE OF PATIENT UNDERGOING ENDOSCOPY**

	S	U	NP	Comments
ASSESSMENT				
1. Identified patient using two identifiers, compared identifiers with MAR.	___	___	___	_____
2. Verified type of procedure scheduled and procedure site with patient.	___	___	___	_____
3. Verified that informed consent was obtained before administering sedation.	___	___	___	_____
4. Determined if GI bleeding was present; observed character of emesis, stool, and NG tube drainage for frank blood.	___	___	___	_____
5. Obtained vital signs and SpO_2/end-tidal CO_2 values.	___	___	___	_____
6. Determined purpose of procedure.	___	___	___	_____
7. Verified that patient was NPO for at least 8 hours for endoscopy of upper GI tract.	___	___	___	_____
8. Verified patient followed a clear liquid diet and completed any ordered bowel-cleansing regimen for lower GI studies.	___	___	___	_____
9. Assessed patient's level of understanding and previous experience with procedure, including any concerns.	___	___	___	_____
PLANNING				
1. Identified expected outcomes.	___	___	___	_____
2. Explained steps of procedure, included sensations to expect, administered preprocedure medication.	___	___	___	_____
IMPLEMENTATION				
1. Performed hand hygiene, applied PPE.	___	___	___	_____
2. Removed patient's eyeglasses, dentures, or other dental appliances.	___	___	___	_____
3. Took time-out to verify patient's name, procedure, and site with patient and team.	___	___	___	_____
4. Ensured IV line was patent, administered IV sedation as ordered.	___	___	___	_____
5. Assisted patient to assume proper position, applied appropriate drape.	___	___	___	_____

Copyright © 2018 by Elsevier Inc. All rights reserved.

	S	U	NP	Comments

6. For upper GI procedures:

   a. Assisted health care provider in spraying the nasopharynx and oropharynx with local anesthetic. — — — _____

   b. Administered atropine if ordered. — — — _____

   c. Positioned suction cannula for easy access in the patient's mouth. — — — _____

7. For lower GI procedures:

   a. Prepared lubricant for fiber optic endoscope. — — — _____

8. Assisted patient throughout procedure by anticipating needs, telling patient what was happening, and suctioning if necessary. — — — _____

9. Placed tissue specimen in proper containers, sealed as needed, dated and initialed all containers, sent to laboratory. — — — _____

10. Assisted patient to return to comfortable position. — — — _____

11. Assisted in disposing of equipment and performing hand hygiene. — — — _____

12. Informed patient not to eat or drink until gag reflex has returned. — — — _____

EVALUATION

1. Monitored vital signs and SpO_2 at appropriate intervals. — — — _____

2. Assessed for level of sedation and LOC. — — — _____

3. Asked patient to describe level of comfort, observed for pain. — — — _____

4. Evaluated emesis or aspirate for frank or occult blood. — — — _____

5. Assessed for return of gag reflex, provided oral hygiene. — — — _____

6. Asked patient to state postprocedure dietary and activity limitations. — — — _____

7. Identified unexpected outcomes. — — — _____

RECORDING AND REPORTING

1. Recorded all pertinent information in the appropriate log. — — — _____

2. Reported onset of bleeding, abdominal pain, dyspnea, and vital sign changes to health care provider. — — — _____

3. Documented your evaluation of patient learning. — — — _____

Copyright © 2018 by Elsevier Inc. All rights reserved.

Student _____   Date _____

Instructor _____   Date _____

PERFORMANCE CHECKLIST SKILL 9.1   **HAND HYGIENE**

	S	U	NP	Comments

ASSESSMENT

1. Inspected surface of hands for breaks or cuts in skin or cuticles, covered lesions with dressing before providing care, determined if lesions were too large to cover.

2. Inspected hands for visible soiling.

3. Inspected condition of nails, ensured nails were short and smooth.

PLANNING

1. Identified expected outcomes.

IMPLEMENTATION

1. Pushed wristwatch and long uniform sleeves above wrists, removed any rings.

2. Used antiseptic hand rub:

   a. Dispensed appropriate amount of product into palm of one hand.

   b. Rubbed hands together, covered all surfaces.

   c. Rubbed hands together until alcohol was dry, allowed hands to dry completely before applying gloves.

3. Used regular or antimicrobial hand soap:

   a. Stood in front of sink, kept hands and uniform away from sink surface.

   b. Turned on water, used faucets or pedal to regulate flow and temperature.

   c. Avoided splashing water against uniform.

   d. Regulated flow of water so temperature was warm.

   e. Wet hands and wrists, kept hands and forearms lower than elbows.

   f. Applied appropriate amount of antiseptic soap, rubbed hands together.

   g. Washed hands properly for at least 15 to 20 seconds, kept fingertips down.

   h. Cleaned under fingernails with nails of other hand or disposable nail cleaner.

Copyright © 2018 by Elsevier Inc. All rights reserved.

	S	U	NP	Comments

i. Rinsed hands and wrists, kept hands down and elbows up. ___ ___ ___ _____

j. Dried hands and wrists thoroughly. ___ ___ ___ _____

k. Discarded paper towel in proper receptacle if used. ___ ___ ___ _____

l. Used clean, dry, paper towel to turn off hand faucet or turned off with foot or knee pedals. ___ ___ ___ _____

m. Applied appropriate lotion to hands. ___ ___ ___ _____

EVALUATION

1. Inspected surface of hands for obvious signs of dirt and other contaminants. ___ ___ ___ _____

2. Inspected hand for dermatitis or cracked skin. ___ ___ ___ _____

3. Asked patient to describe how to wash hands. ___ ___ ___ _____

4. Identified unexpected outcomes. ___ ___ ___ _____

Copyright © 2018 by Elsevier Inc. All rights reserved.

Student _____ Date _____

Instructor _____ Date _____

PERFORMANCE CHECKLIST SKILL 9.2 **CARING FOR PATIENTS UNDER ISOLATION PRECAUTIONS**

	S	U	NP	Comments

ASSESSMENT

1. Assessed patient and reviewed medical history for possible indications for isolation, reviewed precautions for appropriate isolation system. ___ ___ ___ _____

2. Reviewed laboratory test results. ___ ___ ___ _____

3. Reviewed agency policies, considered care measures to be performed under isolation. ___ ___ ___ _____

4. Reviewed nursing care plan notes or conferred with colleagues regarding patient's emotional state, determined if patient and family understood purpose of isolation procedure. ___ ___ ___ _____

5. Assessed whether patient has known latex allergy, referred to agency policies on latex-free care if necessary. ___ ___ ___ _____

PLANNING

1. Identified expected outcomes. ___ ___ ___ _____

IMPLEMENTATION

1. Performed hand hygiene. ___ ___ ___ _____

2. Prepared all equipment to be taken into patient's room. ___ ___ ___ _____

3. Prepared for entrance into isolation room, applied PPE after introduction if possible:

    a. Applied gown and secured. ___ ___ ___ _____

    b. Applied surgical mask or respirator around mouth and nose, had medical evaluation and was fit-tested before using respirator. ___ ___ ___ _____

    c. Applied goggles or eyewear if needed, used side shields if prescription glasses are worn. ___ ___ ___ _____

    d. Applied clean gloves, brought glove cuffs over edge of gown sleeves. ___ ___ ___ _____

4. Entered room, arranged supplies and equipment. ___ ___ ___ _____

5. Explained purpose of isolation and precautions for patient and family to take, offered opportunity to ask questions, instructed patient on TB precautions if necessary. ___ ___ ___ _____

Copyright © 2018 by Elsevier Inc. All rights reserved.

6. Assessed vital signs:

   a. Left equipment in the room if patient is infected with resistant organism.

   b. Disposed of wrapper or cuff in appropriate receptacle.

   c. Used individual thermometers and blood pressure cuffs if available.

7. Administered medications:

   a. Gave oral medication in wrapper or cup.

   b. Cleaned stethoscope thoroughly if to be reused, set aside on a clean surface.

   c. Wore gloves when administering an injection.

   d. Discarded disposable syringe or sheathed needle into designated sharps container.

8. Administered hygiene, encouraged patient to ask questions, provided informal teaching:

   a. Avoided allowing isolation gown to become wet.

   b. Assisted patient in removing gown, discarded in leak-proof linen bag.

   c. Removed linen from bed, avoided contact with isolation gown, placed in leak-proof linen bag.

   d. Provided clean bed linen.

   e. Changed gloves, performed hand hygiene, and regloved if necessary.

9. Disposed of linen, trash, and disposable items securely in bags.

10. Removed all reusable pieces of equipment, cleaned contaminated surfaces with disinfectant.

11. Resupplied room as needed, had staff colleague hand new supplies to you.

12. Left isolation room, removed protective barriers in the proper order:

   a. Removed gloves properly, discarded gloves in proper container.

   b. Removed eyewear properly, discarded in proper container.

   c. Removed gown properly, folded inside out into a bundle, discarded in laundry bag.

   d. Removed mask properly, dropped into trash.

Copyright © 2018 by Elsevier Inc. All rights reserved.

	S	U	NP	Comments

e. Performed hand hygiene. ___ ___ ___ _____

f. Retrieved wristwatch and stethoscope. ___ ___ ___ _____

g. Explained to patient when you plan to return, asked if patient required personal care items, offered entertainment if necessary. ___ ___ ___ _____

h. Disposed of contaminated supplies and equipment appropriately, performed hand hygiene. ___ ___ ___ _____

i. Left room and provided privacy, closed door if necessary. ___ ___ ___ _____

EVALUATION

1. Observed patient's and family's use of isolation precautions when visiting. ___ ___ ___ _____

2. Asked if patient has had chance to discuss health problems, course of treatment, or other topics. ___ ___ ___ _____

3. Asked patient to explain why isolation precautions are necessary. ___ ___ ___ _____

4. Identified unexpected outcomes. ___ ___ ___ _____

RECORDING AND REPORTING

1. Documented procedures and patient's response to isolation, documented patient education. ___ ___ ___ _____

2. Documented type of isolation in use and microorganisms. ___ ___ ___ _____

Copyright © 2018 by Elsevier Inc. All rights reserved.

Student _____ Date _____

Instructor _____ Date _____

PERFORMANCE CHECKLIST PROCEDURAL GUIDELINE 9.1 **CARING FOR PATIENTS WITH MULTIDRUG-RESISTANT ORGANISMS (MDRO) AND CLOSTRIDIUM DIFFICILE**

	S	U	NP	Comments
PROCEDURAL STEPS				
1. Performed hand hygiene.	___	___	___	_____
2. Prepared all equipment needed in patient's room.	___	___	___	_____
3. Applied gown properly before entering room.	___	___	___	_____
4. Applied clean gloves.	___	___	___	_____
5. Explained purpose of contact precautions to patient and family.	___	___	___	_____
6. Provided personal care and treatments.	___	___	___	_____
7. Left room after telling patient when you will return and asking if he or she has questions concerning care.	___	___	___	_____
8. Removed gloves and discarded appropriately.	___	___	___	_____
9. Removed and discarded gown appropriately.	___	___	___	_____
10. Performed hand hygiene, used soap and water to clean hands if patient has *Clostridium difficile* infection.	___	___	___	_____

Copyright © 2018 by Elsevier Inc. All rights reserved.

Student _____ Date _____

Instructor _____ Date _____

PERFORMANCE CHECKLIST SKILL 10.1 **APPLYING AND REMOVING CAP, MASK, AND PROTECTIVE EYEWEAR**

	S	U	NP	Comments

ASSESSMENT

1. Reviewed type of sterile procedure to be performed, consulted agency's policy for use of protection. ___ ___ ___ _____

2. Avoided participating in procedure if you have symptoms of a respiratory infection. ___ ___ ___ _____

3. Assessed patient's risk of infection. ___ ___ ___ _____

PLANNING

1. Identified expected outcomes. ___ ___ ___ _____

2. Prepared equipment, inspected packaging for integrity and exposure to sterilization. ___ ___ ___ _____

IMPLEMENTATION

1. Performed hand hygiene. ___ ___ ___ _____

2. Applied gown appropriately, ensured gown covers all outer garments. ___ ___ ___ _____

3. Applied a cap:

   a. Combed back and secured long hair. ___ ___ ___ _____

   b. Secured hair in place with pins. ___ ___ ___ _____

   c. Applied cap properly, ensured all hair fit under edges of cap. ___ ___ ___ _____

4. Applied a mask:

   a. Ensured metal strip was along the top edge of the mask. ___ ___ ___ _____

   b. Held mask by top strings, kept top edge above bridge of nose. ___ ___ ___ _____

   c. Tied top strings appropriately. ___ ___ ___ _____

   d. Tied lower ties properly with mask under chin. ___ ___ ___ _____

   e. Pinched metal band around bridge of nose. ___ ___ ___ _____

5. Applied protective eyewear:

   a. Applied protective glasses, goggles, or face shield properly, checked that vision was clear. ___ ___ ___ _____

   b. Ensured face shield fit snugly. ___ ___ ___ _____

Copyright © 2018 by Elsevier Inc. All rights reserved.

	S	U	NP	Comments

6. Applied sterile gloves if needed. ___ ___ ___ _____

7. Removed protective barriers:

   a. Removed gloves first if worn, discarded them in the appropriate container. ___ ___ ___ _____

   b. Removed eyewear, avoided placing hands over soiled lens. ___ ___ ___ _____

   c. Removed and discarded gown properly. ___ ___ ___ _____

   d. Removed and discarded mask properly. ___ ___ ___ _____

   e. Grasped outer surface of cap, lifted away from hair. ___ ___ ___ _____

   f. Discarded cap appropriately, performed hand hygiene. ___ ___ ___ _____

EVALUATION

1. Assessed area of body treated for drainage, tenderness, edema, and skin changes. ___ ___ ___ _____

2. Identified unexpected outcomes. ___ ___ ___ _____

Copyright © 2018 by Elsevier Inc. All rights reserved.

Student _____ Date _____

Instructor _____ Date _____

PERFORMANCE CHECKLIST SKILL 10.2 **PREPARING A STERILE FIELD**

	S	U	NP	Comments
ASSESSMENT				
1. Identified patient using two identifiers, compared identifiers with information in MAR.	___	___	___	_____
2. Verified that procedure requires surgical aseptic technique.	___	___	___	_____
3. Assessed patient's comfort, oxygen requirements, and elimination needs before preparation.	___	___	___	_____
4. Instructed patient not to touch work surface or equipment during the procedure.	___	___	___	_____
5. Assessed for latex allergies.	___	___	___	_____
6. Checked sterile package integrity or for sterilization indicator.	___	___	___	_____
7. Anticipated number and variety of supplies needed for procedure.	___	___	___	_____
PLANNING				
1. Identified expected outcomes.	___	___	___	_____
2. Completed all other nursing interventions before procedure.	___	___	___	_____
3. Asked visitors to step out, discouraged movement by assisting staff.	___	___	___	_____
4. Prepared equipment at bedside.	___	___	___	_____
5. Positioned patient comfortably and appropriately with assistance of NAP if necessary.	___	___	___	_____
6. Explained purpose of procedure and importance of sterile technique.	___	___	___	_____
IMPLEMENTATION				
1. Applied PPE as needed.	___	___	___	_____
2. Selected an appropriate workspace above waist level.	___	___	___	_____
3. Performed hand hygiene.	___	___	___	_____

Copyright © 2018 by Elsevier Inc. All rights reserved.

	S	U	NP	Comments

4. Prepared sterile work surface:

   a. Used sterile commercial kit or pack.

     (1) Placed kit or pack on workspace.

     (2) Opened outside cover, removed package and placed on surface.

     (3) Grasped outer surface or tip of outermost flap.

     (4) Opened outermost flap away from body and sterile field.

     (5) Grasped outer surface of edge of first side flap.

     (6) Opened side flap, allowed it to lie flat on table, kept arm away from sterile surface.

     (7) Repeated for second flap.

     (8) Grasped outside border of last flap, stood away from package, folded flap back, allowed it to fall on the table.

   b. Opened a sterile linen-wrapped package.

     (1) Placed package on workspace.

     (2) Removed seal, unwrapped both layers, following same steps as with sterile kit.

     (3) Used open package wrapper as sterile field.

   c. Prepared sterile drape.

     (1) Placed pack containing drape on workspace and opened following same steps as with sterile kit.

     (2) Applied sterile gloves.

     (3) Picked up folded top edge of drape with fingertips of one hand, lifted without touching any object, discarded wrapper with other hand.

     (4) Kept drape above waist and work surface and away from body as unfolded, discarded wrapper with other hand.

     (5) Held drape, positioned bottom half over top half of intended work surface.

     (6) Allowed top half of drape to be placed over bottom half of work surface.

Copyright © 2018 by Elsevier Inc. All rights reserved.

	S	U	NP	Comments

5. Added sterile items to sterile field:

   a. Opened sterile item while holding outside wrapper in nondominant hand. ___ ___ ___ _____

   b. Carefully peeled wrapper over nondominant hand. ___ ___ ___ _____

   c. Placed item on field at an angle, ensured wrapper and arm were not over sterile field. ___ ___ ___ _____

   d. Disposed of outer wrapper. ___ ___ ___ _____

6. Poured sterile solutions:

   a. Verified contents and expiration date of solution. ___ ___ ___ _____

   b. Ensured receptacle was located near workspace edge. ___ ___ ___ _____

   c. Removed sterile seal and cap properly. ___ ___ ___ _____

   d. Poured needed amount of solution properly into container. ___ ___ ___ _____

EVALUATION

1. Observed for break in sterile technique. ___ ___ ___ _____

2. Identified unexpected outcomes. ___ ___ ___ _____

Copyright © 2018 by Elsevier Inc. All rights reserved.

Student _____ Date _____

Instructor _____ Date _____

PERFORMANCE CHECKLIST SKILL 10.3 **STERILE GLOVING**

	S	U	NP	Comments

ASSESSMENT

1. Considered type of procedure to be per-formed, consulted agency policy on use of sterile gloves. ___ ___ ___ _____

2. Considered patient's risk for infection. ___ ___ ___ _____

3. Selected correct size and type of gloves, examined glove package to determine if it was dry and intact with no water stains. ___ ___ ___ _____

4. Inspected condition of hands, determined if presence of lesions prevented participation in a procedure. ___ ___ ___ _____

5. Assessed patient for risk factors before applying latex gloves:

   a. Previous reaction to other items containing latex. ___ ___ ___ _____

   b. Personal history of asthma, contact dermatitis, eczema, urticaria, or rhinitis. ___ ___ ___ _____

   c. History of food allergies. ___ ___ ___ _____

   d. Previous history of adverse reactions during surgery or dental procedure. ___ ___ ___ _____

   e. Previous reaction to latex products. ___ ___ ___ _____

PLANNING

1. Identified expected outcomes. ___ ___ ___ _____

IMPLEMENTATION

1. Applied gloves:

   a. Performed thorough hand hygiene, placed glove package near work area. ___ ___ ___ _____

   b. Removed outer glove wrapper by peeling sides apart. ___ ___ ___ _____

   c. Grasped inner package on appropriate workspace, opened package, kept gloves on inside surface of wrapper. ___ ___ ___ _____

   d. Identified right and left glove, gloved dominant hand first. ___ ___ ___ _____

   e. Grasped glove for dominant hand by touching only glove's inside surface. ___ ___ ___ _____

Copyright © 2018 by Elsevier Inc. All rights reserved.

	S	U	NP	Comments

f. Pulled glove over dominant hand, ensured cuff did not roll up wrist.

—— —— —— ————————

g. Slipped fingers under cuff of second glove with dominant hand.

—— —— —— ————————

h. Pulled second glove over nondominant hand.

—— —— —— ————————

i. Interlocked hands once both gloves were on, held hands away from body until beginning procedure.

—— —— —— ————————

2. Performed procedure.

—— —— —— ————————

3. Removed gloves:

a. Grasped outside of one cuff with other gloved hand, avoided touching wrist.

—— —— —— ————————

b. Pulled glove off by turning it inside out, placed glove in gloved hand.

—— —— —— ————————

c. Placed fingers of bare hand inside remaining glove cuff, peeled glove off inside out and over previously removed glove, discarded both gloves in receptacle.

—— —— —— ————————

d. Performed thorough hand hygiene.

—— —— —— ————————

EVALUATION

1. Assessed patient for signs of infection.

—— —— —— ————————

2. Assessed patient for signs of latex allergy.

—— —— —— ————————

3. Identified unexpected outcomes.

—— —— —— ————————

RECORDING AND REPORTING

1. Recorded any patient response indicating a latex allergy.

—— —— —— ————————

Copyright © 2018 by Elsevier Inc. All rights reserved.

Student _____ Date _____

Instructor _____ Date _____

PERFORMANCE CHECKLIST SKILL 11.1   **USING SAFE AND EFFECTIVE TRANSFER TECHNIQUES**

	S	U	NP	Comments
ASSESSMENT				
1. Identified patient using two identifiers.	___	___	___	_____
2. Performed hand hygiene.	___	___	___	_____
3. Reviewed medical record or assessed patient's physical capacity to transfer and help with transfer, including muscle strength, joint mobility and contracture formation, paralysis or paresis, and bone continuity.	___	___	___	_____
4. Referred to record for most recent weight and height.	___	___	___	_____
5. Assessed for history of weakness, dizziness, or postural hypotension.	___	___	___	_____
6. Assessed record for patient's level of fatigue, activity tolerance, and endurance.	___	___	___	_____
7. Assessed patient's proprioceptive function.	___	___	___	_____
8. Assessed patient's sensory status, including adequacy of vision and hearing and presence of peripheral sensation loss.	___	___	___	_____
9. Assessed patient for pain, measured level of pain, offered prescribed analgesic 30 minutes before transfer.	___	___	___	_____
10. Assessed patient's cognitive status, including ability to follow verbal instructions, short-term memory, recognition of physical deficits and limitations.	___	___	___	_____
11. Assessed patient's level of motivation and eagerness versus unwillingness to be mobile.	___	___	___	_____
12. Assessed previous mode of transfer.	___	___	___	_____
13. Assessed patient's vital signs just before transfer.	___	___	___	_____
14. Determined if lift or transfer device is needed and number of people to help with the transfer, did not start procedure until all caregivers were available.	___	___	___	_____

Copyright © 2018 by Elsevier Inc. All rights reserved.

	S	U	NP	Comments

PLANNING

1. Identified expected outcomes.   S __ U __ NP __ _____

2. Explained to patient how you are going to prepare for transfer and safety precautions to be used, explained benefits and reasons, matched explanation to patient's beliefs regarding health.   __ __ __ _____

3. Provided privacy.   __ __ __ _____

4. Obtained additional devices or caregivers as necessary.   __ __ __ _____

IMPLEMENTATION

1. Performed hand hygiene.   __ __ __ _____

2. Assisted patient to appropriate position.   __ __ __ _____

3. Assisted patient to sit on side of bed, had patient flex and extend feet and move legs up and down, had patient relax until balance is gained, returned patient to bed and checked blood pressure if needed.   __ __ __ _____

4. Transferred patient from bed to chair:

   a. Placed chair in appropriate position facing foot of the bed.   __ __ __ _____

   b. Placed bed in low position where patient's feet are on the floor.   __ __ __ _____

   c. Used additional caregivers or transfer aid as necessary.   __ __ __ _____

   d. Used stand-and-pivot technique with one caregiver if appropriate.

      (1) Applied transfer belt snugly and low; ensured it completely circles waist; avoided placing over lines, tubes, or incisions.   __ __ __ _____

      (2) Helped patient apply nonskid footwear if necessary, placed patient's strong leg on floor with weak foot back.   __ __ __ _____

      (3) Spread feet apart, flexed hips and knees, aligned knees with patient's knees.   __ __ __ _____

      (4) Grasped transfer belt, kept palms along patient's side.   __ __ __ _____

      (5) Rocked patient to standing position on the count of three, ensured body weight is moving with patient's, allowed patient to help by pushing up if not contraindicated.   __ __ __ _____

Copyright © 2018 by Elsevier Inc. All rights reserved.

	S	U	NP	Comments

(6) Maintained stability of patient's weakened leg with own knee. — — — _____

(7) Pivoted on foot farthest from chair. — — — _____

(8) Instructed patient to use armrests on chair for support and ease into chair. — — — _____

(9) Flexed hips and knees while lowering patient. — — — _____

(10) Assessed patient for proper alignment in sitting position, provided support for weakened extremity. — — — _____

e. Used hydraulic lift if patient is unable to cooperate.

(1) Brought lift to bedside and positioned properly. — — — _____

(2) Positioned chair near bed, allowed adequate space. — — — _____

(3) Raised bed to high, flat position; lowered side rail near chair. — — — _____

(4) Positioned second nurse on opposite side of bed. — — — _____

(5) Rolled patient on side away from self. — — — _____

(6) Placed hammock or canvas strips under patient to form sling. — — — _____

(7) Rolled patient toward self as second nurse pulls straps through. — — — _____

(8) Returned patient to supine position, ensured straps are smooth over bed surface and sling supports patient's weight equally. — — — _____

(9) Removed patient's glasses if appropriate. — — — _____

(10) Placed horseshoe base of lift under patient's bed on side with chair. — — — _____

(11) Lowered horizontal bar to proper level, locked valve if required. — — — _____

(12) Attached hooks on chain or strap to holes in sling. — — — _____

(13) Elevated head of bed to appropriate position. — — — _____

(14) Had patient fold arms over chest. — — — _____

(15) Pumped hydraulic handle until patient is raised off bed or used controls to move lift. — — — _____

Copyright © 2018 by Elsevier Inc. All rights reserved.

	S	U	NP	Comments

(16) Raised patient off bed, used steering handle to pull lift as both nurses maneuver patient to chair.

     ____ ____ ____ _____

(17) Rolled base of lift around chair, released check valve slowly, lowered patient into chair.

     ____ ____ ____ _____

(18) Closed check valve as soon as patient is in chair.

     ____ ____ ____ _____

(19) Removed straps, rolled lift out of patient's path.

     ____ ____ ____ _____

(20) Checked patient's sitting alignment, corrected if necessary.

     ____ ____ ____ _____

5. Performed lateral transfer from bed to stretcher:

a. Determined if patient can assist; obtained additional devices, lifts, or caregivers if needed.

     ____ ____ ____ _____

b. Performed lateral transfer with friction-reducing device (slide board or air-assisted device).

(1) Applied clean gloves, lowered head of bed as much as patient can tolerate, ensured bed brakes are locked.

     ____ ____ ____ _____

(2) Crossed patient's arms on chest.

     ____ ____ ____ _____

(3) Lowered side rails, positioned nurses appropriately.

     ____ ____ ____ _____

(4) Fanfolded drawsheet on both sides.

     ____ ____ ____ _____

(5) Logrolled patient on count of three with smooth continuous motion.

     ____ ____ ____ _____

(6) Placed slide board under drawsheet.

     ____ ____ ____ _____

(7) Gently rolled patient back onto slide board.

     ____ ____ ____ _____

(8) Lined up stretcher appropriately lower than bed, locked brakes, instructed patient not to move.

     ____ ____ ____ _____

(9) Repositioned nurses properly, grasped friction-reducing surface.

     ____ ____ ____ _____

(10) Fanfolded drawsheet, two nurses pulled the drawsheet with patient under stretcher while third nurse held slide board in place.

     ____ ____ ____ _____

Copyright © 2018 by Elsevier Inc. All rights reserved.

	S	U	NP	Comments

(11) Positioned patient in center of stretcher, raised head of stretcher if not contraindicated, raised side rails, covered patient with blanket. ___ ___ ___ _____

6. Removed and disposed of gloves, performed hand hygiene. ___ ___ ___ _____

EVALUATION

1. Monitored vital signs, asked if patient felt dizzy or fatigued, asked patient to rate pain on pain scale. ___ ___ ___ _____

2. Noted patient's behavioral response to transfer. ___ ___ ___ _____

3. Asked patient to describe steps in safe transfer. ___ ___ ___ _____

4. Identified unexpected outcomes. ___ ___ ___ _____

RECORDING AND REPORTING

1. Recorded procedure and all pertinent observations in appropriate log. ___ ___ ___ _____

2. Documented evaluation of patient learning. ___ ___ ___ _____

3. Reported transfer ability and help needed to other caregivers, reported progress or remission to rehabilitation staff. ___ ___ ___ _____

Copyright © 2018 by Elsevier Inc. All rights reserved.

Student _____ Date _____

Instructor _____ Date _____

PERFORMANCE CHECKLIST PROCEDURAL GUIDELINE 11.1 **WHEELCHAIR TRANSFER TECHNIQUES**

	S	U	NP	Comments

PROCEDURAL STEPS

1. Performed hand hygiene.

2. Reviewed medical record for patient's weight, height, strength, cognition, pain level, and balance during previous transfer; performed assessment if necessary.

3. Explained steps of transfer to patient.

4. Transferred patient from a wheelchair to bed if patient is cooperative and weight bearing using pivot technique:

   a. Adjusted height of bed to level of the seat of the wheelchair.

   b. Positioned wheelchair properly next to bed, removed armrest nearest to bed.

   c. Locked wheelchair.

   d. Raised footplates.

   e. Placed transfer belt appropriately on patient.

   f. Assisted patient in placing hands on armrests and moving in front of wheelchair.

   g. Stood in front of patient, protected patient during transfer.

   h. Instructed patient to stand on count of three, placed hands under transfer belt and bent knees.

   i. Allowed patient to stand a few seconds, ensured he or she can balance, pivoted with patient, had patient sit on end of mattress.

   j. Placed one arm under patient's shoulder, supported head and neck, placed other arm under patient's knees, postured self properly.

   k. Instructed patient to help lift leg when you move, raised patient as you pivoted, lowered shoulders onto bed, kept own back straight.

   l. Helped patient return to comfortable position in bed.

Copyright © 2018 by Elsevier Inc. All rights reserved.

	S	U	NP	Comments

5. Transferred patient from a wheelchair to bed if patient is non–weight bearing but cooperative using transfer board:

   a. Positioned wheelchair properly next to bed. ___ ___ ___ _____

   b. Removed armrest nearest bed. ___ ___ ___ _____

   c. Locked wheelchair. ___ ___ ___ _____

   d. Raised footplates. ___ ___ ___ _____

   e. Placed transfer belt properly on patient. ___ ___ ___ _____

   f. Positioned seat of chair level with bed if possible, positioned transfer board so patient can slide across it, ensured board will not slip out of place. ___ ___ ___ _____

   g. Stood in front of patient, had patient move to front of wheelchair. ___ ___ ___ _____

   h. Placed own leg outside patient's legs, ensured patient's feet are on the floor, grasped transfer belt, had patient place hands on slide board and mattress. ___ ___ ___ _____

   i. Bent knees, had patient use arms to slide into bed, assisted as needed. ___ ___ ___ _____

   j. Had patient sit on edge of bed. ___ ___ ___ _____

   k. Followed steps 4 j–l when helping patient to comfortable position. ___ ___ ___ _____

6. Performed hand hygiene. ___ ___ ___ _____

7. Monitored vital signs, asked if patient feels dizzy or fatigued. ___ ___ ___ _____

8. Noted patient's behavioral response to transfer. ___ ___ ___ _____

9. Performed hand hygiene. ___ ___ ___ _____

10. Documented patient's ability to tolerate transfer. ___ ___ ___ _____

Copyright © 2018 by Elsevier Inc. All rights reserved.

Student _____ Date _____

Instructor _____ Date _____

PERFORMANCE CHECKLIST SKILL 11.2   **MOVING AND POSITIONING PATIENTS IN BED**

	S	U	NP	Comments

ASSESSMENT

1. Identified patient using at least two identifiers. ___ ___ ___ _____

2. Performed hand hygiene. ___ ___ ___ _____

3. Assessed patient's ROM, body alignment, and level of pain while patient is lying down. ___ ___ ___ _____

4. Assessed for risk factors that contribute to complications of immobility:

   a. Decreased sensation from CVA, spinal cord injury, or neuropathy. ___ ___ ___ _____

   b. Impaired mobility due to traction, arthritis, CVA, spinal cord injury, hip fracture, joint surgery, or other disease processes. ___ ___ ___ _____

   c. Impaired circulation from arterial insufficiency. ___ ___ ___ _____

   d. Age. ___ ___ ___ _____

5. Assessed patient's LOC. ___ ___ ___ _____

6. Assessed patient for pain on a scale of 0 to 10. ___ ___ ___ _____

7. Assessed condition of patient's skin, especially over bony prominences. ___ ___ ___ _____

8. Referred to medical record for patient's most recent height and weight. ___ ___ ___ _____

9. Assessed patient's physical ability to help with moving and positioning. ___ ___ ___ _____

10. Assessed for sensory loss. ___ ___ ___ _____

11. Applied clean gloves to assess for presence of tubes, incisions, and equipment, emptied drainage bags before repositioning, removed and disposed of gloves, performed hand hygiene. ___ ___ ___ _____

12. Assessed motivation of patient and ability of caregivers to participate in moving and positioning. ___ ___ ___ _____

13. Checked health care provider's orders before positioning patient. ___ ___ ___ _____

Copyright © 2018 by Elsevier Inc. All rights reserved.

	S	U	NP	Comments

PLANNING

1. Identified expected outcomes.

2. Offered analgesic 30 minutes before procedure if appropriate.

3. Removed all pillows and devices used in previous position.

4. Obtained extra help as needed.

5. Explained procedure to patient.

IMPLEMENTATION

1. Performed hand hygiene.

2. Provided privacy.

3. Raised bed to comfortable working height.

4. Assisted patient to move up in bed:

   a. If patient can assist:

     (1) Stood at bedside.

     (2) Had patient place feet flat on mattress, grasp rails or trapeze, and lift hips and push legs so body moves up.

   b. If patient can partially assist:

     (1) Encouraged patient to help using friction-reducing device.

     (2) Obtained slide board or additional caregivers if necessary.

     (3) Positioned patient and nurses appropriately.

     (4) Removed pillow from under head and placed at head of bed.

     (5) Turned patient side to side to place friction-reducing device under drawsheet, positioned patient appropriately.

     (6) Positioned nurses grasping drawsheet and device properly.

     (7) Flexed hips and knees, shift weight to move patient up in bed.

   c. If patient is unable to assist:

     (1) Obtained appropriate caregivers and devices to reposition safely.

5. Positioned patient ensuring correct body alignment, protected pressure area:

   a. Determined if patient can assist using previous steps.

Copyright © 2018 by Elsevier Inc. All rights reserved.

	S	U	NP	Comments

b. Moved patient up in bed using previous steps. ___ ___ ___ _____

c. Positioned patient in supported semi-Fowler's or Fowler's position.

   (1) Elevated head of bed if not contra-indicated. ___ ___ ___ _____

   (2) Rested head on small pillow. ___ ___ ___ _____

   (3) Used pillows to support arms and hands if necessary. ___ ___ ___ _____

   (4) Positioned small pillows under back, thighs, and calves. ___ ___ ___ _____

d. Positioned hemiplegic patient in supported semi-Fowler's or Fowler's position.

   (1) Elevated head of bed appropriately. ___ ___ ___ _____

   (2) Positioned patient in Fowler's position as straight as possible. ___ ___ ___ _____

   (3) Positioned head on small pillow, avoided hyperextension of neck. ___ ___ ___ _____

   (4) Provided support for involved arm and hand. ___ ___ ___ _____

   (5) Placed rolled blanket along patient's legs. ___ ___ ___ _____

   (6) Supported feet in dorsiflexion with therapeutic boots or splints. ___ ___ ___ _____

e. Positioned patient in supported supine position.

   (1) Placed patient supine with head of bed flat. ___ ___ ___ _____

   (2) Placed rolled towel under lumbar area of back. ___ ___ ___ _____

   (3) Placed pillow under upper shoulders, neck, and head. ___ ___ ___ _____

   (4) Placed trochanter rolls or sandbags parallel to patient's thighs. ___ ___ ___ _____

   (5) Placed patient's feet in therapeutic boots or splints. ___ ___ ___ _____

   (6) Placed pillows under forearms, kept upper arms parallel to patient's body. ___ ___ ___ _____

   (7) Placed rolls under patient's hands. ___ ___ ___ _____

f. Positioned hemiplegic patient in supine position.

   (1) Placed head of bed flat. ___ ___ ___ _____

Copyright © 2018 by Elsevier Inc. All rights reserved.

	S	U	NP	Comments

(2) Placed small pillow under shoulder or affected side.

(3) Positioned affected arm properly away from body.

(4) Placed folded towel under hip of involved side.

(5) Flexed affected knee 30 degrees and supported on a pillow or blanket.

(6) Supported feet with soft pillows at right angle to leg.

g. Positioned patient in 30-degree lateral (side-lying) position (one nurse).

(1) Lowered head of bed as low as patient can tolerate.

(2) Lowered side rail, positioned patient on appropriate side of bed.

(3) Raised side rail, went to opposite side of bed.

(4) Flexed patient's knee, positioned self for better leverage.

(5) Rolled patient onto side toward self.

(6) Placed pillow under patient's head and neck.

(7) Placed hands under patient's dependent shoulder, brought shoulder blade forward.

(8) Positioned arms properly, supported appropriately.

(9) Placed hands under dependent hip, brought hip forward to appropriate angle.

(10) Placed small tuck-back pillow behind patient's back.

(11) Placed pillow under semiflexed upper leg.

(12) Placed sandbags parallel to plantar surface of dependent foot, used ankle-foot orthotic on feet if necessary.

h. Positioned patient in Sims' (semi-prone) position.

(1) Lowered head of bed completely.

Copyright © 2018 by Elsevier Inc. All rights reserved.

	S	U	NP	Comments

(2) Place patient supine on appropriate side of bed.

    —— —— —— ————————

(3) Moved to other side of bed, turned patient on side, positioned patient properly in lateral position.

    —— —— —— ————————

(4) Placed small pillow under patient's head.

    —— —— —— ————————

(5) Placed pillow under flexed upper arm, supported arm appropriately.

    —— —— —— ————————

(6) Placed pillow under flexed upper legs, supported leg appropriately.

    —— —— —— ————————

(7) Placed sandbags parallel to plantar surface of foot.

    —— —— —— ————————

  i. Logrolled patient (three nurses).

(1) Placed small pillow between patient's knees.

    —— —— —— ————————

(2) Crossed patient's arms on chest.

    —— —— —— ————————

(3) Positioned nurses appropriately.

    —— —— —— ————————

(4) Fanfolded drawsheet alongside patient.

    —— —— —— ————————

(5) Ensured all nurses were grasping drawsheet properly, rolled patient as a unit in smooth, continuous motion.

    —— —— —— ————————

(6) Ensured nurses place pillows along length of patient for support.

    —— —— —— ————————

(7) Leaned patient back as a unit.

    —— —— —— ————————

6. Performed hand hygiene.

    —— —— —— ————————

EVALUATION

1. Assessed patient's body alignment, position, and level of comfort.

    —— —— —— ————————

2. Measured ROM.

    —— —— —— ————————

3. Observed for areas of erythema or breakdown involving skin.

    —— —— —— ————————

4. Asked patient to describe steps for moving up in bed.

    —— —— —— ————————

5. Identified unexpected outcomes.

    —— —— —— ————————

RECORDING AND REPORTING

1. Recorded time and position change, observations, and devices needed in appropriate log.

    —— —— —— ————————

2. Documented evaluation of patient learning.

    —— —— —— ————————

3. Reported observations at change of shift and documented in appropriate log.

    —— —— —— ————————

Copyright © 2018 by Elsevier Inc. All rights reserved.

Student _____   Date _____

Instructor _____   Date _____

PERFORMANCE CHECKLIST SKILL 12.1 **PROMOTING EARLY ACTIVITY AND EXERCISE**

	S	U	NP	Comments
ASSESSMENT				
1. Identified patient using two identifiers.	___	___	___	_____
2. Reviewed patient's medical history for conditions that could influence or contraindicate mobility, reviewed health care provider's orders for early mobility to exercise program, obtained physician clearance for outpatient exercise.	___	___	___	_____
3. Gathered baseline assessment of vital signs and oxygen saturation.	___	___	___	_____
4. Assessed patient's pain level on a scale of 1 to 10.	___	___	___	_____
5. Assessed patient's beliefs and values regarding health status and confidence in capabilities to perform exercise.	___	___	___	_____
6. Implemented Inpatient Early Mobility Protocol.	___	___	___	_____
7. Performed safety screening (MOVE):				
a. Assessed patient's myocardial stability.	___	___	___	_____
b. Assessed oxygenation status.	___	___	___	_____
c. Assessed for vasopressor activity.	___	___	___	_____
d. Assessed patient's response to verbal commands.	___	___	___	_____
8. Performed outpatient assessment:				
a. Identified patient's activity/exercise history.	___	___	___	_____
b. Asked patient about enjoyment of and beliefs about ability to exercise.	___	___	___	_____
c. Determined if patient has social support.	___	___	___	_____
d. Determined if patient has access to exercise area.	___	___	___	_____
e. Considered factors negatively associated with adult participation in activity.	___	___	___	_____
f. Had patient rate level of quality of life.	___	___	___	_____

Copyright © 2018 by Elsevier Inc. All rights reserved.

	S	U	NP	Comments

PLANNING

1. Identified expected outcomes.

2. Consulted physical therapist for role in both inpatient and outpatient activities.

3. Explained benefits and reasons for activity/ exercise, including patient's beliefs and values regarding recovery and health.

4. Explained fall prevention precautions in place.

5. Scheduled ambulation around patient's other activities.

IMPLEMENTATION

1. Implemented Early Progressive Mobility Protocol at appropriate level for patient's abilities:

   a. For Level 1, initiated passive ROM exercises, turned and sat patient up at appropriate intervals, obtained OT consultation if needed.

   b. For Level 2, added sitting patient on side of bed or in chair, consulted OT for strengthening program.

   c. For Level 3, added sitting on edge of bed unsupported and active transfer to chair.

   d. For Level 4, initiated ambulation, applied gait belt if needed, increased ambulation time and distance daily.

2. Initiated outpatient exercise and activity program:

   a. Initiated appropriate exercise program with help of physical therapist.

   b. Recommended strength training.

   c. Included activities to improve cardiovascular health.

   d. Recommended balance exercises, ensured patient has something to hold onto if her or she becomes unstable.

   e. Recommended patient perform cool-down stretches.

EVALUATION

1. Measured vital signs and oxygen saturation during activity, compared findings with baseline.

2. Evaluated patient's pain using 0 to 10 scale.

3. Evaluated patient's level of confidence in performing exercises after appropriate level is attained.

Copyright © 2018 by Elsevier Inc. All rights reserved.

	S	U	NP	Comments

4. Asked patient to explain why warm-up and cool-down are important.   ____ ____ ____ _____

5. Identified unexpected outcomes.   ____ ____ ____ _____

RECORDING AND REPORTING

1. Recorded results of screening, type of exercise, assessments, and patient tolerance in appropriate log.   ____ ____ ____ _____

2. Documented evaluation of patient learning.   ____ ____ ____ _____

3. Reported signs indicative of exercise intolerance to health care provider.   ____ ____ ____ _____

Copyright © 2018 by Elsevier Inc. All rights reserved.

Student _____ Date _____

Instructor _____ Date _____

PERFORMANCE CHECKLIST PROCEDURAL GUIDELINE 12.1 **PERFORMING RANGE-OF-MOTION EXERCISES**

	S	U	NP	Comments

PROCEDURAL STEPS

1. Identified patient using at least two identifiers. ____ ____ ____ _____

2. Reviewed patient's chart for physical assessment findings, health care provider's orders, medical diagnosis, medical history, and progress. ____ ____ ____ _____

3. Obtained data on patient's baseline joint function, observed for obvious limitations. ____ ____ ____ _____

4. Determined patient's or caregiver's readiness to learn, explained rationales for ROM exercises, described and demonstrated exercises to be performed. ____ ____ ____ _____

5. Assessed patient's level of comfort, administered analgesic before exercise if necessary. ____ ____ ____ _____

6. Performed hand hygiene, wore clean gloves if wound drainage or lesions are present. ____ ____ ____ _____

7. Assisted patient to comfortable position. ____ ____ ____ _____

8. Supported joints properly while performing passive ROM exercise. ____ ____ ____ _____

9. Observed patient performing ROM activities. ____ ____ ____ _____

10. Removed gloves, performed hand hygiene. ____ ____ ____ _____

11. Measured joint motion as needed. ____ ____ ____ _____

12. Evaluated patient's pain level during exercise. ____ ____ ____ _____

13. Asked patient to describe exercises he or she can do at home. ____ ____ ____ _____

14. Documented exercises performed and patient tolerance in the appropriate log. ____ ____ ____ _____

Copyright © 2018 by Elsevier Inc. All rights reserved.

Student _____ Date _____

Instructor _____ Date _____

PERFORMANCE CHECKLIST PROCEDURAL GUIDELINE 12.2 **MONITORING PATIENT ON A CONTINUOUS PASSIVE MOTION MACHINE**

	S	U	NP	Comments

PROCEDURAL STEPS

1. Reviewed medical record, assessed nature of patient's condition and ROM limits, ensured order designates cycles per minute and time on machine. ___ ___ ___ _____

2. Assessed CPM machine for electrical safety, notified electrical safety department if problem was suspected. ___ ___ ___ _____

3. Assessed setup of the machine before placing on bed. ___ ___ ___ _____

4. Identified patient using at least two identifiers. ___ ___ ___ _____

5. Performed hand hygiene. ___ ___ ___ _____

6. Assessed patient's pain level to establish a baseline. ___ ___ ___ _____

7. Assessed patient's vitals to establish baseline for exercise tolerance. ___ ___ ___ _____

8. Assessed patient's knowledge about CPM and ability and willingness to learn about CPM machine. ___ ___ ___ _____

9. Explained procedure and demonstrate CPM machine. ___ ___ ___ _____

10. Helped patient to comfortable supine position. ___ ___ ___ _____

11. Applied clean gloves if wound drainage is present. ___ ___ ___ _____

12. Placed elastic compression stockings on patient if ordered. ___ ___ ___ _____

13. Placed CPM machine on bed, set limits of flexion and extension and speed control, turned machine on for a cycle. ___ ___ ___ _____

14. Stopped CPM machine in extension and placed padding on it. ___ ___ ___ _____

15. Supported patient's affected joint, placed extremity in CPM machine frame. ___ ___ ___ _____

16. Adjusted CPM to patient's extremity. ___ ___ ___ _____

17. Secured patient's extremity loosely with Velcro straps. ___ ___ ___ _____

Copyright © 2018 by Elsevier Inc. All rights reserved.

	S	U	NP	Comments

18. Started machine, checked degree of flexion in flexed position, observed patient for two full cycles.

19. Asked if patient feels comfortable, evaluated patient severity on pain scale.

20. Ensured power switch is within patient's reach, instructed patient on when to turn machine off and notify nurse.

21. Discarded gloves, performed hand hygiene.

22. Asked patient to explain purpose of CPM machine.

23. Inspected skin in contact with machine for breakdown.

24. Checked patient's alignment and positioning at appropriate intervals.

25. Evaluated patient for pain, provided analgesic if necessary.

26. Observed patient and CPM machine with each increase in flexion and extension.

27. Recorded patient's tolerance and all pertinent information in the appropriate log.

28. Reported as resistance to ROM, increased pain, or swelling, heat, or redness in joint.

Copyright © 2018 by Elsevier Inc. All rights reserved.

Student _____   Date _____

Instructor _____   Date _____

PERFORMANCE CHECKLIST PROCEDURAL GUIDELINE 12.3 **APPLYING GRADUATED COMPRESSION (ELASTIC) STOCKINGS AND SEQUENTIAL COMPRESSION DEVICE**

	S	U	NP	Comments
PROCEDURAL STEPS				
1. Reviewed medical record for order for SCDs or graduated compression stockings.	___	___	___	_____
2. Identified patient using at least two identifiers.	___	___	___	_____
3. Assessed patient for risk factors for developing DVT.	___	___	___	_____
4. Assessed for contraindications for use of elastic stockings or SCDs	___	___	___	_____
5. Assessed condition of patient's skin and circulation to the legs, palpated pedal pulses, noted palpable veins, inspected skin over lower extremities.	___	___	___	_____
6. Obtained health care provider's order.	___	___	___	_____
7. Assessed patient's or caregiver's knowledge of previous use of compression stockings.	___	___	___	_____
8. Explained procedure and reason for applying stockings/SCDs.	___	___	___	_____
9. Positioned patient appropriately.	___	___	___	_____
10. Performed hand hygiene, bathed and dried patient's legs, performed hand hygiene again.	___	___	___	_____
11. Applied graduated compression stockings:				
a. Measured patient's leg, determined proper stocking size.	___	___	___	_____
b. Applied small amount of powder or cornstarch to legs if appropriate.	___	___	___	_____
c. Turned stocking inside out.	___	___	___	_____
d. Placed patient's toes into foot of stocking, ensured stocking is smooth.	___	___	___	_____
e. Slid remaining stocking over patient's foot, ensured foot fits into toe-and-heel positioning.	___	___	___	_____
f. Slid stocking over patient's calf until fully extended, ensured stocking is smooth.	___	___	___	_____

Copyright © 2018 by Elsevier Inc. All rights reserved.

	S	U	NP	Comments

g. Instructed patient not to roll stockings partially down, to avoid wrinkles and crossing legs, and to avoid elevating legs while sitting.   ____ ____ ____ _____

12. Applied SCD sleeve(s):

a. Removed SCD sleeve from plastic, unfolded and flattened.   ____ ____ ____ _____

b. Arranged SCD sleeve properly under patient's leg.   ____ ____ ____ _____

c. Placed patient's leg on SCD sleeve, lined up ankle with ankle marking.   ____ ____ ____ _____

d. Positioned back of knee with opening on the sleeve.   ____ ____ ____ _____

e. Wrapped SCD sleeve securely around patient's leg, checked fit.   ____ ____ ____ _____

f. Attached SCD sleeve connector to mechanical unit, lined up arrows on connector and mechanical unit.   ____ ____ ____ _____

g. Turned unit on, monitored function through one full cycle of inflation and deflation.   ____ ____ ____ _____

13. Positioned patient comfortably, performed hand hygiene.   ____ ____ ____ _____

14. Removed elastic stockings or SCD sleeves at least once per shift.   ____ ____ ____ _____

15. Evaluated skin integrity and circulation to patient's lower extremities.   ____ ____ ____ _____

16. Educated patient/caregiver about core of elastic stockings and DVT precautions.   ____ ____ ____ _____

17. Asked patient to describe why he or she is wearing elastic stockings.   ____ ____ ____ _____

18. Documented condition of lower extremities, application of stockings/SCD, and patient education and response in appropriate record.   ____ ____ ____ _____

Copyright © 2018 by Elsevier Inc. All rights reserved.

Student _____ Date _____

Instructor _____ Date _____

PERFORMANCE CHECKLIST PROCEDURAL GUIDELINE12.4 **ASSISTING WITH AMBULATION (WITHOUT ASSIST DEVICES)**

	S	U	NP	Comments

PROCEDURAL STEPS

1. Reviewed medical record for patient's most recent activity experience, recorded weight.
   ___ ___ ___ _____

2. Reviewed medical record for history or risks of orthostatic hypotension.
   ___ ___ ___ _____

3. Reviewed health care provider's orders for activity, noted mobility or weight-bearing restrictions.
   ___ ___ ___ _____

4. Determined best time to ambulate, scheduled around other activities.
   ___ ___ ___ _____

5. Checked patient's environment for barriers or safety risks.
   ___ ___ ___ _____

6. Identified patient using at least two identifiers.
   ___ ___ ___ _____

7. Performed hand hygiene.
   ___ ___ ___ _____

8. Assessed patient's readiness to ambulate:

   a. Assessed baseline vitals.
   ___ ___ ___ _____

   b. Assessed ROM and muscle strength of lower extremities in bed if necessary.
   ___ ___ ___ _____

   c. Asked if patient is tired or experiencing pain, determined source and severity of pain, administered analgesic if necessary.
   ___ ___ ___ _____

9. Assessed patient's level of response to commands, views regarding health, and willingness to participate in activity.
   ___ ___ ___ _____

10. Assessed patient for any deficit that may affect his or her ability to follow instructions.
    ___ ___ ___ _____

11. Had chair or wheelchair nearby if necessary.
    ___ ___ ___ _____

12. Explained to patient how to prepare for ambulation, explained benefits and reasons for activity, considered patient's beliefs and values regarding health.
    ___ ___ ___ _____

Copyright © 2018 by Elsevier Inc. All rights reserved.

	S	U	NP	Comments

13. Assisted patient from a supine position to side of bed:

   a. Raised head of bed, placed bed in low position, placed nonskid footwear on patient. ____ ____ ____ _____

   b. Stood on appropriate side of bed, turned patient onto side facing self. ____ ____ ____ _____

   c. Stood opposite patient's hips, turned to face patient and far corner of bed. ____ ____ ____ _____

   d. Placed feet in wide base of support. ____ ____ ____ _____

   e. Placed arm properly under patient's shoulder, placed other arm around patient's thighs. ____ ____ ____ _____

   f. Moved patient's legs and feet over side of bed, pivoted weight to allow patient's upper legs to swing down, elevated patient's trunk to upright position. ____ ____ ____ _____

14. Allowed patient to sit for a few minutes, flexed and extended patient's feet and moved legs up and down, checked blood pressure if necessary, had patient relax and breathe if he or she feels dizzy, returned patient to bed if necessary. ____ ____ ____ _____

15. Applied gait belt appropriately, held belt properly once patient stands. ____ ____ ____ _____

16. Helped patient to standing position with shoulders back, assessed ability to bear weight and balance. ____ ____ ____ _____

17. Returned patient to bed or chair immediately if he or she is unsteady, obtained additional help. ____ ____ ____ _____

18. Placed IV pole on side of infusion, instructed patient to push pole while walking. ____ ____ ____ _____

19. Emptied drainage bag if necessary, ensured bag is carried appropriately and that there is no tension on tubing. ____ ____ ____ _____

20. Decided with patient how far to ambulate. ____ ____ ____ _____

21. Stood on appropriate side of patient and slightly behind. ____ ____ ____ _____

22. Grasped gait belt, supported patient appropriately through first few steps. ____ ____ ____ _____

23. Assessed strength and balance before continuing. ____ ____ ____ _____

24. Positioned patient between self and wall, encouraged use of handrail. ____ ____ ____ _____

Copyright © 2018 by Elsevier Inc. All rights reserved.

	S	U	NP	Comments
25. Observed how patient walks, evaluated activity tolerance.	___	___	___	_____
26. Reacted if patient starts to fall:				
a. Grasped gait belt with both hands.	___	___	___	_____
b. Stood with feet apart for support.	___	___	___	_____
c. Pulled patient against self, slid patient down leg slowly to floor, did not risk personal injury.	___	___	___	_____
d. Bent knees and lowered body with patient.	___	___	___	_____
e. Stayed with patient until help arrives.	___	___	___	_____
27. Returned patient to comfortable position in bed or chair, performed hand hygiene.	___	___	___	_____
28. Recorded time and distance ambulated, changes in vitals, and patient's tolerance in the appropriate log.	___	___	___	_____

Copyright © 2018 by Elsevier Inc. All rights reserved.

Student _____ Date _____

Instructor _____ Date _____

PERFORMANCE CHECKLIST SKILL 12.2 **ASSISTING WITH USE OF CANES, WALKERS, AND CRUTCHES**

	S	U	NP	Comments
ASSESSMENT				
1. Identified patient using at least two identifiers.	___	___	___	_____
2. Completed assessment steps in Procedural Guideline 12.4, steps 1–5, 7–11.	___	___	___	_____
3. Determined patient's or caregiver's understanding of type of device being used.	___	___	___	_____
4. Assessed degree of assistance patient needs with physical therapist's input.	___	___	___	_____
PLANNING				
1. Identified expected outcomes.	___	___	___	_____
2. Explained the patient how to prepare for ambulation and the benefits of activity, considered patient's education level and beliefs regarding recovery.	___	___	___	_____
3. Explained and demonstrated specific gait technique to patient or caregiver.	___	___	___	_____
4. Checked for appropriate height and fit of cane or crutch.	___	___	___	_____
5. Ensured ambulation device had rubber tips.	___	___	___	_____
IMPLEMENTATION				
1. Performed hand hygiene.	___	___	___	_____
2. Asked patient to report any tingling or numbness in upper torso.	___	___	___	_____
3. Helped patient to side of bed.	___	___	___	_____
4. Allowed patient to sit for a few minutes, flexed and extended feet, moved lower legs, asked if he or she feels dizzy, had patient take deep breaths until dizziness subsides.	___	___	___	_____
5. Applied gait belt properly.	___	___	___	_____
6. Had patient stand at bedside, ensured device is correct size, assessed patient's ability to bear weight and balance.	___	___	___	_____
7. Returned patient immediately to chair or bed if necessary.	___	___	___	_____
8. Decided with patient how far to ambulate.	___	___	___	_____

Copyright © 2018 by Elsevier Inc. All rights reserved.

	S	U	NP	Comments

9. Implemented ambulation around patient's other activities.   ___ ___ ___ _____

10. Helped patient walk with cane:

  a. Had patient hold cane on strong side.   ___ ___ ___ _____

  b. Directed patient to place cane appropriately forward, keeping weight on both legs.   ___ ___ ___ _____

  c. Instructed patient to advance leg even with cane.   ___ ___ ___ _____

  d. Had patient advance strong leg properly past cane.   ___ ___ ___ _____

  e. Had patient move involved leg even with strong leg.   ___ ___ ___ _____

  f. Repeated sequence as patient tolerates; once tolerated, had patient advance cane and weak leg together.   ___ ___ ___ _____

11. Helped patient crutch walk by using appropriate crutch gait:

  a. Instructed patient in use of the four-point gait.

    (1) Began in tripod position, placed crutch tips in front of foot, ensured patient's weight was on handgrips.   ___ ___ ___ _____

    (2) Moved right crutch forward.   ___ ___ ___ _____

    (3) Moved left foot forward to level of left crutch.   ___ ___ ___ _____

    (4) Moved left crutch forward.   ___ ___ ___ _____

    (5) Moved right foot forward to level of right crutch.   ___ ___ ___ _____

    (6) Repeated above sequence.   ___ ___ ___ _____

  b. Instructed patient in use of the three-point gait.

    (1) Began in tripod position.   ___ ___ ___ _____

    (2) Advanced both crutches and affected leg.   ___ ___ ___ _____

    (3) Moved weight-bearing leg forward, stepping on foot.   ___ ___ ___ _____

    (4) Repeated sequence.   ___ ___ ___ _____

  c. Instructed patient in use of the two-point gait.

    (1) Began in tripod position.   ___ ___ ___ _____

    (2) Moved left cutch and right foot forward.   ___ ___ ___ _____

Copyright © 2018 by Elsevier Inc. All rights reserved.

	S	U	NP	Comments

(3) Moved right crutch and left foot forward. ___ ___ ___ _____

(4) Repeated sequence. ___ ___ ___ _____

d. Instructed patient in use of the swing-to gait.

    (1) Began in tripod position. ___ ___ ___ _____

    (2) Moved crutches forward. ___ ___ ___ _____

    (3) Lifted and swung legs to crutches, let crutches support body weight. ___ ___ ___ _____

    (4) Repeated steps. ___ ___ ___ _____

e. Instructed patient in use of the swing-through gait.

    (1) Began in tripod position. ___ ___ ___ _____

    (2) Moved both crutches forward. ___ ___ ___ _____

    (3) Lifted and swung legs through and beyond crutches. ___ ___ ___ _____

    (4) Repeated previous steps. ___ ___ ___ _____

12. Helped patient climb stairs with a railing with crutches:

a. Began in tripod position. ___ ___ ___ _____

b. Transferred body weight to crutches. ___ ___ ___ _____

c. Positioned patient with handrail on side of strong leg. ___ ___ ___ _____

d. Supported weight evenly between crutch and handrail. ___ ___ ___ _____

e. Placed some weight on crutches and stepped up with strong leg, allowed patient to regain balance. ___ ___ ___ _____

f. Straightened strong knee and lifted body weight up to stair. ___ ___ ___ _____

g. Repeated sequence until patient reaches top of stairs, observed patient's balance and level of fatigue. ___ ___ ___ _____

h. Had patient ascend stairs from a seated position if necessary, moving crutches up stairs as he or she goes. ___ ___ ___ _____

13. Helped patient descend stairs with a railing with crutches:

a. Began in tripod position. ___ ___ ___ _____

b. Transferred body weight. ___ ___ ___ _____

c. Had patient hold handrail on strong side. ___ ___ ___ _____

Copyright © 2018 by Elsevier Inc. All rights reserved.

	S	U	NP	Comments

d. Bent strong knee, moved crutch and involved leg down a step.

e. Supported weight evenly between handrail and crutch, ensured patient has good balance.

f. Brought involved leg down to step, cautioned patient not to hop.

g. Had patient descend steps from sitting position if necessary, moving crutches down as he or she goes.

14. Helped patient ambulate with walker:

   a. Had patient stand straight in center of walker and grasp handgrips.

   b. Had patient move walker forward and move involved leg followed by strong leg, instructed patient not to advance leg past front of walker.

   c. Instructed patient properly on how to advance if weakness was present.

   d. Instructed patient not to climb stairs with walker unless walker is specifically designed for steps.

15. Assisted patient to comfortable position in bed or chair after ambulation.

16. Performed hand hygiene.

EVALUATION

1. Obtained patient's vital signs, observed skin color, asked about patient's level of comfort and energy level.

2. Evaluated patient's subjective statements regarding experience.

3. Evaluated gait of patient, observed body alignment in standing position and balance.

4. Asked patient and caregiver to describe the importance of a gait belt.

5. Identified unexpected outcomes.

RECORDING AND REPORTING

1. Recorded pertinent information in the appropriate log.

2. Documented evaluation of patient learning.

3. Reported any injury sustained, alteration in vital signs, or inability to ambulate to health care provider.

Copyright © 2018 by Elsevier Inc. All rights reserved.

Student _____ Date _____

Instructor _____ Date _____

PERFORMANCE CHECKLIST PROCEDURAL GUIDELINE 13.1　**SELECTION OF PRESSURE-REDISTRIBUTED SUPPORT SURFACE**

	S	U	NP	Comments

PROCEDURAL STEPS

1. Assessed patient's risk for skin breakdown using a risk assessment tool.

2. Assessed patient's existing pressure injuries.

3. Assessed patient's level of comfort using a pain scale.

4. Determined the need for pressure-reduction surface, placed at-risk patient on a pressure-reduction surface.

5. Identified patient factors when selecting appropriate surface:

   a. Assessed if patient needed pressure redistribution.

   b. Assessed if surface was needed for short- or long-term care.

   c. Assessed potential comfort level achieved by the surface.

   d. Assessed if patient, family, and caregiver were adherent to repositioning; assessed if they were aware a support surface should never replace repositioning.

   e. Assessed if support surface had potential to interfere with patient's independent functioning.

   f. Assessed patient's financial limitations.

   g. Assessed environmental limitations in the home if necessary.

   h. Assessed durability of the product.

   i. Assessed if patient needed pressure-relief surfaces in a chair/wheelchair and if caregiver had been instructed on appropriate inflation of device.

Copyright © 2018 by Elsevier Inc. All rights reserved.

	S	U	NP	Comments

6. Chose appropriate surface:

   a. Selected nonpowered support surface if patient can reposition without putting weight on the pressure injury or bottoming out.

   b. Selected powered support surface when appropriate.

   c. Selected high-specification foam for high-risk patients.

   d. Selected air-fluidized bed when appropriate.

   e. Selected low-air-loss bed for appropriate patients in intensive care.

   f. Selected support surface that supplied airflow when necessary.

   g. Selected support surface that provides airflow when excessive moisture is a potential risk.

7. Checked agency policy regarding implementing a support surface:

   a. Obtained a health care provider's orders.

   b. Consulted with case manager or social worker to help with patient's financial eligibility and terms and length of third-party reimbursement.

   c. Consulted with agency home care or discharge planning if device was anticipated for long-term use.

8. Performed hand hygiene, applied clean gloves, inspected condition of the skin regularly to evaluate changes in skin and effectiveness of therapy.

9. Inspected existing pressure injuries for evidence of healing.

10. Observed for side effects.

11. Documented pressure injury risk assessment and skin assessment in patient record, documented surface selected and patient response.

12. Documented support surface selected and patient response to surface.

Copyright © 2018 by Elsevier Inc. All rights reserved.

Student _____ Date _____

Instructor _____ Date _____

PERFORMANCE CHECKLIST SKILL 13.1 **PLACING A PATIENT ON A SUPPORT SURFACE**

	S	U	NP	Comments
ASSESSMENT				
1. Identified patient using two identifiers, compared identifiers with information in MAR.	___	___	___	_____
2. Performed hand hygiene.	___	___	___	_____
3. Determined patient's risk for pressure ulcer formation properly.	___	___	___	_____
4. Performed skin assessment, especially over dependent sites and bony prominences.	___	___	___	_____
5. Assessed patient's level of comfort.	___	___	___	_____
6. Assessed patient's understanding of purpose of support surface.	___	___	___	_____
7. Verified health care provider's orders for type of support surface.	___	___	___	_____
PLANNING				
1. Identified expected outcomes.	___	___	___	_____
2. Explained purpose of mattress and method of application to patient and caregiver.	___	___	___	_____
IMPLEMENTATION				
1. Provided privacy.	___	___	___	_____
2. Performed hand hygiene, applied clean gloves, obtained assistance as needed.	___	___	___	_____
3. Applied support surface to bed or prepared alternative bed, kept sharp objects away from air mattress:				
a. Replaced mattress.				
(1) Applied mattress to bed frame after removing hospital mattress.	___	___	___	_____
(2) Applied sheet over mattress, kept linens between surfaces to a minimum.	___	___	___	_____
b. Prepared an air mattress/overlay.				
(1) Applied deflated mattress flat over bed mattress.	___	___	___	_____
(2) Brought any plastic strips or flaps around corners of bed mattress.	___	___	___	_____

Copyright © 2018 by Elsevier Inc. All rights reserved.

	S	U	NP	Comments

(3) Attached connector on air mattress to inflation device, inflated mattress to proper air pressure.

— — — _____

(4) Placed sheet over air mattress, eliminated all wrinkles.

— — — _____

(5) Checked air pumps to be sure pressure cycle alternates.

— — — _____

(6) Assisted patient with transferring in and out of bed.

— — — _____

c. Used an air-surface bed.

(1) Obtained and placed linen on bed.

— — — _____

(2) Placed switch in the "prevention" mode.

— — — _____

4. Positioned patient comfortably as desired over support position, repositioned routinely.

— — — _____

5. Removed and disposed of gloves and performed hand hygiene.

— — — _____

EVALUATION

1. Reassessed patient's risk for pressure ulcer formation at routine intervals.

— — — _____

2. Inspected and compared condition of patient's skin every 8 hours to determine changes in skin integrity, pressure ulcer status, and effectiveness of support surface.

— — — _____

3. Asked patient to rate comfort.

— — — _____

4. Evaluated functioning of support surface periodically.

— — — _____

5. Asked patient to explain why he or she is on a special bed.

— — — _____

6. Identified unexpected outcomes.

— — — _____

RECORDING AND REPORTING

1. Recorded all pertinent information, patient teaching, and validation of understanding in appropriate log.

— — — _____

2. Documented evaluation of patient and caregiver learning.

— — — _____

3. Reported evidence of pressure ulcer formation to nurse in charge or health care provider.

— — — _____

Copyright © 2018 by Elsevier Inc. All rights reserved.

Student _____ Date _____

Instructor _____ Date _____

PERFORMANCE CHECKLIST SKILL 13.2 · **PLACING A PATIENT ON A SPECIAL BED**

	S	U	NP	Comments
ASSESSMENT				
1. Identified patient using two identifiers, compared identifiers with information on MAR.	___	___	___	_____
2. Performed hand hygiene.	___	___	___	_____
3. Determined patient's risk for pressure ulcer formation, assessed for risk factors for pressure injuries.	___	___	___	_____
4. Identified if patient would benefit from air-suspension therapy or air-fluidized therapy.	___	___	___	_____
5. Inspected condition of skin, noted appearance of existing injury and determined stage of injury.	___	___	___	_____
6. Assessed patient's comfort level.	___	___	___	_____
7. Verified health care provider's order for type of support surface.	___	___	___	_____
8. Reviewed patient's serum electrolyte levels if available.	___	___	___	_____
9. Assessed risk for complications from air-fluidized bed.	___	___	___	_____
PLANNING				
1. Identified expected outcomes.	___	___	___	_____
2. Explained purpose of mattress and method of application to patient and caregiver.	___	___	___	_____
3. Reviewed instructions provided by manufacturer.	___	___	___	_____
4. Obtained additional personnel if needed.	___	___	___	_____
5. Premedicated approximately 30 minutes before transfer if needed.	___	___	___	_____
IMPLEMENTATION				
1. Provided privacy.	___	___	___	_____
2. Performed hand hygiene, applied clean gloves if necessary, obtained assistance if necessary.	___	___	___	_____
3. Transferred patient to bed using appropriate transfer techniques, did not attempt transfer without assistance.	___	___	___	_____

Copyright © 2018 by Elsevier Inc. All rights reserved.

	S	U	NP	Comments

4. Turned bed on once patient has been transferred, regulated temperature.

_____ _____ _____ _____

5. Positioned patient to ROM exercises as appropriate.

_____ _____ _____ _____

6. Turned on Instaflate settings to turn patient, position bedpans, or perform therapies; used foam wedges with air-fluidized bed. Released Instaflate once procedure is completed.

_____ _____ _____ _____

7. Used bed's special features as needed.

_____ _____ _____ _____

8. Assessed effectiveness of pressure-relief mattress or seat cushion.

_____ _____ _____ _____

9. Removed and disposed of gloves, performed hand hygiene.

_____ _____ _____ _____

EVALUATION

1. Reassessed patient's risk of pressure injury formation at routine intervals.

_____ _____ _____ _____

2. Inspected condition of patient's skin periodically, determined changes in skin integrity and effectiveness of support surface.

_____ _____ _____ _____

3. Asked patient to rate level of comfort.

_____ _____ _____ _____

4. Evaluated functioning of support surface periodically.

_____ _____ _____ _____

5. Asked patient to describe why bed is turned laterally and how he or she feels.

_____ _____ _____ _____

6. Identified unexpected outcomes.

_____ _____ _____ _____

RECORDING AND REPORTING

1. Recorded pertinent information in appropriate log, recorded patient teaching and validation of understanding in nurses' notes.

_____ _____ _____ _____

2. Documented evaluation of patient and caregiver learning.

_____ _____ _____ _____

3. Reported changes in condition of skin, level of orientation, and electrolyte levels to health care provider.

_____ _____ _____ _____

Copyright © 2018 by Elsevier Inc. All rights reserved.

Student _____ Date _____

Instructor _____ Date _____

PERFORMANCE CHECKLIST SKILL 14.1 **FALL PREVENTION IN HEALTH CARE AGENCIES**

	S	U	NP	Comments

ASSESSMENT

1. Identified patient using two identifiers. ____ ____ ____ _____

2. Assessed patient's fall risks. ____ ____ ____ _____

3. Assessed patient's pain using appropriate rating scale. ____ ____ ____ _____

4. Determined if patient had history of recent falls or other injuries in the home, assessed previous falls following SPLATT. ____ ____ ____ _____

5. Reviewed patient's medication history, assessed OTC medications and herbal products, assessed for polypharmacy. ____ ____ ____ _____

6. Assessed patient for fear of falling. ____ ____ ____ _____

7. Performed TGUG test if patient is able to ambulate. ____ ____ ____ _____

8. Assessed condition of equipment. ____ ____ ____ _____

9. Assessed patient's history for osteoporosis, anticoagulant therapy, history of previous fracture, and recent chest or abdominal surgery. ____ ____ ____ _____

10. Used a patient-centered approach, determined what patient knew about risks for falling and fall prevention. ____ ____ ____ _____

11. Applied color-coded wristband if patient at risk for falling. ____ ____ ____ _____

12. Assessed level of comfort, fatigue, boredom, mental status, or level of engagement in patient in a wheelchair. ____ ____ ____ _____

PLANNING

1. Identify expected outcomes. ____ ____ ____ _____

2. Gathered equipment, performed hand hygiene. ____ ____ ____ _____

3. Explained plan, discussed reasons patient is at risk for falling, included caregivers, provided privacy. ____ ____ ____ _____

Copyright © 2018 by Elsevier Inc. All rights reserved.

	S	U	NP	Comments

IMPLEMENTATION

1. Conducted hourly rounds on all patients, determined status of pain and need for related items, provided pain relief intervention.

2. Adjusted bed to low position with wheels locked, placed padded mats on the exit side of the bed.

3. Encouraged patient to wear proper footwear.

4. Oriented patient to surroundings, call light, and routines to expect:

   a. Provided patient's hearing aid and glasses, ensured each is functioning and clean, referred to health care provider if necessary.

   b. Placed call light/bed control within patient's reach, explained and demonstrated how to turn system on and off, had patient perform return demonstration.

   c. Explained to patient and family when and why to use call system, provided clear instructions regarding mobility restrictions.

5. Taught safe use of side rails:

   a. Explained to patient and family reasons for using side rails.

   b. Checked agency policy regarding side rail use.

6. Made patient's environment safe:

   a. Removed excess equipment, supplies, and furniture from rooms and halls.

   b. Kept floors clear, coiled and secured other cords or tubing.

   c. Coiled and secured excess cords and tubing.

   d. Cleaned all spills promptly, managed wet floor signs appropriately.

   e. Ensured adequate glare-free lighting, used a night light.

   f. Had assistive devices located on exit side of bed.

   g. Arranged necessary items within patient's reach.

   h. Secured locks on beds, stretchers, and wheelchairs.

7. Provided comfort measures, offered ordered analgesics for patient experiencing pain.

154

Copyright © 2018 by Elsevier Inc. All rights reserved.

	S	U	NP	Comments

8. Interventions for patients at moderate to high risk:

   a. Prioritized call light responses. ____ ____ ____ _____

   b. Established elimination schedule, used bedside commode when appropriate. ____ ____ ____ _____

   c. Stayed with patient during toileting. ____ ____ ____ _____

   d. Placed patients in Geri chair or wheelchair with a wedge cushion, used wheelchair only for transport. ____ ____ ____ _____

   e. Used a low bed. ____ ____ ____ _____

   f. Activated bed alarm for patient. ____ ____ ____ _____

   g. Conferred with physical therapist on feasibility of training activities. ____ ____ ____ _____

   h. Used sitters or restraints only when absolutely necessary. ____ ____ ____ _____

9. Had patient wear gait belt while ambulating, walked along patient's strong side. ____ ____ ____ _____

10. Ensured safe use of wheelchair:

   a. Ensured wheelchair is correct fit for patient. ____ ____ ____ _____

   b. Transferred patient to wheelchair.

      (1) Determined help needed to transfer patient to wheelchair, positioned wheelchair properly. ____ ____ ____ _____

      (2) Placed wedge cushion in chair. ____ ____ ____ _____

      (3) Locked brakes on both wheels. ____ ____ ____ _____

      (4) Raised footplates before transfer, lowered and placed patient's feet on footplates when he or she is seated. ____ ____ ____ _____

      (5) Had patient sit all the way back in seat, applied seatbelt if necessary. ____ ____ ____ _____

      (6) Backed wheelchair into and out of elevator or door. ____ ____ ____ _____

   c. Managed patient's pain, provided alternative sitting position. ____ ____ ____ _____

11. Removed unnecessary supplies, performed hand hygiene. ____ ____ ____ _____

EVALUATION

1. Asked patient/caregiver to identify patient's fall risks. ____ ____ ____ _____

2. Asked patient/caregiver to describe fall prevention interventions. ____ ____ ____ _____

Copyright © 2018 by Elsevier Inc. All rights reserved.

	S	U	NP	Comments
3. Evaluated patient's ability to use assistive devices.	——	——	——	_____
4. Evaluated motor, sensory, and cognitive status; reviewed if any falls or injuries had occurred.	——	——	——	_____
5. Asked patient to explain why he or she is at a higher fall risk.	——	——	——	_____
6. Identified unexpected outcomes.	——	——	——	_____

RECORDING AND REPORTING

	S	U	NP	Comments
1. Reported specific risks to patient's safety and measures taken to minimize risks.	——	——	——	_____
2. Documented evaluation of patient learning.	——	——	——	_____
3. Documented description of any falls by witnesses, included baseline assessment, injuries reported, treatments, follow-up care, and safety precautions taken after fall.	——	——	——	_____

Copyright © 2018 by Elsevier Inc. All rights reserved.

Student _____ Date _____

Instructor _____ Date _____

PERFORMANCE CHECKLIST SKILL 14.2 **DESIGNING A RESTRAINT-FREE ENVIRONMENT**

	S	U	NP	Comments
ASSESSMENT				
1. Assessed patient's medical history for dementia, depression, and risk factors for wandering.	___	___	___	_____
2. Assessed patient's behavior, balance, gait, vision, hearing, bowel/bladder routine, level of pain, electrolyte and blood count values, and presence of orthostatic hypotension.	___	___	___	_____
3. Reviewed prescribed medications for interactions and untoward effects.	___	___	___	_____
4. Assessed patient's or caregiver's knowledge of condition and prescribed treatments.	___	___	___	_____
5. Assessed cognitive decline using MMSE for patients who wander or have known dementia.	___	___	___	_____
6. Assessed the degree of wandering behavior using RAWS.	___	___	___	_____
7. Asked family or friends about patient's usual communication style and cues for patients with dementia.	___	___	___	_____
8. Inspected condition of any therapeutic medical devices.	___	___	___	_____
PLANNING				
1. Identified expected outcomes.	___	___	___	_____
IMPLEMENTATION				
1. Oriented patient and family to surroundings, introduced staff, explained all treatments and procedures, ensured patient was able to read your name badge.	___	___	___	_____
2. Assigned same staff to care for patient as often as possible, encouraged friends and families to stay with patient, obtained agency volunteers if needed.	___	___	___	_____
3. Placed patient in room that is easily accessible to caregivers.	___	___	___	_____
4. Ensured patient has sensory aid devices, ensured all devices were functioning.	___	___	___	_____
5. Provided visual and auditory stimuli meaningful to patient.	___	___	___	_____

Copyright © 2018 by Elsevier Inc. All rights reserved.

	S	U	NP	Comments

6. Anticipated patient's basic needs as quickly as possible, conducted hourly rounds.

7. Provided scheduled ambulation, chair activity, and toileting; organized treatments so patient had uninterrupted periods throughout the day.

8. Positioned catheters and tubes/drains out of patient view, camouflaged IV site, covered visible catheters or feeding tubes/drains.

9. Eliminated stressors that may encourage wandering.

10. Used stress-reduction techniques including back rub, massage, and guided imagery.

11. Used diversional activities, ensured patient had interest in the chosen activity, involved a family member in the activity if possible.

12. Positioned patient on a wedge cushion, applied a wraparound belt.

13. Used pressure-sensitive bed or chair pad with alarms:

    a. Explained use of device to patient and family.

    b. Positioned device under patient's mid-to-low back or under buttocks.

    c. Tested alarm by applying and releasing pressure.

14. Placed electronic monitoring bracelet on wrist of patient with dementia.

15. Placed patient in bed enclosure system.

16. Consulted with therapists for activities that provide stimulation and exercise.

17. Minimized invasive treatments as much as possible.

EVALUATION

1. Monitored patient's behavior routinely.

2. Observed patient for any injuries.

3. Observed patient's behavior toward staff, visitors, and other patients.

4. Asked caregivers to describe ways in which they can help reduce patient wandering.

5. Identified unexpected outcomes.

Copyright © 2018 by Elsevier Inc. All rights reserved.

	S	U	NP	Comments

RECORDING AND REPORTING

1. Recorded restraint alternatives attempted, patient behaviors that related to cognitive status, and interventions in appropriate log.   ____ ____ ____ _____

2. Documented evaluation of patient learning.   ____ ____ ____ _____

Copyright © 2018 by Elsevier Inc. All rights reserved.

Student _____ Date _____

Instructor _____ Date _____

PERFORMANCE CHECKLIST SKILL 14.3 **APPLYING PHYSICAL RESTRAINTS**

	S	U	NP	Comments

ASSESSMENT

1. Identified patient using two identifiers. ___ ___ ___ _____

2. Assessed for underlying causes of agitation and cognitive impairment:

   a. Assessed for life-threatening physiological impairments. ___ ___ ___ _____

   b. Assessed for respiratory impairment, neurological impairment, fever and sepsis, hypoglycemia and hyperglycemia, alcohol and substance withdrawal, and fluid and electrolyte imbalance. ___ ___ ___ _____

   c. Notified health care provider of change in mental status or compromised physiologic status. ___ ___ ___ _____

   d. Obtained baseline or premorbid cognitive function from caregivers. ___ ___ ___ _____

   e. Established whether patient has history of dementia or depression. ___ ___ ___ _____

   f. Reviewed medications that cause risk for falling for interactions and adverse effects. ___ ___ ___ _____

   g. Reviewed current laboratory values. ___ ___ ___ _____

3. Assessed patient's current behavior, assessed whether patient creates risk to other patients. ___ ___ ___ _____

4. If restraint alternatives failed, conferred with health care provider, reviewed agency policies regarding restraints; obtained health care provider's orders for purpose, type, location, and duration of restraint; determined if signed consent was needed. ___ ___ ___ _____

5. Reviewed manufacturer instructions for restraint application, determined most appropriate size of restraint. ___ ___ ___ _____

PLANNING

1. Identified expected outcomes. ___ ___ ___ _____

2. Gathered equipment, performed hand hygiene. ___ ___ ___ _____

3. Explained what you plan to do and why, provided privacy. ___ ___ ___ _____

Copyright © 2018 by Elsevier Inc. All rights reserved.

IMPLEMENTATION

	S	U	NP	Comments
1. Adjusted bed to proper height, lowered side rail on side of patient contact, ensured patient is comfortable and positioned properly.	___	___	___	_____
2. Inspected area where restraint is to be placed, noted nearby tubing, assessed condition of skin, sensation, adequacy of circulation, and range of joint motion.	___	___	___	_____
3. Padded skin and bony prominences that will be under restraint.	___	___	___	_____
4. Applied proper size restraint:				
a. Mitten restraint: Placed hand in mitten, ensured straps are around wrist.	___	___	___	_____
b. Elbow restraint: Inserted patient's arm so that elbow joint rested against padded area, kept joint extended.	___	___	___	_____
c. Belt restraint: Had patient sit properly, applied belt over clothes, placed restraint around waist, removed wrinkles in clothing, brought ties through slots in belt, had patient lie down in bed and roll to side, ensured straps are properly secured to bed frame, applied restraint net if necessary.	___	___	___	_____
d. Extremity restraint: Wrapped restraint with soft part toward skin, secured with Velcro straps, ensured restraint is not too tight.	___	___	___	_____
5. Attached restraint straps to appropriate part of bedframe, ensured straps were secured.	___	___	___	_____
6. Secured restraints with appropriate buckle, ensured buckle is out of patient reach.	___	___	___	_____
7. Inserted two fingers under secured restraint, assessed proper placement of restraint.	___	___	___	_____
8. Removed restraints at least every 2 hours, assessed patient each time, obtained assistance and removed restraints one at a time if necessary.	___	___	___	_____
9. Secured call light or intercom within reach.	___	___	___	_____
10. Left bed or chair with wheels locked, kept bed in lowest position.	___	___	___	_____
11. Performed hand hygiene.	___	___	___	_____

Copyright © 2018 by Elsevier Inc. All rights reserved.

	S	U	NP	Comments

EVALUATION

1. Evaluated patient's condition for signs of injury regularly, used visual checks if needed. ⎯⎯ ⎯⎯ ⎯⎯ ⎯⎯⎯⎯⎯⎯⎯⎯⎯⎯⎯

2. Evaluated patient's need for toileting, nutrition, and hygiene, released restraints at least every 2 hours. ⎯⎯ ⎯⎯ ⎯⎯ ⎯⎯⎯⎯⎯⎯⎯⎯⎯⎯⎯

3. Evaluated patient for any complications of immobility. ⎯⎯ ⎯⎯ ⎯⎯ ⎯⎯⎯⎯⎯⎯⎯⎯⎯⎯⎯

4. Evaluated patient within 1 to 4 hours or found someone trained in CMS requirements to do so. ⎯⎯ ⎯⎯ ⎯⎯ ⎯⎯⎯⎯⎯⎯⎯⎯⎯⎯⎯

5. Ensured health care provider assessed patient 24 hours after initiation of restraint. ⎯⎯ ⎯⎯ ⎯⎯ ⎯⎯⎯⎯⎯⎯⎯⎯⎯⎯⎯

6. Observed catheters and drainage tubes routinely. ⎯⎯ ⎯⎯ ⎯⎯ ⎯⎯⎯⎯⎯⎯⎯⎯⎯⎯⎯

7. Observed patient's behavior and presence of restraint. ⎯⎯ ⎯⎯ ⎯⎯ ⎯⎯⎯⎯⎯⎯⎯⎯⎯⎯⎯

8. Asked patient to describe reason for restraints. ⎯⎯ ⎯⎯ ⎯⎯ ⎯⎯⎯⎯⎯⎯⎯⎯⎯⎯⎯

9. Identified unexpected outcomes. ⎯⎯ ⎯⎯ ⎯⎯ ⎯⎯⎯⎯⎯⎯⎯⎯⎯⎯⎯

RECORDING AND REPORTING

1. Recorded nursing interventions and restraint alternatives tried in appropriate log. ⎯⎯ ⎯⎯ ⎯⎯ ⎯⎯⎯⎯⎯⎯⎯⎯⎯⎯⎯

2. Documented evaluation of patient learning. ⎯⎯ ⎯⎯ ⎯⎯ ⎯⎯⎯⎯⎯⎯⎯⎯⎯⎯⎯

3. Reported all pertinent information about restraint in the appropriate log. ⎯⎯ ⎯⎯ ⎯⎯ ⎯⎯⎯⎯⎯⎯⎯⎯⎯⎯⎯

Copyright © 2018 by Elsevier Inc. All rights reserved.

Student _____ Date _____

Instructor _____ Date _____

	S	U	NP	Comments

PROCEDURAL STEPS

1. Reviewed agency guidelines for rapid response to emergency, understood nursing responsibilities.

2. Demonstrated knowledge of location of fire alarms, emergency equipment, SDS forms, eyewash stations, and exit routes.

3. Assessed patient's mental status and ability to ambulate, transfer, and move to anticipate evacuation procedures.

4. Remained alert to situations that increase risk for fire, checked patient's room for hazards.

5. Remained aware of which patients were on oxygen.

6. Inspected equipment for current maintenance sticker, checked electrical equipment for basic safety features, knew agency policy for reporting unsafe equipment.

7. Fire safety:

   a. Followed RACE acronym.

     (1) Rescued patient from immediate injury.

     (2) Activated fire alarm, followed agency policy for alerting staff.

     (3) Contained fire by closing doors and windows, turning off oxygen and equipment, and placing wet towels along base of doors.

     (4) Evacuated patients.

       (a) Directed ambulatory patients to a safe area.

       (b) Maintained respiratory status of patient on life support manually until removed from fire area.

       (c) Moved bedridden patients by stretcher, bed, or wheelchair.

Copyright © 2018 by Elsevier Inc. All rights reserved.

	S	U	NP	Comments

(d) Moved patient who cannot walk appropriately using blanket, two-person swing, or "back-strap" method. ___ ___ ___ _____

b. Extinguished fire using appropriate fire extinguisher, followed PASS acronym. ___ ___ ___ _____

c. Ensured fire doors are not blocked. ___ ___ ___ _____

8. Electrical safety:

a. Unplugged electrical source and assessed for presence of pulse after patient received a shock, checked for presence of water on the floor. ___ ___ ___ _____

b. Provided appropriate interventions, instituted emergency resuscitation if needed. ___ ___ ___ _____

c. Notified emergency personnel and patient's health care provider. ___ ___ ___ _____

d. Obtained vitals and assessed skin for signs of thermal injury if patient had pulse and remained alert. ___ ___ ___ _____

9. Chemical safety:

a. Attended to any exposed person, treated splashes to the eyes immediately, removed contact lenses if necessary. ___ ___ ___ _____

b. Notified persons in immediate area of spill, evacuated nonessential personnel. ___ ___ ___ _____

c. Referred to SDS, turned off electrical and heat sources if necessary. ___ ___ ___ _____

d. Avoided breathing vapors, applied respirator if necessary. ___ ___ ___ _____

e. Used appropriate PPE to clean up spill. ___ ___ ___ _____

f. Disposed of any materials used in cleanup as hazardous waste. ___ ___ ___ _____

10. Followed agency policy for reporting sentinel event. ___ ___ ___ _____

Copyright © 2018 by Elsevier Inc. All rights reserved.

Student _____ Date _____

Instructor _____ Date _____

PERFORMANCE CHECKLIST SKILL 14.4 **SEIZURE PRECAUTIONS**

	S	U	NP	Comments

ASSESSMENT

1. Assessed patient's seizure history and knowledge of precipitating factors; asked patient to describe frequency, presence and type of aura, and body parts affected; used family as a resource if needed. ___ ___ ___ _____

2. Assessed for medical and surgical conditions. ___ ___ ___ _____

3. Assessed medication history, assessed patient's adherence to drug levels if test results were available. ___ ___ ___ _____

4. Inspected patient's environment for potential safety hazards if seizure occurred; kept bed low and side rails up. ___ ___ ___ _____

5. Assessed patient's individual and cultural perspective about meaning of seizures and their treatment. ___ ___ ___ _____

PLANNING

1. Identified expected outcomes. ___ ___ ___ _____

2. Informed patient and caregiver that patient is on seizure precautions. ___ ___ ___ _____

IMPLEMENTATION

1. Kept bed in lowest position with side rails up, padded rails if needed, had oral suction and oxygen equipment ready for use. ___ ___ ___ _____

2. Placed patient in a room close to nurses' station or in a room with a video monitor if necessary. ___ ___ ___ _____

3. Partial or general seizure response:

   a. Positioned patient safely.

      (1) Guided patient to floor, protected head appropriately, turned patient onto side with head tilted forward, did not lift patient during seizure. ___ ___ ___ _____

      (2) Turned patient in bed on side and raised side rails. ___ ___ ___ _____

Copyright © 2018 by Elsevier Inc. All rights reserved.

	S	U	NP	Comments

b. Noted time seizure began, called for help, had health care provider notified immediately, had staff bring emergency cart, cleared surrounding area of furniture, provided airway protection and gas exchange. —— —— —— _____

c. Kept patient in side-lying position, supported head, and kept it flexed slightly forward. —— —— —— _____

d. Did not restrain patient, held limbs loosely if necessary, loosened restrictive clothing. —— —— —— _____

e. Did not force any object into patient's mouth. —— —— —— _____

f. Provided privacy, had staff control flow of visitors. —— —— —— _____

g. Observed sequence and timing of seizure activity, noted all relevant behaviors. —— —— —— _____

h. Assessed vital signs and reoriented patient after patient regained consciousness, explained what happened and answered patient's questions, stayed with patient until fully awake. —— —— —— _____

4. Status epilepticus:

a. Followed steps 3a–3c to stabilize airway and called emergency team. —— —— —— _____

b. Assisted health care provider with intubation if necessary. —— —— —— _____

c. Accessed oxygen and suction equipment, kept airway patent. —— —— —— _____

d. Ensured others were measuring vitals and blood glucose at appropriate intervals. —— —— —— _____

e. Suctioned patient's airway and ensured any oral airway stayed in correct position. —— —— —— _____

f. Kept patient in appropriate position with side rails up and bed in lowest position. —— —— —— _____

5. Reoriented and reassured patient, explained what happened, provided time for patient to express feelings and concerns, placed call light within reach, instructed patient not to get out of bed without help. —— —— —— _____

6. Cleaned up patient care area, disposed of used supplies, performed hand hygiene. —— —— —— _____

Copyright © 2018 by Elsevier Inc. All rights reserved.

	S	U	NP	Comments

EVALUATION

1. Checked vital signs and oxygen saturation every 15 minutes, maintained patent airway.

2. Rechecked blood glucose per health care provider order.

3. Examined patient for injury, included oral cavity and extremities.

4. Evaluated patient's mental status, encouraged him or her to verbalize feelings.

5. Helped health care provider conduct neurologic examination, collected any ordered blood tests.

6. Identified unexpected outcomes.

RECORDING AND REPORTING

1. Recorded observations of the seizure, including type of seizure activity and sequence of events, in the appropriate log.

2. Recorded treatments administered.

3. Alerted health care provider immediately.

Copyright © 2018 by Elsevier Inc. All rights reserved.

Student _____ Date _____

Instructor _____ Date _____

_____

PERFORMANCE CHECKLIST SKILL 15.1 **CARE OF A PATIENT AFTER BIOLOGICAL EXPOSURE**

_____

	S	U	NP	Comments
ASSESSMENT				
1. Performed hand hygiene, applied proper PPE.	——	——	——	_____
2. Identified patient using at least two identifiers.	——	——	——	_____
3. Conducted focused health history and physical examination, reviewed history of patient's presenting symptoms, determined if pattern exists.	——	——	——	_____
4. Measured patient's vital signs, included pain assessment.	——	——	——	_____
5. Reviewed results of diagnostic tests, consulted with health care provider.	——	——	——	_____
6. Assessed patient for health risks that complicated the effects of exposure to a biologic agent.	——	——	——	_____
7. Stayed calm, assessed patient's immediate psychological response after exposure.	——	——	——	_____
8. Identified all patient contacts before patient leaves the emergency department.	——	——	——	_____
9. Identified resources available.	——	——	——	_____
PLANNING				
1. Identified expected outcomes.	——	——	——	_____
2. Dispensed timely and accurate information.	——	——	——	_____
IMPLEMENTATION				
1. Continued wearing PPE, followed transmission-based isolation precautions.	——	——	——	_____
2. Decontaminated if indicated, had patient remove clothes and place in a biohazard bag, cut garments off instead of pulling them over the patient's head, instructed patient to shower thoroughly with soap and water.	——	——	——	_____
3. Administered appropriate antibiotics/antitoxins.	——	——	——	_____
4. Administered immunizations.	——	——	——	_____
5. Administered fluid and nutrition therapy.	——	——	——	_____
6. Administered oxygen therapy.	——	——	——	_____
7. Provided supportive care.	——	——	——	_____

Copyright © 2018 by Elsevier Inc. All rights reserved.

	S	U	NP	Comments

8. Removed most heavily contaminated items first, peeled off gown and gloves and disposed, performed hand hygiene, removed face shield properly and disposed, removed goggles and mask and disposed, performed hand hygiene.   ___ ___ ___ _____

9. Counseled patient and family on acute and potential long-term psychological effects of exposure, offered access to counselors, supported survivors of a disaster by identifying resources.   ___ ___ ___ _____

EVALUATION

1. Observed for improved airway maintenance, breathing, circulation, LOC, and neurologic functioning.   ___ ___ ___ _____

2. Evaluated vital signs and level of pain.   ___ ___ ___ _____

3. Inspected condition of patient's skin, noted character of lesions.   ___ ___ ___ _____

4. Asked patient, "How do you feel right now?" Checked level of orientation and ability to conduct conversation.   ___ ___ ___ _____

5. Identified unexpected outcomes.   ___ ___ ___ _____

RECORDING AND REPORTING

1. Reported suspected cases of biological incident to health care provider or ED officer.   ___ ___ ___ _____

2. Used disaster checklists to record patient status data, treatment administered, and response to treatment or comfort measures.   ___ ___ ___ _____

3. Reported any unexpected outcome to health care provider.   ___ ___ ___ _____

Copyright © 2018 by Elsevier Inc. All rights reserved.

Student _____   Date _____

Instructor _____   Date _____

PERFORMANCE CHECKLIST SKILL 15.2   **CARE OF A PATIENT AFTER CHEMICAL EXPOSURE**

	S	U	NP	Comments
ASSESSMENT				
1. Performed hand hygiene, applied proper PPE.	___	___	___	_____
2. Identified patient using at least two identifiers.	___	___	___	_____
3. Observed for presence of liquid on patient's skin or clothing and for odor, determined severity of exposure.	___	___	___	_____
4. Assessed patient for preexisting medical conditions that will complicate effects of toxic exposure.	___	___	___	_____
5. Calmly assessed patient's immediate psychological response following exposure.	___	___	___	_____
6. Identified resources available.	___	___	___	_____
PLANNING				
1. Identified expected outcomes.	___	___	___	_____
2. Explained care to patient and family, explained your role, oriented patient to location and activities, asked how patient was feeling, assured patient that a medical professional would see the patient shortly.	___	___	___	_____
IMPLEMENTATION				
1. Continued wearing PPE applied during assessment.	___	___	___	_____
2. Provided privacy.	___	___	___	_____
3. Decontaminated patient:				
a. Acted quickly, avoided touching contaminated parts of clothing.	___	___	___	_____
b. Removed all of patient's clothing, cut garments off.	___	___	___	_____
c. Used large amounts of soap and water to wash patient thoroughly.	___	___	___	_____
d. Rinsed eyes with water if necessary, removed contacts if needed, washed eyeglasses and reapplied them.	___	___	___	_____
4. Disposed of patient's contaminated clothing in sealed biohazard bag, placed in another plastic bag and sealed.	___	___	___	_____

Copyright © 2018 by Elsevier Inc. All rights reserved.

	S	U	NP	Comments

5. Initiated treatment for chemical agent using appropriate chemical agent protocol. ____ ____ ____ _____

6. Established airway if needed, administered oxygen therapy. ____ ____ ____ _____

7. Controlled bleeding. ____ ____ ____ _____

8. Established IV access, administered fluid and nutritional therapy. ____ ____ ____ _____

9. Provided supportive care. ____ ____ ____ _____

10. Removed most heavily contaminated items first, peeled off gown and gloves and discarded, performed hand hygiene, removed face shield properly and discarded, removed goggles and mask and discarded appropriately, performed hand hygiene. ____ ____ ____ _____

11. Counseled patient and family on acute and potential long-term psychological effect of exposure, offered access to trained counselors. ____ ____ ____ _____

EVALUATION

1. Observed status of airway maintenance, breathing, circulation, LOC, and neurologic functioning; assessed vital signs. ____ ____ ____ _____

2. Asked patient to rate level of pain on a scale of 0 to 10. ____ ____ ____ _____

3. Inspected condition of skin, noted extent of blistering. ____ ____ ____ _____

4. Evaluated patient's level of orientation, ability to problem solve, and perception of condition. ____ ____ ____ _____

5. Identified unexpected outcomes. ____ ____ ____ _____

RECORDING AND REPORTING

1. Reported suspected cases of a toxic chemical event to health care provider or emergency officer. ____ ____ ____ _____

2. Recorded in nurses' notes patient's status, decontamination and treatment procedures, and response to treatment/comfort measures. ____ ____ ____ _____

3. Reported any unexpected outcome to health care provider in charge. ____ ____ ____ _____

Copyright © 2018 by Elsevier Inc. All rights reserved.

Student _____ Date _____

Instructor _____ Date _____

PERFORMANCE CHECKLIST SKILL 15.3 **CARE OF A PATIENT AFTER RADIATION EXPOSURE**

	S	U	NP	Comments
ASSESSMENT				
1. Performed hand hygiene, applied proper PPE.	——	——	——	_____
2. Identified patient using at least two identifiers.	——	——	——	_____
3. Assessed patient's symptoms by performing a focused physical examination.	——	——	——	_____
4. Measured patient's vital signs, included assessment of pain.	——	——	——	_____
5. Assessed patient for preexisting medical conditions that would complicate effects of radiologic exposure.	——	——	——	_____
6. Determined patient's allergies.	——	——	——	_____
7. Assessed individual psychological response to radiologic event, ask how patient feels, determined level of orientation.	——	——	——	_____
8. Identified resources available.	——	——	——	_____
PLANNING				
1. Identified expected outcomes.	——	——	——	_____
2. Explained care to patient and family, explained role, oriented to location and activities, explained what patient had experienced, asked how patient was feeling, assured patient that medical personnel would see the patient shortly.	——	——	——	_____
IMPLEMENTATION				
1. Performed hand hygiene.	——	——	——	_____
2. Continued wearing PPE applied during assessment.	——	——	——	_____
3. Provided privacy.	——	——	——	_____
4. Decontaminated patient:				
a. Removed patient's clothing.	——	——	——	_____
b. Washed patient's skin thoroughly with soap and water, took care not to abrade or irritate skin, did not allow radioactive material to be incorporated into wounds.	——	——	——	_____
c. Had radiation technician resurvey patient after washing, rewashed if necessary.	——	——	——	_____

172

Copyright © 2018 by Elsevier Inc. All rights reserved.

	S	U	NP	Comments

d. Isolated and covered areas of skin still positive for radiation by using a plastic bag or wrap.

5. Isolated and covered areas of skin still positive for radiation by using a plastic bag or wrap.

6. Prepared for obtaining a CBC, urinalysis, fecal specimen, and swabs of body orifices.

7. Treated symptoms according to ordinary treatment practices, provided IV fluid support, antidiarrheal therapies, antiemetic medication, and potassium iodine tablets.

8. Removed most heavily contaminated items first, peeled off gown and gloves and discarded, performed hand hygiene, removed face shield properly and discarded, removed goggles and mask and discarded appropriately. Performed hand hygiene.

9. Counseled patient and family on psychological effects of exposure, offered access to trained counselors.

EVALUATION

1. Observed skin integrity, fluid balance, respiratory and GI status, LOC, and neurologic functioning, looked for improvement of other radiologic agent–specific symptoms, evaluated vital signs.

2. Monitored CBC and other laboratory tests.

3. Evaluated patient's LOC, orientation, and ability to relate events; asked if patient remembers what occurred; observed patient's affect.

4. Identified unexpected outcomes.

RECORDING AND REPORTING

1. Recorded in nurses' notes patient's status and response to treatment/comfort measures.

2. Reported presence of open wound and any suspected radioactive fragment to health care provider in charge.

3. Reported any unexpected outcomes to health care provider.

Copyright © 2018 by Elsevier Inc. All rights reserved.

Student _____ Date _____

Instructor _____ Date _____

PERFORMANCE CHECKLIST SKILL 16.1 **PAIN ASSESSMENT AND BASIC COMFORT MEASURES**

	S	U	NP	Comments

ASSESSMENT

1. Identified patient using two identifiers. ___ ___ ___ _____

2. Assessed patient's risk for pain. ___ ___ ___ _____

3. Asked patient if he or she is in pain, used appropriate language for patient's values, obtained an interpreter if necessary. ___ ___ ___ _____

4. Performed hand hygiene. Examined site of patient's pain, inspected ROM of joints involved, percussed and auscultated to help identify abnormalities, determined cause of pain, auscultated abdomen before palpation. ___ ___ ___ _____

5. Assessed physical, behavioral, and emotional signs and symptoms of pain. ___ ___ ___ _____

6. Assessed characteristics of pain, followed agency policy regarding frequency of assessment, used PQRSTU pain assessment. ___ ___ ___ _____

7. Assessed patient's medical history for successful pain relief therapies. ___ ___ ___ _____

8. Assessed patient's response to previous pharmacological interventions, determined if analgesic side effects are likely. ___ ___ ___ _____

9. Assessed for allergies to medications. ___ ___ ___ _____

PLANNING

1. Identified expected outcomes. ___ ___ ___ _____

IMPLEMENTATION

1. Performed hand hygiene, applied clean gloves if indicated. ___ ___ ___ _____

2. Prepared patient's environment with proper temperature, lighting, and sound to allow rest. ___ ___ ___ _____

3. Taught patient how to use pain-rating scale. ___ ___ ___ _____

4. Set pain-intensity goal with patient when able. ___ ___ ___ _____

5. Administered pain-relieving medications per health care provider's orders. ___ ___ ___ _____

6. Removed or reduced painful stimuli by assisting patient to comfortable position and repositioning linens, bandages, tubes, and equipment as needed. ___ ___ ___ _____

Copyright © 2018 by Elsevier Inc. All rights reserved.

	S	U	NP	Comments

7. Taught patient how to splint over painful site using pillow or hand:

    a. Explained purpose of splinting. ____ ____ ____ _____

    b. Placed pillow or blanket over site, assisted patient to place hands firmly over area of discomfort. ____ ____ ____ _____

    c. Had patient hold area firmly while coughing, deep breathing, and turning. ____ ____ ____ _____

8. Reduced or eliminated emotional factors that increase pain experiences:

    a. Offered information that reduces anxiety. ____ ____ ____ _____

    b. Offered patient opportunity to pray. ____ ____ ____ _____

    c. Spent time to allow patient to talk about pain. ____ ____ ____ _____

9. If used, removed and disposed of gloves, performed hand hygiene. ____ ____ ____ _____

EVALUATION

1. Asked patient to describe level of relief within 1 hour of intervention. ____ ____ ____ _____

2. Compared patient's current pain with personally set pain-intensity goal. ____ ____ ____ _____

3. Compared patient's ability to function and perform ADLs before and after pain interventions. ____ ____ ____ _____

4. Observed patient's nonverbal behaviors. ____ ____ ____ _____

5. Evaluated for analgesic side effects. ____ ____ ____ _____

6. Asked patient to explain when to use previous techniques for pain relief. ____ ____ ____ _____

7. Identified unexpected outcomes. ____ ____ ____ _____

RECORDING AND REPORTING

1. Recorded and reported character of pain before intervention, therapies used, and patient response in appropriate log. ____ ____ ____ _____

2. Documented evaluation of patient learning. ____ ____ ____ _____

3. Recorded inadequate pain relief, reduction in patient function, adverse side effects from pain interventions, and any patient or family education. ____ ____ ____ _____

Copyright © 2018 by Elsevier Inc. All rights reserved.

Student _____ Date _____

Instructor _____ Date _____

PERFORMANCE CHECKLIST SKILL 16.2 **PATIENT-CONTROLLED ANALGESIA**

	S	U	NP	Comments
ASSESSMENT				
1. Checked accuracy and completeness of each MAR.	___	___	___	_____
2. Reviewed drug reference or consulted with pharmacist if necessary.	___	___	___	_____
3. Identified patient using two identifiers, compared identifiers with information on MAR.	___	___	___	_____
4. Performed hand hygiene, assessed severity and character of patient's pain using appropriate pain scale.	___	___	___	_____
5. Assessed environment for factors that could contribute to pain.	___	___	___	_____
6. Assessed for conditions that predisposed patient to unwanted effects from opioids.	___	___	___	_____
7. Applied clean gloves, assessed patency of IV access and surrounding tissue for inflammation or swelling.	___	___	___	_____
8. Inspected incision if patient had had surgery, palpated area for tenderness, used sterile gloves if necessary. Removed gloves and performed hand hygiene.	___	___	___	_____
9. Checked medical record for history of drug allergies and typical reactions.	___	___	___	_____
10. Assessed patient's knowledge and perceived effectiveness of previous pain management strategies.	___	___	___	_____
PLANNING				
1. Identified expected outcomes.	___	___	___	_____
2. Collected appropriate equipment and provided privacy.	___	___	___	_____
IMPLEMENTATION				
1. Performed hand hygiene.	___	___	___	_____
2. Obtained PCA analgesic, checked label of medication twice.	___	___	___	_____
3. Identified patient using two identifiers, compared with information on MAR.	___	___	___	_____

Copyright © 2018 by Elsevier Inc. All rights reserved.

4. Compared MAR with name of medication on drug cartridge at bedside, had a second RN confirm health care provider's orders and correct setup of PCA.

5. Explained purpose of PCA and demonstrated function of PCA to patient and family:

   a. Explained type of medication in PCA device.

   b. Explained how device administers medication when needed and minimized side effects from analgesia.

   c. Explained that self-dosing aids in repositioning, walking or coughing, and deep breathing.

   d. Explained dose and type ordered, lockout interval, and dosage limits.

   e. Demonstrated how to push medication demand button on PCA device.

   f. Instructed patient to notify nurse for possible side effects, problems in attaining pain relief, changes in severity or location, alarms sounding, or questions.

6. Applied clean gloves, checked infuser and patient-control module for accurate labeling or evidence of leaking.

7. Positioned patient comfortably, ensured venipuncture or central line site is accessible.

8. Inserted drug cartridge into infusion device and primed tubing.

9. Attached needleless adapter to tubing adapter of patient-controlled module.

10. Wiped injection port of main IV line with alcohol.

11. Inserted needleless adapter into injection port nearest patient.

12. Secured connection with tape and anchored PCA tubing, labeled tubing.

13. Programmed computerized PCA pump as ordered, had second nurse check setting.

14. Administered loading dose of analgesia if prescribed.

15. Discarded gloves and supplies in appropriate containers, disposed of cassette or syringe in appropriate manner, performed hand hygiene.

Copyright © 2018 by Elsevier Inc. All rights reserved.

	S	U	NP	Comments

16. Had patient demonstrate use of PCA system if currently in pain; had patient verbally repeat instructions given earlier if not currently in pain. ___ ___ ___ _____

17. Ensured venipuncture line or central line site is protected and rechecked before leaving. ___ ___ ___ _____

18. Discontinued PCA:

   a. Checked health care provider order for discontinuation, obtained necessary information from pump for documentation. ___ ___ ___ _____

   b. Performed hand hygiene, applied clean gloves, turned off pump, disconnected PCA tubing but maintained IV access. ___ ___ ___ _____

   c. Disposed of empty cartridge, tubing, and gloves according to agency policy. ___ ___ ___ _____

EVALUATION

1. Evaluated patient's pain intensity following treatments and procedures. ___ ___ ___ _____

2. Observed patient for nausea or pruritus. ___ ___ ___ _____

3. Monitored patient's level of sedation, vital signs, and pulse oximetry every 1 to 2 hours for 12 hours or more often if necessary. ___ ___ ___ _____

4. Had patient demonstrate dose delivery. ___ ___ ___ _____

5. Evaluated number of attempts, delivery of demand doses, and basal dose if ordered. ___ ___ ___ _____

6. Observed patient initiate self-care. ___ ___ ___ _____

7. Asked patient to describe steps to activate the PCA. ___ ___ ___ _____

8. Identified unexpected outcomes. ___ ___ ___ _____

RECORDING AND REPORTING

1. Recorded all pertinent information in appropriate log. ___ ___ ___ _____

2. Recorded regular assessment on patient response to analgesia on the appropriate form. ___ ___ ___ _____

3. Documented evaluation of patient learning. ___ ___ ___ _____

Copyright © 2018 by Elsevier Inc. All rights reserved.

Student _____ Date _____

Instructor _____ Date _____

PERFORMANCE CHECKLIST SKILL 16.3   **EPIDURAL ANALGESIA**

	S	U	NP	Comments
ASSESSMENT				
1. Identified patient using two identifiers, compared identifiers with information on MAR.	___	___	___	_____
2. Assessed if patient has completed informed consent and is aware of risks and benefits of epidural analgesia.	___	___	___	_____
3. Verified health care provider's order against MAR.	___	___	___	_____
4. Performed hand hygiene, assessed patient's pain level and character of pain, obtained interpreter if necessary.	___	___	___	_____
5. Checked to see if patient recently received anticoagulants.	___	___	___	_____
6. Assessed if patient routinely takes herbal medication, documented complete list.	___	___	___	_____
7. Assessed for history of drug allergies.	___	___	___	_____
8. Assessed patient's sedation level.	___	___	___	_____
9. Assessed rate, pattern, and depth of respirations; assessed pulse oximetry; assessed blood pressure and temperature.	___	___	___	_____
10. Assessed initial motor and sensory function of lower extremities.	___	___	___	_____
11. Performed hand hygiene, inspected catheter insertion site for signs of infection, applied sterile gloves if necessary.	___	___	___	_____
12. Followed catheter tubing and checked connection site with IV tubing, verified catheter is appropriately attached to patient's skin, removed gloves and performed hand hygiene.	___	___	___	_____
13. Checked patency of IV tubing, checked infusion pump for proper calibration and operation.	___	___	___	_____

Copyright © 2018 by Elsevier Inc. All rights reserved.

	S	U	NP	Comments

PLANNING

1. Identified expected outcomes.

2. Explained purpose and function of epidural analgesia and expectations of patient during procedure, demonstrated how to use pump on demand.

IMPLEMENTATION

1. Placed patient receiving an epidural analgesia close to nurses' station.

2. Reidentified patient using at least two identifiers, compared against information on MAR.

3. Performed hand hygiene, prepared analgesic following "six rights" of medication administration.

4. Attached "epidural line" label to infusion tubing at the appropriate time, ensured there are *no Y-ports*.

5. Compared MAR with medication container at bedside.

6. Applied clean gloves, administered infusion with help of anesthesia provider:

   a. Administered continuous infusion.

     (1) Attached container of medication to pump tubing, primed tubing.

     (2) Inserted tubing into infusion pump, attached distal end of tubing to antibacterial filter, connected to epidural catheter using aseptic technique.

     (3) Checked infusion pump for proper calibration and operation.

     (4) Taped all connections, started infusion.

   b. Administered bolus dose of analgesic via infusion pump.

     (1) Performed steps 6a (1 to 4) while helping anesthesia provider, adjusted infusion pumping setting for maximum bolus size, initiated pump to deliver ordered bolus.

   c. Administered dose on demand.

     (1) Performed steps 6a (1 to 4) while helping anesthesia provider, set pump for lock-out time.

180

Copyright © 2018 by Elsevier Inc. All rights reserved.

	S	U	NP	Comments

(2) Had patient initiate demand dose as needed.

7. Explained that nurses will monitor patient's response to analgesia routinely, instructed patient on signs and problems to report.

8. Kept IV line patent for 24 hours after epidural analgesia has ended.

9. Removed and disposed of gloves, performed hand hygiene.

10. Checked for presence of therapeutic anticoagulation before removal of epidural catheter, checked agency policy if necessary.

EVALUATION

1. Evaluated patient's pain severity and character of pain.

2. Evaluated blood pressure and heart rate, pulse oximetry, and sedation level, measured at appropriate intervals.

3. Helped patient when changing positions.

4. Evaluated catheter insertion site every 2 to 4 hours for infection, noted character of drainage.

5. Inspected epidural site for disruption or displacement of catheter.

6. Observed for pruritus, informed patient that this is a side effect and not an allergic response.

7. Observed for nausea, vomiting, and presence of headache.

8. Monitored I&O, assessed for bladder distention, observed for frequency or urgency of urination, consulted health care provider for possible need for intermittent catheterization.

9. Evaluated for motor weakness or numbness and tingling of lower extremities.

10. Asked patient to describe which side effects to discuss with nurses.

11. Identified unexpected outcomes.

RECORDING AND REPORTING

1. Recorded pertinent specific information in the appropriate log.

2. Obtained and recorded pump readout with appropriate frequency with continuous or demand infusion.

Copyright © 2018 by Elsevier Inc. All rights reserved.

	S	U	NP	Comments
3. Recorded regular periodic assessments of patient's status in appropriate logs.	___	___	___	_____
4. Reported any adverse reactions or complications to health care provider immediately.	___	___	___	_____
5. Documented evaluation of patient learning.	___	___	___	_____

Copyright © 2018 by Elsevier Inc. All rights reserved.

Student _____ Date _____

Instructor _____ Date _____

	S	U	NP	Comments
ASSESSMENT				
1. Identified patient using at least two identifiers, compared identifiers with information on MAR.	___	___	___	_____
2. Performed hand hygiene, applied clean gloves, assessed dressing and site of catheter insertion.	___	___	___	_____
3. Ensured catheter tubing is correctly labeled, ensured catheter connection is secure, notified surgeon if catheter is detached.	___	___	___	_____
4. Performed a complete pain assessment.	___	___	___	_____
5. Reviewed surgeon's operative report for position of catheter.	___	___	___	_____
6. Compared label on device to MAR or health care provider's order.	___	___	___	_____
7. Assessed for blood backing up in tubing, stopped infusion, notified health care provider if present, removed gloves, performed hand hygiene.	___	___	___	_____
8. Determined level of extremity activity that patient can perform.	___	___	___	_____
9. Confirmed patient's allergies, assessed for signs of local anesthetic toxicity.	___	___	___	_____
10. Assessed patient's and caregiver's knowledge of infusion pump.	___	___	___	_____
PLANNING				
1. Identified expected outcomes.	___	___	___	_____
IMPLEMENTATION				
1. Performed hand hygiene, used caution when repositioning patient.	___	___	___	_____
2. Connected catheter to smaller pump on discharge if necessary.	___	___	___	_____
3. Taught patient or caregiver what to observe and how to removed catheter at home:				
a. Explained how to perform hand hygiene and apply clean gloves.	___	___	___	_____
b. Had patient assume a relaxed position.	___	___	___	_____

Copyright © 2018 by Elsevier Inc. All rights reserved.

	S	U	NP	Comments

c. Applied clean gloves, had patient or caregiver lift adhesive dressing and remove tape. ___ ___ ___ _____

d. Directed patient or caregiver to place gauze over site, grasp catheter close to skin, and pull out with a steady motion. ___ ___ ___ _____

e. Had patient or caregiver observe for mark on end of catheter tip, held sterile gauze over site for at least 2 minutes. ___ ___ ___ _____

f. Washed skin to remove surgical soap or adhesive, applied Band-Aid. ___ ___ ___ _____

g. Placed catheter in bag using standard precautions, reminded patient to bring to health care provider at follow-up visit, removed and disposed of gloves, performed hand hygiene. ___ ___ ___ _____

h. Explained to patient that any remaining numbness should go away within 24 hours. ___ ___ ___ _____

4. Reminded patient or caregiver of follow-up appointment with surgeon. ___ ___ ___ _____

EVALUATION

1. Asked patient to rate pain intensity at rest and with activity. ___ ___ ___ _____

2. Observed for signs of adverse drug reactions, reported signs immediately. ___ ___ ___ _____

3. Observed patient's position, mobility, relaxation, participation in ADLs, and any nonverbal behaviors. ___ ___ ___ _____

4. Inspected condition of surgical dressing. ___ ___ ___ _____

5. Inspected catheter exit site during follow-up visit. ___ ___ ___ _____

6. Asked patient to explain steps to remove catheter. ___ ___ ___ _____

7. Identified unexpected outcomes. ___ ___ ___ _____

RECORDING AND REPORTING

1. Recorded drug, concentration, date inserted, and type of demand feature in the appropriate log. ___ ___ ___ _____

2. Recorded location of catheter, patient's pain rating, response to anesthetic and additional comfort measure given in nurses' notes. ___ ___ ___ _____

3. Recorded additional analgesics necessary to control pain. ___ ___ ___ _____

Copyright © 2018 by Elsevier Inc. All rights reserved.

	S	U	NP	Comments
4. Recorded any adverse reaction to local anesthetic.	___	___	___	_____
5. Reported damp dressing/displaced catheter to surgeon.	___	___	___	_____
6. Documented evaluation of patient learning.	___	___	___	_____

Copyright © 2018 by Elsevier Inc. All rights reserved.

Student _____ Date _____

Instructor _____ Date _____

PERFORMANCE CHECKLIST SKILL 16.5 **NONPHARMACOLOGICAL PAIN MANAGEMENT**

	S	U	NP	Comments

ASSESSMENT

1. Assessed patient's language level and values regarding alternative pain relief, identified descriptive terms to use during relaxation or guided imagery.   ___ ___ ___ _____

2. Assessed character of pain, including severity and underlying cause.   ___ ___ ___ _____

3. Assessed facial expressions, nonverbal indications of discomfort, body position and movement, and patient's self-report.   ___ ___ ___ _____

4. Performed hand hygiene, applied gloves if necessary, examined site of pain by visual inspection, palpation, and range of motion of involved joints.   ___ ___ ___ _____

5. Assessed character of patient's respirations.   ___ ___ ___ _____

6. Reviewed health care provider's orders for pain relief.   ___ ___ ___ _____

7. Assessed patient's understanding of pain and willingness to receive nonpharmacological pain-relief measures.   ___ ___ ___ _____

8. Assessed patient's preferred activities.   ___ ___ ___ _____

9. Assessed patient's preferred type of image.   ___ ___ ___ _____

10. Reviewed restrictions in patient's mobility or positioning.   ___ ___ ___ _____

PLANNING

1. Identified expected outcomes.   ___ ___ ___ _____

2. Explained purpose of technique and what is expected of patient, explained pain rating scale.   ___ ___ ___ _____

3. Set pain-intensity goals with patient.   ___ ___ ___ _____

4. Planned time to perform technique when patient was able to concentrate.   ___ ___ ___ _____

5. Administered analgesic 30 minutes before implementing a nonpharmacological therapy.   ___ ___ ___ _____

IMPLEMENTATION

1. Performed hand hygiene, prepared patient's environment.   ___ ___ ___ _____

Copyright © 2018 by Elsevier Inc. All rights reserved.

	S	U	NP	Comments

2. Massaged patient:

   a. Performed hand hygiene. ____ ____ ____ _____

   b. Placed patient in appropriate, comfortable position. ____ ____ ____ _____

   c. Adjusted bed to comfortable working height, lowered side rail, draped patient to expose only area to be massaged. ____ ____ ____ _____

   d. Turned on music to patient's preference. ____ ____ ____ _____

   e. Ensured patient was not allergic to lotion, warmed lotion. ____ ____ ____ _____

   f. Chose stroke technique based on desired effect or body part. ____ ____ ____ _____

   g. Encouraged patient to breathe deeply and relax during massage. ____ ____ ____ _____

   h. Stood behind patient, stimulated scalp and temples. ____ ____ ____ _____

   i. Used friction to rub muscles at base of head while supporting patient's head. ____ ____ ____ _____

   j. Massaged hands and arms properly with patient in supine position. ____ ____ ____ _____

   k. Massaged neck appropriately after determining patient had no neck injury that contraindicated manipulation. ____ ____ ____ _____

   l. Massaged back appropriately. ____ ____ ____ _____

   m. Massaged feet appropriately. ____ ____ ____ _____

   n. Told patient massage was ending. ____ ____ ____ _____

   o. Instructed patient to inhale deeply and exhale when procedure was complete, cautioned patient to move slowly after resting a few minutes. ____ ____ ____ _____

   p. Wiped excess lotion or oil from patient's body with bath towel. ____ ____ ____ _____

   q. Returned bed to low position, raised side rails, performed hand hygiene. ____ ____ ____ _____

3. Performed progressive relaxation with deep breathing:

   a. Had patient assume comfortable sitting position. ____ ____ ____ _____

   b. Instructed patient to close eyes and take several slow, deep breaths. ____ ____ ____ _____

   c. Explained feeling of deep breathing versus normal or shallow breathing. ____ ____ ____ _____

Copyright © 2018 by Elsevier Inc. All rights reserved.

	S	U	NP	Comments

d. Explained feeling of both abdomen and chest rising and falling with deep breathing. ___ ___ ___ _____

e. Observed patient, cautioned against hyperventilation. ___ ___ ___ _____

f. Coached patient to locate areas of muscle tension and to alternate tightening and relaxing muscle groups.

   (1) Instructed patient to tighten muscles during inhalation and relax during exhalation. ___ ___ ___ _____

   (2) Asked patient to enjoy relaxed feeling, allow mind to drift, had patient breathe deeply. ___ ___ ___ _____

   (3) Explained that patient may feel different sensations during relaxation. ___ ___ ___ _____

   (4) Had patient continue slow deep breaths. ___ ___ ___ _____

   (5) Had patient inhale, exhale, and then move slowly after resting. ___ ___ ___ _____

4. Took patient through guided imagery:

  a. Directed patient through exercise while focusing on an image.

   (1) Instructed patient to imagine that inhaled air is a ball of healing energy. ___ ___ ___ _____

   (2) Instructed patient to imagine inhaled air travels to area of pain. ___ ___ ___ _____

  b. Directed imagery if needed.

   (1) Asked patient to imagine a pleasant place such as beach or mountains. ___ ___ ___ _____

   (2) Directed patient to experience all sensory aspects of the restful place. ___ ___ ___ _____

   (3) Directed patient to continue slow, deep, rhythmic breathing. ___ ___ ___ _____

   (4) Directed patient to count to three, inhale, and open eyes, suggested patient initially move slowly. ___ ___ ___ _____

  c. Provided patient time to practice exercise without interruption. ___ ___ ___ _____

5. Performed distraction technique:

  a. Directed patient's attention away from pain with distraction techniques such as music, pleasant memories, meaningful conversation, or other activities. ___ ___ ___ _____

6. Took patient through guided imagery. ___ ___ ___ _____

Copyright © 2018 by Elsevier Inc. All rights reserved.

	S	U	NP	Comments

EVALUATION

1. Observed character of respirations, body position, facial expression, tone of voice, mood, mannerisms, or verbalization of discomfort.

2. Asked patient to rate comfort level on pain scale.

3. Observed patient perform pain-control measures.

4. Asked patient about techniques he or she would like to try.

5. Identified unexpected outcomes.

RECORDING AND REPORTING

1. Recorded pertinent information in the appropriate log, incorporated pain-relief measures into nursing care plan.

2. Reported patient's response to nonpharmacological interventions to staff at change of shift.

3. Documented evaluation of patient learning.

4. Reported unusual responses to techniques to nurse in charge or health care provider.

Copyright © 2018 by Elsevier Inc. All rights reserved.

Student _____ Date _____

Instructor _____ Date _____

PERFORMANCE CHECKLIST SKILL 17.1 **SUPPORTING PATIENTS AND FAMILIES IN GRIEF**

	S	U	NP	Comments

ASSESSMENT

1. Sat near patient in a quiet, private location; established quiet presence and eye contact if appropriate.

2. Considered individual patient while communicating, applied principals of plain language and health literacy.

3. Listened carefully; observed patient responses, used open communication.

4. Determined meaning of loss to patient and specifics, used open-ended questions.

5. Combined knowledge of grief theory with observation of patient behaviors, validated observations with patient.

6. Encouraged patient to describe loss and impact on daily life.

7. Asked patient to describe coping strategies that patient uses often.

8. Assessed family caregiver's unique needs and resources.

9. Assessed patient's spiritual needs and resources.

PLANNING

1. Identified expected outcomes.

IMPLEMENTATION

1. Showed empathetic understanding of patient's strengths and needs.

2. Offered information about patient's illness, clarified misunderstandings, used culturally appropriate language.

3. Helped patient in achieving short-term goals.

4. Provided frequent opportunities for patient and family to express concerns, maintained attention.

5. Educated and supported patient and family, discussed procedures, plan of care, and anticipated changes, used team to support patient's needs.

190

Copyright © 2018 by Elsevier Inc. All rights reserved.

	S	U	NP	Comments

6. Instructed patient in relaxation strategies, including mindfulness, guided imagery, meditation, hand massage, and healing touch. ____ ____ ____ _____

7. Encouraged visits with loved ones, life review, or projects (e.g., looking at photos, journaling). ____ ____ ____ _____

8. Facilitated patient's religious practices and connections with community, made referral to a spiritual care provider if appropriate. ____ ____ ____ _____

EVALUATION

1. Noted patient descriptions of relationships and activities with others. ____ ____ ____ _____

2. Observed patient's behaviors during ongoing interactions. ____ ____ ____ _____

3. Elicited patient perceptions of benefit gained from coping interventions. ____ ____ ____ _____

4. Discussed progress toward performing routine activities at home. ____ ____ ____ _____

5. Identified unexpected outcomes. ____ ____ ____ _____

RECORDING AND REPORTING

1. Recorded interventions, noted patient's verbal and nonverbal responses in the appropriate log. ____ ____ ____ _____

2. Reported patient's grief reactions to interdisciplinary team, noted behaviors affecting health outcomes. ____ ____ ____ _____

Copyright © 2018 by Elsevier Inc. All rights reserved.

Student _____ Date _____

Instructor _____ Date _____

PERFORMANCE CHECKLIST SKILL 17.2 **SYMPTOM MANAGEMENT AT THE END OF LIFE**

	S	U	NP	Comments

ASSESSMENT

1. Identified patient using at least two identifiers. ___ ___ ___ _____

2. Asked patient to describe symptoms in his or her own words, used open-ended prompts. ___ ___ ___ _____

3. Allowed sufficient time for patient to describe symptoms, encouraged patient to say more, assessed patient's ability to cooperate with procedure and collect specimen. ___ ___ ___ _____

4. Assessed patient's emotional health, used standardized anxiety tool if necessary. ___ ___ ___ _____

5. Assessed patient's pain severity or observed for patient symptoms. ___ ___ ___ _____

6. Performed hand hygiene. ___ ___ ___ _____

7. Assessed for feeling of breathlessness, respiratory rate, breathing patterns, and lung sounds, assessed for presence of airway secretions. ___ ___ ___ _____

8. Observed the condition of the skin. ___ ___ ___ _____

9. Inspected patient's oral cavity. ___ ___ ___ _____

10. Assessed bowel function:

    a. Determined usual bowel elimination pattern and effectiveness of bowel-management routines. ___ ___ ___ _____

    b. Assessed for presence of fecal impaction if patient is passing liquid stool. ___ ___ ___ _____

    c. Reviewed medication regimens known to cause constipation. ___ ___ ___ _____

    d. Identified typical food and fluid intake over 1 week and activity levels. ___ ___ ___ _____

11. Assessed urinary elimination and ability to control urination, assessed for skin breakdown if incontinent. ___ ___ ___ _____

12. Assessed patient's appetite, ability to swallow, and for presence of nausea or vomiting. ___ ___ ___ _____

13. Assessed daily food and fluid intake in relation to patient's condition and preferences. ___ ___ ___ _____

Copyright © 2018 by Elsevier Inc. All rights reserved.

	S	U	NP	Comments

14. Assessed fatigue using a descriptive scale, asked if fatigue has limited patient's ability to perform desired activities.   ____ ____ ____ _____

15. Assessed for terminal delirium in patient near death:

   a. Considered if patient has pain, nausea, dyspnea, full bladder or bowel, poor sleep patterns, anxiety, or joint pain from immobility.   ____ ____ ____ _____

   b. Reviewed medical record for hyperglycemia, hypoglycemia, hyponatremia, or dehydration.   ____ ____ ____ _____

   c. Reviewed patient's medications.   ____ ____ ____ _____

   d. Determined if patient had unresolved emotional or spiritual issues.   ____ ____ ____ _____

PLANNING
1. Identified expected outcomes.   ____ ____ ____ _____

IMPLEMENTATION
1. Performed hand hygiene.   ____ ____ ____ _____

2. Provided pain relief, used multimodal interventions:

   a. Administered ordered analgesics and adjuvants, conferred with health care provider on dosing schedule.   ____ ____ ____ _____

   b. Provided nonpharmacological interventions, including mindfulness, relaxation, and guided imagery.   ____ ____ ____ _____

   c. Provided patient and family education on causes and patterns of pain and safety of opioid use, explained interventions.   ____ ____ ____ _____

   d. Reassessed pain 1 hour after administration of medication or alternative therapy.   ____ ____ ____ _____

3. Provided general comfort measures:

   a. Provided bath and skin care based on patient's preferences and hygiene needs.   ____ ____ ____ _____

   b. Provided eye care, used artificial tears if necessary.   ____ ____ ____ _____

   c. Repositioned frequently, did not position on tubes or other objects.   ____ ____ ____ _____

4. Provided oral hygiene after meals, at bedtime, and or more frequently in mouth-breathing or unconscious patient:

   a. Used appropriate oral rinses.   ____ ____ ____ _____

Copyright © 2018 by Elsevier Inc. All rights reserved.

	S	U	NP	Comments

b. Moistened lips with nonpetroleum balm.   ___ ___ ___ _____

5. Initiated a bowel-management regimen to reduce risk for constipation or diarrhea:

    a. Gave patient fluids he or she enjoys if tolerated, did not force fluid intake near end of life.   ___ ___ ___ _____

    b. Encouraged physical activity if tolerated.   ___ ___ ___ _____

    c. Administered daily stool softener or laxative.   ___ ___ ___ _____

    d. Provided low-residue diet in case of diarrhea.   ___ ___ ___ _____

6. Managed urinary incontinence appropriately.   ___ ___ ___ _____

7. Offered patient favorite foods as he or she desires, did not overly encourage patient to eat, treated nausea appropriately.   ___ ___ ___ _____

8. Managed fatigue:

    a. Helped patient identify valued tasks and helped to conserve energy for those tasks, eliminated extra steps in activities.   ___ ___ ___ _____

    b. Explained care activities before performing, included patient in setting the daily schedule.   ___ ___ ___ _____

    c. Discussed with patient easy ways to incorporate exercise into daily activities.   ___ ___ ___ _____

9. Supported patient's breathing efforts:

    a. Positioned patient for comfort.   ___ ___ ___ _____

    b. Elevated head and turned from side to side to drain secretions, suctioned only if necessary.   ___ ___ ___ _____

    c. Provided ordered antimuscarinic medications.   ___ ___ ___ _____

    d. Stayed with patients experiencing dyspnea or air hunger, administered opioids or anxiolytics as prescribed, kept room cool with low humidity.   ___ ___ ___ _____

10. Managed restlessness:

    a. Kept patient's room quiet with soft lighting and comfortable temperature, offered family opportunities to maintain close contact, encouraged music, prayer, or reading from patient's favorite book.   ___ ___ ___ _____

Copyright © 2018 by Elsevier Inc. All rights reserved.

	S	U	NP	Comments

b. Used least-sedating pharmacological means possible to control restlessness, consulted with interdisciplinary team, discontinued nonessential education, used appropriate delivery routes.

——— ——— ——— ————————————

11. Managed anxiety through counseling and supportive therapy, consulted with prescribing health care provider, offered other counseling services.

——— ——— ——— ————————————

EVALUATION

1. Asked patient to rate pain and evaluate pain characteristics, assessed behavior in nonverbal patients.

——— ——— ——— ————————————

2. Asked patient to describe mouth comfort, inspected oral cavity.

——— ——— ——— ————————————

3. Evaluated frequency of defecation, inspected feces.

——— ——— ——— ————————————

4. Observed skin condition.

——— ——— ——— ————————————

5. Asked patient to rate fatigue and compared with baseline, observed for fatigue or shortness of breath.

——— ——— ——— ————————————

6. Observed patient's respiratory patterns, asked patient if breathing was easy and comfortable.

——— ——— ——— ————————————

7. Observed patient's behavior, asked family to report on patient's behavior, noted level of restlessness.

——— ——— ——— ————————————

8. Asked patient to describe what the numbers on the pain scale mean.

——— ——— ——— ————————————

9. Identified unexpected outcomes.

——— ——— ——— ————————————

RECORDING AND REPORTING

1. Recorded detailed description of patient's symptoms in appropriate log, used consisted descriptors for comparison.

——— ——— ——— ————————————

2. Documented evaluation of patient learning.

——— ——— ——— ————————————

3. Recorded types of interventions used and patient's response in nurses' notes, noted successful interventions in care plan.

——— ——— ——— ————————————

4. Reported unexpected new symptoms or uncontrolled existing symptoms to health care provider.

——— ——— ——— ————————————

Copyright © 2018 by Elsevier Inc. All rights reserved.

Student _____ Date _____

Instructor _____ Date _____

PERFORMANCE CHECKLIST SKILL 17.3   **CARE OF A BODY AFTER DEATH**

	S	U	NP	Comments

ASSESSMENT

1. Asked health care provider to establish time of death, determined if autopsy had been requested, observed any special precautions required.

2. Determined if family were present and if they had been informed of the death, identified patient's surrogate.

3. Determined if patient's surrogate had been asked about organ and tissue donation, validated that donation request for had been signed, notified organ request team per agency policy.

4. Provided family members and friends a private place to gather, allowed them time to ask questions or discuss grief.

5. Asked family members if they had requests for viewing or preparation of the body, determined if they wished to be present or assist with care of the body.

6. Contacted a support person to stay with family not assisting in preparation of the body, implemented a bereavement care plan in a timely manner.

7. Consulted health care providers' orders for special care directives or specimens to be collected.

8. Performed hand hygiene, applied PPE.

9. Assessed the general condition of the body, noted presence of dressings, tubes, and medical equipment.

PLANNING

1. Identified expected outcomes.

2. Placed body in an appropriate position in a private room, moved roommate to another location if necessary.

3. Ensured patient has been pronounced dead by a hospital authority and that forms are appropriately filled out.

Copyright © 2018 by Elsevier Inc. All rights reserved.

	S	U	NP	Comments

4. Directed NAP to gather equipment and arrange at bedside.

___ ___ ___ _____

IMPLEMENTATION

1. Helped family members notify others of the death, notified mortuary, discussed plans for postmortem care.

___ ___ ___ _____

2. Consulted agency policy guidelines for care of the body if patient had made tissue donation.

___ ___ ___ _____

3. Performed hand hygiene, applied PPE.

___ ___ ___ _____

4. Identified patient using two identifiers, tagged body as directed.

___ ___ ___ _____

5. Removed indwelling devices, disconnected and capped IV lines, did not remove indwelling devices if autopsy is to be done.

___ ___ ___ _____

6. Cleaned mouth, cleaned and replaced dentures as soon as possible, sent dentures with body in a clearly labeled cup to mortuary, closed mouth with a rolled-up towel if appropriate.

___ ___ ___ _____

7. Placed pillow under head, positioned appropriately, checked agency policy regarding need to secure hands and feet, used only circular gauze bandaging.

___ ___ ___ _____

8. Closed eyes gently, left open if culturally appropriate.

___ ___ ___ _____

9. Groomed and arranged hair in preferred style, removed clips, pins, and rubber bands, did not shave patient.

___ ___ ___ _____

10. Washed soiled body parts, allowed family assistance if necessary.

___ ___ ___ _____

11. Removed soiled dressings, replaced with clean dressings, used paper tape and circular gauze.

___ ___ ___ _____

12. Placed absorbent pad under buttocks.

___ ___ ___ _____

13. Placed a clean gown on the body.

___ ___ ___ _____

14. Identified personal belongings that stay with the body and those to be given to the family.

___ ___ ___ _____

15. Placed clean sheet appropriately over body if family requested a viewing, removed medical equipment from room, provided appropriate lighting and chairs.

___ ___ ___ _____

16. Allowed family time alone with body, encouraged goodbyes and appropriate religious rituals.

___ ___ ___ _____

17. Removed linens and gown after viewing, placed body in shroud provided by agency.

___ ___ ___ _____

Copyright © 2018 by Elsevier Inc. All rights reserved.

	S	U	NP	Comments

18. Placed identification label on outside of the shroud, followed policy for marking a body that poses infectious risks, removed and disposed of PPE and performed hand hygiene.   ____ ____ ____ _____

19. Arranged prompt transportation of the body to mortuary or morgue.   ____ ____ ____ _____

EVALUATION

1. Observed family members', friends', and significant others' responses to loss.   ____ ____ ____ _____

2. Noted appearance and condition of patient's skin during preparation of body.   ____ ____ ____ _____

3. Identified unexpected outcomes.   ____ ____ ____ _____

RECORDING AND REPORTING

1. Recorded time of death in appropriate log, described any resuscitative measures, noted name of professional certifying the death.   ____ ____ ____ _____

2. Recorded any special preparation of the body for autopsy or donation, noted who made the request.   ____ ____ ____ _____

3. Recorded name of mortuary and names of family consulted at time of death.   ____ ____ ____ _____

4. Recorded on appropriate log personal articles left on body, noted how belongings were handled and who received them, secured signature as required.   ____ ____ ____ _____

5. Recorded time body was transported and its destination, noted location of identification tags.   ____ ____ ____ _____

Copyright © 2018 by Elsevier Inc. All rights reserved.

Student _____ Date _____

Instructor _____ Date _____

PERFORMANCE CHECKLIST SKILL 18.1   **COMPLETE OR PARTIAL BED BATH**

	S	U	NP	Comments
ASSESSMENT				
1. Identified patient using at least two identifiers.	___	___	___	_____
2. Performed hand hygiene, assessed environment for safety.	___	___	___	_____
3. Assessed patient's fall risk status if bathing out of bed or self-bath was to be performed.	___	___	___	_____
4. Assessed patient's tolerance for bathing.	___	___	___	_____
5. Assessed patient's cognitive and functional status, observed patient's response if dementia is suspected.	___	___	___	_____
6. Assessed patient's visual status, ability to sit without support, hand grasp, and ROM of extremities.	___	___	___	_____
7. Assessed for presence of position of external medical equipment.	___	___	___	_____
8. Assessed patient's bathing preferences.	___	___	___	_____
9. Asked if patient had noticed any problems related to condition of skin and genitalia.	___	___	___	_____
10. Assessed condition of patient's skin before or during bathing, noted presence of dryness or excessive moisture.	___	___	___	_____
11. Identified risks for skin impairment.	___	___	___	_____
12. Assessed patient's comfort using a pain scale.	___	___	___	_____
13. Assessed patient's knowledge and perceptions of skin hygiene.	___	___	___	_____
14. Reviewed orders for specific precautions concerning patient's movement or positioning, confirmed with patient allergies to bath products.	___	___	___	_____
PLANNING				
1. Identified expected outcomes.	___	___	___	_____
2. Explained procedure, asked patient for suggestions on how to prepare supplies and how much of bath patient wishes to complete.	___	___	___	_____
3. Adjusted room temperature and ventilation, provided privacy.	___	___	___	_____

Copyright © 2018 by Elsevier Inc. All rights reserved.

	S	U	NP	Comments

4. Prepared equipment and placed supplies on bedside table, ensured call light is within reach and bed is low and locked if it is necessary to leave the room.

    ___ ___ ___ _____

IMPLEMENTATION

1. Offered patient bedpan or urinal, applied clean gloves as needed, provided towel and moist washcloth.

    ___ ___ ___ _____

2. Performed hand hygiene, applied new clean gloves.

    ___ ___ ___ _____

3. Raised bed to working height, lowered side rail, assisted patient to appropriate position.

    ___ ___ ___ _____

4. Placed bath blanket over patient, removed top sheet while patient held blanket, placed soiled linen in laundry bag.

    ___ ___ ___ _____

5. Removed patient's gown or pajamas:

  a. Unsnapped sleeves to remove gown.

    ___ ___ ___ _____

  b. Began removal on unaffected side if an extremity was injured.

    ___ ___ ___ _____

  c. Removed gown properly if patient had IV line and gown has no snaps.

    ___ ___ ___ _____

6. Raised side rail, positioned bed at appropriate height while filling basin with warm water, positioned basin and supplies on over-bed table, had patient check water temperature.

    ___ ___ ___ _____

7. Lowered side rail, removed pillow if allowed, raised head of bed appropriately, placed towel under patient's head and over chest.

    ___ ___ ___ _____

8. Washed face:

  a. Asked if patient was wearing contact lenses, removed if appropriate.

    ___ ___ ___ _____

  b. Formed mitt with washcloth, immersed in water and wrung out thoroughly.

    ___ ___ ___ _____

  c. Washed patient's eyes properly, used clean area of cloth for each eye, soaked crusts on eyelids before attempting removal, dried eyes.

    ___ ___ ___ _____

  d. Asked if patient preferred soap on face; washed, rinsed, and dried face and neck; asked male patient if he wanted to be shaved.

    ___ ___ ___ _____

  e. Provided eye care for unconscious patient.

    (1) Instilled eyedrops or ointment per orders.

    ___ ___ ___ _____

Copyright © 2018 by Elsevier Inc. All rights reserved.

	S	U	NP	Comments
(2) Kept eyelids closed in absence of blink reflex, closed eye before placing eye patch or shield, did not tape eyelid.	___	___	___	_____

9. Washed upper extremities and trunk, changed bathwater if necessary:

   a. Removed bath blanket from patient's arm closest to you, placed bath towel lengthwise under arm, bathed properly with water and soap.   ___ ___ ___ _____

   b. Raised and supported arm, washed and dried axilla, applied deodorant if appropriate.   ___ ___ ___ _____

   c. Moved to other side of bed, repeated steps with other arm.   ___ ___ ___ _____

   d. Covered patient's chest with bath towel, folded bath blanket down to umbilicus, bathed chest properly, rinsed and dried well.   ___ ___ ___ _____

10. Washed hands and nails:

    a. Folded bath towel on bed, placed basin on towel, allowed hand to soak before cleaning nails, dried hand well, repeated on other side.   ___ ___ ___ _____

11. Checked temperature of bathwater, changed water if necessary.   ___ ___ ___ _____

12. Washed abdomen:

    a. Placed bath towel over chest and abdomen; folded bath blanket down to just above pubic region; bathed, rinsed, and dried abdomen; paid attention to skinfolds; dried well. ___ ___ ___ _____

    b. Applied clean gown, dressed affected side first, waited until end of bath if appropriate.   ___ ___ ___ _____

13. Washed lower extremities:

    a. Covered chest and abdomen with bath blanket, exposed near leg by folding blanket toward midline, ensured other leg and perineum remain draped, placed towel under leg. ___ ___ ___ _____

    b. Washed leg properly; assessed for signs of redness, swelling, or leg pain.   ___ ___ ___ _____

    c. Cleansed foot, made sure to bathe between toes, cleaned and filed nails, dried feet.   ___ ___ ___ _____

Copyright © 2018 by Elsevier Inc. All rights reserved.

	S	U	NP	Comments

d. Raised side rail, moved to opposite side, repeated steps to wash other leg, applied lotion to both feet, removed towel.

e. Covered patient with bath blanket, raised side rail, changed bathwater.

14. Washed back:

a. Applied clean gloves, lowered side rail, assisted patient to proper position, placed towel along patient's side.

b. Enclosed any fecal matter in toilet tissue, removed with disposable wipes.

c. Kept patient draped by sliding bath blanket over shoulders and thighs during bathing; washed, rinsed, and dried back properly, paid attention to folds of buttocks and anus.

d. Cleansed buttocks and anus; washed front to back; cleansed, rinsed, and dried areas thoroughly; placed clean absorbent pad under patient's buttocks if needed.

15. Provided perineal care while patient is supine.

16. Massaged patient's back if desired.

17. Applied body lotion and topical moisturizing agents to skin.

18. Removed and disposed of gloves, performed hand hygiene before helping patient finish grooming.

19. Checked function and position of internal devices.

20. Replaced top linen before removing bath blanket, applied gloves if linen is soiled, made bed if appropriate.

21. Placed bed in low locked position, raised side rails appropriately, ensured patient is comfortable with call light and personal possessions within reach.

22. Disinfected, rinsed, and dried basin appropriately.

23. Performed hand hygiene, left room.

EVALUATION

1. Observed skin, especially areas that were previously showing signs of breakdown; inspected areas normally exposed to pressure.

2. Observed ROM during bathing.

Copyright © 2018 by Elsevier Inc. All rights reserved.

	S	U	NP	Comments
3. Asked patient to rate comfort.	____	____	____	_____
4. Asked if patient feels tired.	____	____	____	_____
5. Asked patient to explain why bathing daily is important.	____	____	____	_____
6. Identified unexpected outcomes.	____	____	____	_____

RECORDING AND REPORTING

	S	U	NP	Comments
1. Recorded procedure and observations, included amount of patient participation and how patient tolerated procedure in the appropriate log.	____	____	____	_____
2. Reported evidence of alterations in skin integrity, break in suture line, or increased wound secretions to nurse in charge or health care provider, provided special skin care if necessary.	____	____	____	_____

Copyright © 2018 by Elsevier Inc. All rights reserved.

Student _____ Date _____

Instructor _____ Date _____

PERFORMANCE CHECKLIST PROCEDURAL GUIDELINE 18.1   **PERINEAL CARE**

	S	U	NP	Comments

PROCEDURAL STEPS

1. Identified patient using at least two identifiers.   ___ ___ ___ _____

2. Assessed environment for safety.   ___ ___ ___ _____

3. Assembled supplies, provided privacy, explained procedure and importance of preventing infection.   ___ ___ ___ _____

4. Performed hand hygiene, applied clean gloves, placed basin of warm water and cleansing solution on over-bed table.   ___ ___ ___ _____

5. Performed perineal care for a female:

   a. Allowed patient to cleanse perineum on her own if able.   ___ ___ ___ _____

   b. Assisted patient in assuming proper position, noted restrictions in patient's positioning, placed waterproof pad under patient's buttocks.   ___ ___ ___ _____

   c. Draped patient appropriately with bath blanket.   ___ ___ ___ _____

   d. Folded outer corners of blanket around patient's thighs, lifted lower tip of blanket to expose perineum.   ___ ___ ___ _____

   e. Washed and dried patient's upper thighs.   ___ ___ ___ _____

   f. Washed labia majora, retracted labia from thigh with nondominant hand, used dominant hand to wash skinfolds, wiped front to back, repeated on opposite side with separate section of washcloth, rinsed and dried area thoroughly.   ___ ___ ___ _____

   g. Separated labia, washed urethral meatus and vaginal orifice front to back, used separate section of cloth for each stroke, avoided tension on indwelling catheter if present.   ___ ___ ___ _____

   h. Rinsed and dried area thoroughly, used front-to-back method.   ___ ___ ___ _____

   i. Poured warm water over perineal area and dried thoroughly if patient uses a bedpan.   ___ ___ ___ _____

204

Copyright © 2018 by Elsevier Inc. All rights reserved.

	S	U	NP	Comments

j. Folded lower corner of bath blanket down, asked patient to assume comfortable position.

    ____   ____   ____   _____

6. Performed perineal care for a male:

   a. Allowed patient to cleanse perineum on his own if able.

    ____   ____   ____   _____

   b. Assisted patient to supine position, noted restrictions in mobility.

    ____   ____   ____   _____

   c. Folded lower half of bath blanket up to expose upper thighs, washed and dried thighs.

    ____   ____   ____   _____

   d. Covered thighs with bath towels, raised blanket to expose genitalia, raised penis, placed bath towel underneath, retracted foreskin if present, deferred procedure if patient had an erection.

    ____   ____   ____   _____

   e. Washed tip of penis first, cleansed outwards, discarded washcloth, repeated until penis was clean, rinsed and dried thoroughly.

    ____   ____   ____   _____

   f. Returned foreskin to its natural position.

    ____   ____   ____   _____

   g. Had patient abduct legs, cleansed shaft of penis and scrotum, paid attention to underlying surfaces and folds, rinsed and dried thoroughly.

    ____   ____   ____   _____

   h. Folded bath blanket over patient's perineum, assisted patient to comfortable position.

    ____   ____   ____   _____

7. Avoided placing tension on an indwelling catheter.

    ____   ____   ____   _____

8. Observed perineal area for any irritation, redness, or drainage that persisted after hygiene.

    ____   ____   ____   _____

9. Disposed of gloves in receptacle, performed hand hygiene.

    ____   ____   ____   _____

10. Asked patient to describe genital hygiene procedures.

    ____   ____   ____   _____

Copyright © 2018 by Elsevier Inc. All rights reserved.

Student _____ Date _____

Instructor _____ Date _____

PERFORMANCE CHECKLIST PROCEDURAL GUIDELINE 18.2 **USE OF DISPOSABLE BED BATH, TUB, OR SHOWER**

	S	U	NP	Comments

PROCEDURAL STEPS

1. Identified patient using at least two identifiers.   —   —   —   _____

2. Assessed environment for safety, provided privacy.   —   —   —   _____

3. Assessed degree of help patient will need for bathing, fall and skin breakdown risks, and presence of allergies.   —   —   —   _____

4. Performed hand hygiene, applied clean gloves.   —   —   —   _____

5. Arranged supplies at bedside if necessary, prepared other equipment in bathroom or shower room.   —   —   —   _____

6. Bathed patient using bathing cloths:

   a. Adjusted room temperature and ventilation, provided privacy.   —   —   —   _____

   b. Positioned patient appropriately, draped patient with bath blanket to cover areas of body not being cleaned.   —   —   —   _____

   c. Helped patient remove old gown.   —   —   —   _____

   d. Warmed bathing cloths in a microwave not used for food preparation.   —   —   —   _____

   e. Washed patients face and eyes with water.   —   —   —   _____

   f. Used all six bathing cloths in the appropriate order, positioned patient and draping properly.   —   —   —   _____

   g. Massaged skin with CHG cloth, told patient skin may feel sticky for a few minutes.   —   —   —   _____

   h. Ensures soiled areas are cleansed thoroughly.   —   —   —   _____

   i. Allowed to air dry.   —   —   —   _____

   j. Used only CHG-compatible products if additional moisturizer is needed.   —   —   —   _____

   k. Disposed of leftover cloths, helped patient to comfortable position, assisted in applying clean gown.   —   —   —   _____

206

Copyright © 2018 by Elsevier Inc. All rights reserved.

	S	U	NP	Comments

7. Bathed patient using tub bath or shower:

a. Assessed patient's fall risk status, reviewed orders for precautions concerning patient's movement or positioning.

b. Scheduled use of shower or tub.

c. Checked tub or shower for cleanliness, used cleaning techniques per agency policy, placed rubber mat on tub or shower bottom, placed skid-proof bath mat or towel on floor in front of tub or shower.

d. Place hygiene and toiletry items within easy reach of the tub.

e. Demonstrated how to use call signal, placed "occupied" sign on bathroom door, closed door.

f. Filled bathtub halfway with warm water, checked temperature, had patient test water, adjusted as necessary, explained faucet controls, did not use bath oil.

g. Turned shower on and adjusted temperature if patient was taking a shower, used seat or tub chair if available.

h. Instructed patient that he or she could stay in the tub no longer than 20 minutes, checked on patient every 5 minutes, removed and disposed of gloves, performed hand hygiene.

i. Applied clean gloves, returned to bathroom when patient signals, knocked before entering.

j. Drained tub for unsteady patient before patient attempted to get out, placed bath towel over patient's shoulders, assisted patient as needed, assisted with drying, had a shower chair available if possible.

k. Assisted patient as needed in donning clothing.

l. Assisted patient to room and comfortable position, left call light in reach.

m. Cleaned tub or shower, removed soiled linen, placed in the dirty linen bag, discarded disposable equipment appropriately, placed "unoccupied" sign on bathroom door, returned supplies to storage.

n. Removed and disposed of gloves, performed hand hygiene.

Copyright © 2018 by Elsevier Inc. All rights reserved.

	S	U	NP	Comments

8. Evaluated condition of patient's skin, paid attention to areas that were previously soiled or showing signs of breakdown.

9. Asked patient to rate level of fatigue and comfort.

Copyright © 2018 by Elsevier Inc. All rights reserved.

Student _____ Date _____

Instructor _____ Date _____

PERFORMANCE CHECKLIST SKILL 18.2   **ORAL HYGIENE**

	S	U	NP	Comments
ASSESSMENT				
1. Identified patient using at least two identifiers.	___	___	___	_____
2. Assessed environment for safety.	___	___	___	_____
3. Performed hand hygiene, applied clean gloves.	___	___	___	_____
4. Instructed patient not to bite down, inspected integrity of lips, teeth, buccal mucosa, gums, palate, and tongue.	___	___	___	_____
5. Identified presence of common oral problems.	___	___	___	_____
6. Removed gloves and performed hand hygiene.	___	___	___	_____
7. Reviewed medical record, assessed risk for oral hygiene problems.	___	___	___	_____
8. Determined patient's oral hygiene practices.	___	___	___	_____
9. Assessed patient's ability to grasp and manipulate toothbrush.	___	___	___	_____
PLANNING				
1. Identified expected outcomes.	___	___	___	_____
2. Gathered equipment and supplies.	___	___	___	_____
3. Explained procedure to patient, discussed preferences regarding use of hygiene aids.	___	___	___	_____
IMPLEMENTATION				
1. Performed hand hygiene, provided privacy.	___	___	___	_____
2. Arranged supplies on bedside table within easy reach.	___	___	___	_____
3. Raised bed to working height, raised HOB and lowered side rail, assisted patient to appropriate position.	___	___	___	_____
4. Placed a towel over patient's chest.	___	___	___	_____
5. Performed hand hygiene, applied clean gloves.	___	___	___	_____
6. Applied toothpaste to brush, held brush over emesis basin, poured water over toothpaste.	___	___	___	_____
7. Allowed patient to assist, held brush properly, brushed teeth properly.	___	___	___	_____
8. Had patient hold brush appropriately and brush tongue, avoided initiating gag reflex.	___	___	___	_____

Copyright © 2018 by Elsevier Inc. All rights reserved.

	S	U	NP	Comments
9. Allowed patient to rinse mouth with water and spit into basin, observed patient's brushing technique, taught importance of brushing twice a day.	—	—	—	_____
10. Had patient rinse teeth with antiseptic mouthwash and spit in basin.	—	—	—	_____
11. Helped wipe patient's mouth.	—	—	—	_____
12. Allowed patient to floss or flossed patient properly, instructed patient on importance of flossing.	—	—	—	_____
13. Allowed patient to rinse mouth with cool water and spit in basin, assisted wiping patient's mouth, applied moisturizing lubricant to lips.	—	—	—	_____
14. Assisted patient to comfortable position, removed basin and over-bed table, raised side rail and lowered bed to original position.	—	—	—	_____
15. Wiped off over-bed table, discarded soiled linen, removed soiled gloves, returned equipment to proper place.	—	—	—	_____
16. Performed hand hygiene.	—	—	—	_____

EVALUATION

	S	U	NP	Comments
1. Asked patient if any area of oral cavity feels uncomfortable or irritated.	—	—	—	_____
2. Applied clean gloves, inspected condition of oral cavity, performed hand hygiene.	—	—	—	_____
3. Observed patient brushing and flossing.	—	—	—	_____
4. Asked patient to describe proper hygiene techniques and recommended frequency.	—	—	—	_____
5. Identified unexpected outcomes.	—	—	—	_____

RECORDING AND REPORTING

	S	U	NP	Comments
1. Recorded procedure and noted condition of oral cavity in appropriate log.	—	—	—	_____
2. Reported bleeding, pain, or presences of lesions to nurse in charge or health care provider.	—	—	—	_____

Copyright © 2018 by Elsevier Inc. All rights reserved.

Student _____   Date _____

Instructor _____   Date _____

PERFORMANCE CHECKLIST PROCEDURAL GUIDELINE 18.3   **CARE OF DENTURES**

	S	U	NP	Comments
PROCEDURAL STEPS				
1. Identified patient using at least two identifiers.	___	___	___	_____
2. Assessed environment for safety.	___	___	___	_____
3. Performed hand hygiene.	___	___	___	_____
4. Asked patient if dentures fit, if gum or mucous membrane tenderness or irritation occurred, asked about denture care and product preferences.	___	___	___	_____
5. Determined if patient could clean dentures independently.	___	___	___	_____
6. Positioned patient comfortably or helped patient to sink.	___	___	___	_____
7. Filled emesis basin with tepid water or filled sink appropriately.	___	___	___	_____
8. Applied clean gloves.	___	___	___	_____
9. Removed dentures properly if patient was unable to do so independently, placed dentures in emesis basin or sink.	___	___	___	_____
10. Applied cleaning agent to brush, brushed surfaces of dentures appropriately.	___	___	___	_____
11. Rinsed thoroughly in tepid water.	___	___	___	_____
12. Applied adhesive to undersurface if appropriate.	___	___	___	_____
13. Assisted patient with insertion of dentures if necessary, asked if dentures felt comfortable.	___	___	___	_____
14. Stored dentures properly if requested, kept denture cup in a secure place, labeled cup with patient's name.	___	___	___	_____
15. Disposed of supplies, removed and discarded gloves, and performed hand hygiene.	___	___	___	_____
16. Returned patient to a comfortable position, left call light in reach.	___	___	___	_____

Copyright © 2018 by Elsevier Inc. All rights reserved.

Student _____ Date _____

Instructor _____ Date _____

PERFORMANCE CHECKLIST SKILL 18.3   **PERFORMING MOUTH CARE FOR AN UNCONSCIOUS OR DEBILITATED PATIENT**

	S	U	NP	Comments
ASSESSMENT				
1. Identified patient using at least two identifiers.	—	—	—	_____
2. Assessed environment for safety.	—	—	—	_____
3. Performed hand hygiene, applied clean gloves.	—	—	—	_____
4. Assessed for presence of gag reflex.	—	—	—	_____
5. Inspected condition of oral cavity.	—	—	—	_____
6. Removed gloves, performed hand hygiene.	—	—	—	_____
7. Assessed patient's risk for oral hygiene problems.	—	—	—	_____
8. Assessed patient's respirations or oxygen saturation.	—	—	—	_____
PLANNING				
1. Identified expected outcomes.	—	—	—	_____
2. Gathered equipment and supplies.	—	—	—	_____
3. Explained procedure to patient and family.	—	—	—	_____
IMPLEMENTATION				
1. Provided privacy.	—	—	—	_____
2. Performed hand hygiene, applied clean gloves.	—	—	—	_____
3. Placed towel on over-bed table, arranged equipment, turned on suction machine and connected tubing if necessary.	—	—	—	_____
4. Raised bed to appropriate height, lowered side rail, positioned patient appropriately.	—	—	—	_____
5. Placed towel under patient's head and basin under chin.	—	—	—	_____
6. Removed dentures or partial plates if present.	—	—	—	_____
7. Inserted oral airway if necessary, inserted when patient was relaxed if possible, did not use force.	—	—	—	_____

Copyright © 2018 by Elsevier Inc. All rights reserved.

	S	U	NP	Comments

8. Cleaned mouth using moistened brush, applied toothpaste or used solution to loosen crusts, suctioned accumulated secretions. Moistened brush with CHG solution to rinse, brushed tongue, repeated rinsing several times. ___ ___ ___ _____

9. Applied thin layer of water-soluble moisturizer to lips. ___ ___ ___ _____

10. Informed patient that procedure was completed, returned patient to comfortable and safe position. ___ ___ ___ _____

11. Left call light in reach. ___ ___ ___ _____

12. Cleaned equipment and returned to proper place, placed soiled linen in proper receptacle. ___ ___ ___ _____

13. Removed and disposed gloves in proper receptacle, performed hand hygiene. ___ ___ ___ _____

EVALUATION

1. Applied clean gloves, inspected oral cavity. ___ ___ ___ _____

2. Asked debilitated patient if mouth feels clean. ___ ___ ___ _____

3. Asked caregiver to explain how to prevent choking while providing mouth care. ___ ___ ___ _____

4. Identified unexpected outcomes. ___ ___ ___ _____

RECORDING AND REPORTING

1. Recorded procedure, appearance of oral cavity, presence of gag reflex, and patient's response in appropriate log. ___ ___ ___ _____

2. Documented evaluation of patient learning. ___ ___ ___ _____

3. Reported unusual findings to nurse in charge or health care provider. ___ ___ ___ _____

Copyright © 2018 by Elsevier Inc. All rights reserved.

Student _____ Date _____

Instructor _____ Date _____

PERFORMANCE CHECKLIST PROCEDURAL GUIDELINE 18.4   **HAIR CARE—COMBING AND SHAVING**

	S	U	NP	Comments

PROCEDURAL STEPS

1. Identified patient using at least two identifiers. ____ ____ ____ _____

2. Performed hand hygiene, inspected condition of hair and scalp, inspected for presence of infestation, applied clean gloves if necessary then performed hand hygiene after inspection. ____ ____ ____ _____

3. Assessed patient's hair-care and shaving product preferences. ____ ____ ____ _____

4. Assessed if patient had bleeding tendency before shaving, reviewed history, medications, and laboratory values. ____ ____ ____ _____

5. Assessed patient's ability to manipulate comb, brush, or razor. ____ ____ ____ _____

6. Gathered equipment at patient's bedside, explained intent to provide hair/beard care, asked patient to explain steps used in his or her care routine, asked patient to indicate if he or she is uncomfortable. ____ ____ ____ _____

7. Positioned patient appropriately with head elevated. ____ ____ ____ _____

8. Provided privacy, arranged supplies at bedside, adjusted lighting. ____ ____ ____ _____

9. Performed hand hygiene, applied clean gloves. ____ ____ ____ _____

10. Combed and brushed patient's hair:

    a. Parted hair into two sections and then two more. ____ ____ ____ _____

    b. Brushed or combed hair from scalp to ends. ____ ____ ____ _____

    c. Moistened hair with water, conditioner, or detangler before combing. ____ ____ ____ _____

    d. Moved fingers through hair to loosen larger tangles. ____ ____ ____ _____

    e. Combed hair appropriately, shaped and styled hair. ____ ____ ____ _____

Copyright © 2018 by Elsevier Inc. All rights reserved.

	S	U	NP	Comments

11. Shaved patient with a disposable razor:

   a. Placed bath towel over patient's chest and shoulders.

   b. Ran warm water in washbasin, checked water temperature.

   c. Placed washcloth in basin, wrung thoroughly, applied cloth over patient's face for several seconds.

   d. Applied shaving cream to patient's face; smoothed evenly over sides of face, chin, and under nose.

   e. Held razor properly in dominant hand, shaved patient properly, checked if patient felt comfortable.

   f. Dipped razor blade in water as shaving cream accumulated.

   g. Rinsed face with warm, moist washcloth after all facial hair was shaved.

   h. Dried face thoroughly, applied aftershave lotion if desired.

12. Shaved patient with an electric razor:

   a. Placed bath towel over patient's chest and shoulders.

   b. Applied skin conditioner or preshave preparation.

   c. Turned razor on, shaved patient appropriately.

   d. Applied aftershave lotion as desired after completing shave.

13. Performed mustache and beard care:

   a. Placed bath towel over patient's chest and shoulders.

   b. Gently combed mustache and beard.

   c. Allowed patient to use mirror and direct trimming.

   d. Removed towel after completing.

14. Helped patient assume comfortable position, left call light in reach.

15. Returned usable equipment to proper place, discarded soiled linen in dirty laundry bag, performed hand hygiene.

Copyright © 2018 by Elsevier Inc. All rights reserved.

	S	U	NP	Comments

16. Asked patient how hair and scalp feel. ___ ___ ___ _____

17. Inspected condition of skin, looked for areas of bleeding and dryness. ___ ___ ___ _____

18. Asked patient if face feels clean and comfortable. ___ ___ ___ _____

19. Asked patient to explain risks of using a razor and what to watch for with a bleeding tendency. ___ ___ ___ _____

Copyright © 2018 by Elsevier Inc. All rights reserved.

Student _____ Date _____

Instructor _____ Date _____

PERFORMANCE CHECKLIST PROCEDURAL GUIDELINE 18.5 **HAIR CARE—SHAMPOOING**

	S	U	NP	Comments

PROCEDURAL STEPS

1. Inspected hair and scalp before shampooing, determined if special treatments were necessary, applied gloves and/or gown if necessary. ___ ___ ___ _____

2. Ensured there are no contraindications to procedure. ___ ___ ___ _____

3. Identified patient using at least two identifiers. ___ ___ ___ _____

4. Assessed environment for safety. ___ ___ ___ _____

5. Explained procedure to patient simply. ___ ___ ___ _____

6. Performed hand hygiene, assembled equipment at bedside. ___ ___ ___ _____

7. Provided privacy, raised bed to working height and lowered side rails. ___ ___ ___ _____

8. Shampooed bed-bound patient with shampoo board:

   a. Applied clean gloves, placed waterproof pad under patient's shoulders, neck, and head. ___ ___ ___ _____

   b. Placed shampoo board under patient's head and washbasin under end of spout; ensured spout extends beyond edge of mattress. ___ ___ ___ _____

   c. Placed towel under patient's neck and bath towel over patient's shoulders. ___ ___ ___ _____

   d. Brushed and combed patient's hair. ___ ___ ___ _____

   e. Asked patient to hold towel or washcloth over eyes. ___ ___ ___ _____

   f. Tested water temperature, poured water over hair until completely wet, applied hydrogen peroxide to dissolve any blood clots, rinsed hair with saline, applied small amount of shampoo. ___ ___ ___ _____

   g. Worked up lather with both hands, started at hairline and worked toward neck, lifted head slightly to wash back of head, shampooed sides of head, massaged scalp by applying pressure with fingertips. ___ ___ ___ _____

Copyright © 2018 by Elsevier Inc. All rights reserved.

	S	U	NP	Comments

h. Rinsed hair with water, ensured water drained into basin, repeated rinsing until free of soap.

    ___ ___ ___ _____

i. Applied conditioner or crème rinse if requested, rinsed hair thoroughly.

    ___ ___ ___ _____

j. Wrapped patient's head in bath towel, dried patient's face with cloth, dried off any moisture along neck or shoulders.

    ___ ___ ___ _____

k. Dried patient's hair and scalp, used second towel if necessary.

    ___ ___ ___ _____

l. Combed hair to remove tangles, dried hair with a dryer if desired.

    ___ ___ ___ _____

m. Applied oil preparation or conditioner to hair if desired.

    ___ ___ ___ _____

n. Conditioned and combed out coarse, curly hair appropriately with wide-tooth comb.

    ___ ___ ___ _____

o. Assisted patient to comfortable position, completed styling of hair, left call light in reach.

    ___ ___ ___ _____

p. Disposed of and stored supplies, removed gloves and performed hand hygiene.

    ___ ___ ___ _____

9. Shampooed patient with disposable shampoo product:

a. Positioned patient properly, applied clean gloves.

    ___ ___ ___ _____

b. Combed hair to remove tangles or debris.

    ___ ___ ___ _____

c. Opened package, applied cap, secured all hair beneath cap.

    ___ ___ ___ _____

d. Massaged head through cap, checked fitting of cap.

    ___ ___ ___ _____

e. Massaged according to directions on package, added time to massage as necessary.

    ___ ___ ___ _____

f. Discarded cap in trash.

    ___ ___ ___ _____

g. Towel dried hair if desired, brushed or combed patient's hair.

    ___ ___ ___ _____

h. Removed gloves, performed hand hygiene.

    ___ ___ ___ _____

i. Helped patient to comfortable position, ensured call light was within reach.

    ___ ___ ___ _____

10. Inspected condition of hair and scalp.

    ___ ___ ___ _____

11. Asked patient to explain how to reduce risk of exposure to lice.

    ___ ___ ___ _____

218

Copyright © 2018 by Elsevier Inc. All rights reserved.

Student _____ Date _____

Instructor _____ Date _____

PERFORMANCE CHECKLIST SKILL 18.4 **PERFORMING NAIL AND FOOT CARE**

	S	U	NP	Comments
ASSESSMENT				
1. Identified patient using at least two identifiers.	___	___	___	_____
2. Assessed environment for safety.	___	___	___	_____
3. Performed hand hygiene, applied clean gloves, inspected all surfaces of fingers, toes, feet, and nails; paid attention to areas of dryness, inflammation, or cracking; inspected socks for stains.	___	___	___	_____
4. Assessed circulation to extremities bilaterally, removed gloves and performed hand hygiene.	___	___	___	_____
5. Observed patient's walking gait, asked if patient has pain while walking.	___	___	___	_____
6. Asked if patient had history of leg pain on walking that is relieved by rest.	___	___	___	_____
7. Asked patient about use of nail polish and polish remover.	___	___	___	_____
8. Assessed type of footwear patient wears.	___	___	___	_____
9. Identified patient's risk for foot or nail problems.	___	___	___	_____
10. Assessed for use of home remedies.	___	___	___	_____
11. Assessed patient's ability to care for nails or feet.	___	___	___	_____
PLANNING				
1. Identified expected outcomes.	___	___	___	_____
2. Gathered equipment and supplies.	___	___	___	_____
3. Explained procedure to patient.	___	___	___	_____
4. Obtained health care provider's orders for cutting nails, obtained order for podiatry consultation if needed.	___	___	___	_____
IMPLEMENTATION				
1. Performed hand hygiene and applied gloves.	___	___	___	_____
2. Provided privacy.	___	___	___	_____
3. Assisted patient to appropriate position, placed bath mat on floor under patient's feet or placed waterproof pad on mattress as appropriate.	___	___	___	_____

Copyright © 2018 by Elsevier Inc. All rights reserved.

	S	U	NP	Comments

4. Filled washbasin with warm water, tested temperature, placed basin on floor or on pad, had patient immerse feet. ___ ___ ___ _____

5. Adjusted over-bed table to low position, placed over patient's lap. ___ ___ ___ _____

6. Filled emesis basin with warm water, placed basin on towel on over-bed table, tested water temperature. ___ ___ ___ _____

7. Instructed patient to place fingers in basin, placed arms in comfortable position. ___ ___ ___ _____

8. Allowed patient's feet and nails to soak for 10 minutes unless contraindicated. ___ ___ ___ _____

9. Cleaned under fingernails with plastic applicator stick while fingers are immersed. ___ ___ ___ _____

10. Cleaned around cuticles with a soft brush. ___ ___ ___ _____

11. Removed emesis basin, dried fingers thoroughly. ___ ___ ___ _____

12. Checked agency policy, trimmed nails properly, filed sharp corners off nails. ___ ___ ___ _____

13. Moved over-bed table away from patient, scrubbed callused areas of feet with washcloth. ___ ___ ___ _____

14. Cleaned between toes, used washcloth. ___ ___ ___ _____

15. Dried feet, trimmed nails following step 12. ___ ___ ___ _____

16. Applied lotion to feet and hands, rubbed in thoroughly. ___ ___ ___ _____

17. Helped patient to comfortable position, left call light in reach. ___ ___ ___ _____

18. Sanitized equipment and returned to proper place, disposed of emery boards and soiled linen appropriately, removed gloves and performed hand hygiene. ___ ___ ___ _____

EVALUATION

1. Inspected nails, areas between fingers and toes, and skin surfaces. ___ ___ ___ _____

2. Had patient stand and walk to rate any pain if possible. ___ ___ ___ _____

3. Observed patient's walk after foot and nail care. ___ ___ ___ _____

4. Asked patient to explain how to protect feet from infection. ___ ___ ___ _____

5. Identified unexpected outcomes. ___ ___ ___ _____

Copyright © 2018 by Elsevier Inc. All rights reserved.

	S	U	NP	Comments
RECORDING AND REPORTING				
1. Recorded procedure and observations in medical record.	___	___	___	_____
2. Reported areas of discomfort, any breaks in skin, or ulcerations to nurse in charge or health care provider.	___	___	___	_____
3. Documented evaluation of patient learning.	___	___	___	_____

Copyright © 2018 by Elsevier Inc. All rights reserved.

Student _____ Date _____

Instructor _____ Date _____

PERFORMANCE CHECKLIST PROCEDURAL GUIDELINE 18.6 **MAKING AN OCCUPIED BED**

	S	U	NP	Comments

PROCEDURAL STEPS

1. Reviewed medical records and assessed restrictions in mobility/positioning of patient.

2. Organized supplies and provided privacy.

3. Assessed environment for safety.

4. Performed hand hygiene, applied gloves if necessary.

5. Explained procedure to patient.

6. Raised bed to working height, lowered HOB as tolerated, removed call light.

7. Lowered side rails, loosened all top linen, removed bedspread and blanket and disposed of appropriately.

8. Covered patient with clean bath blanket, pulled sheet out from under blanket appropriately, discarded sheet appropriately.

9. Positioned patient on far side, turned onto side and facing away from self, obtained help from another caregiver if necessary.

10. Assessed to make sure there is no tension on external medical devices.

11. Loosened bottom linens, rolled cloth pads, drawsheet, and bottom sheet toward patient, tucked old linen under patient's back, removed and discarded any disposable pads.

12. Cleaned, disinfected, and dried mattress surface if necessary.

13. Applied clean linens to exposed half of bed, placed new mattress pad and bottom sheet appropriately.

14. If bottom sheet is flat, mitered top corner at HOB appropriately.

15. Tucked remaining sheet under mattress, rolled drawsheet on top of bottom sheet, tucked under patient without touching old linen.

16. Added waterproof pad, kept clean and soiled linen separate, kept linen under patient flat.

Copyright © 2018 by Elsevier Inc. All rights reserved.

	S	U	NP	Comments

17. Asked patient to roll toward self over layers of linen and not to raise the hips, stressed need to stay aligned, kept patient covered. ___ ___ ___ _____

18. Raised side rails, moved to opposite side of bed, had patient roll away from self over all linens. ___ ___ ___ _____

19. Loosened edges of soiled linen from under mattress, removed soiled linen properly. ___ ___ ___ _____

20. Held linen away from body and placed it in laundry bag. ___ ___ ___ _____

21. Cleaned, disinfected, and dried other half of mattress as needed. ___ ___ ___ _____

22. Pulled clean mattress pad, sheet, drawsheet, and pad out from beneath patient, smoothed all linen, helped patient to comfortable position. ___ ___ ___ _____

23. Made corners of bottom sheet appropriately. ___ ___ ___ _____

24. Grasped remaining edge of flat sheet, leaned back and pulled while tucking excess linen under mattress, avoided lifting mattress. ___ ___ ___ _____

25. Smoothed drawsheet and waterproof pads, ensured bed surface is wrinkle free. ___ ___ ___ _____

26. Placed top sheet properly over patient. ___ ___ ___ _____

27. Placed bed blanket properly over patient, raised side rail. ___ ___ ___ _____

28. Went to other side of bed, lowered side rail, spread sheet and blanket evenly. ___ ___ ___ _____

29. Had patient hold sheet and blanket while bath blanket is removed, discarded linen. ___ ___ ___ _____

30. Went to other side of bed, lowered side rail, spread sheet and blanket evenly. ___ ___ ___ _____

31. Made cuff properly. ___ ___ ___ _____

32. Made horizontal toe pleat at bottom of bed. ___ ___ ___ _____

33. Tucked remaining sheet and blanket appropriately under mattress. ___ ___ ___ _____

34. Made modified mitered corner with top sheet and blanket. ___ ___ ___ _____

35. Repeated steps 33 and 34 on other side. ___ ___ ___ _____

36. Changed pillowcase, supported patient's head, did not hold pillow against uniform, ensured pillow corners fit before repositioning under patient's head. ___ ___ ___ _____

Copyright © 2018 by Elsevier Inc. All rights reserved.

	S	U	NP	Comments

37. Placed call light within patient's reach, returned bed to low and locked position, raised side rail.
___ ___ ___ _____

38. Placed all linen in dirty bag, removed and disposed of gloves.
___ ___ ___ _____

39. Organized patient's room, performed hand hygiene.
___ ___ ___ _____

40. Inspected patient during procedure for areas of skin irritation, observed patient for signs of fatigue, dyspnea, and pain.
___ ___ ___ _____

Copyright © 2018 by Elsevier Inc. All rights reserved.

Student _____ Date _____

Instructor _____ Date _____

PERFORMANCE CHECKLIST PROCEDURAL GUIDELINE 18.7 **MAKING AN UNOCCUPIED BED**

	S	U	NP	Comments
PROCEDURAL STEPS				
1. Performed hand hygiene, arranged supplies at bedside.	___	___	___	_____
2. Assessed environment for safety.	___	___	___	_____
3. Provided privacy, transferred patient to bedside chair.	___	___	___	_____
4. Lowered side rails, raised bed to comfortable working height.	___	___	___	_____
5. Applied clean gloves if necessary, removed all linen and placed in laundry bag, avoided touching linen to uniform or shaking linen.	___	___	___	_____
6. Straightened mattress, wiped with washcloth moistened in antiseptic solution, dried thoroughly.	___	___	___	_____
7. Applied all bottom linen on one side:				
a. Ensured fitted sheet is smooth over mattress, fit corners on both ends, OR	___	___	___	_____
b. Placed flat sheet over mattress, mitered corners ad tucked remaining part of sheet under mattress.	___	___	___	_____
c. Applied drawsheet or waterproof pad properly if needed.	___	___	___	_____
8. Moved to opposite side of bed, repeated step 7.	___	___	___	_____
9. Placed top sheet over bed and folded out properly.	___	___	___	_____
10. Stood on side at foot of bed, lifted mattress to tuck top sheet and blanket under.	___	___	___	_____
11. Made modified mitered corner with top sheet, blanket, and spread.	___	___	___	_____
12. Made cuff properly.	___	___	___	_____
13. Lifted mattress to tuck top sheet, blanket, and spread under mattress, ensured toe pleats are not pulled out.	___	___	___	_____
14. Made modified mitered corner with top sheet, blanket, and spread.	___	___	___	_____

Copyright © 2018 by Elsevier Inc. All rights reserved.

	S	U	NP	Comments

15. Moved to other side of bed, spread linen out evenly, made cuff with top sheet and blanket, made modified corner at foot of bed.   ___ ___ ___ _____

16. Applied clean pillowcase.   ___ ___ ___ _____

17. Placed call light within patient's reach, returned bed to lowest position, helped patient into bed.   ___ ___ ___ _____

18. Placed linen bag in dirty laundry bag, removed and disposed of gloves.   ___ ___ ___ _____

19. Arranged and organized patient's room, performed hand hygiene.   ___ ___ ___ _____

Copyright © 2018 by Elsevier Inc. All rights reserved.

Student _____ Date _____

Instructor _____ Date _____

PERFORMANCE CHECKLIST PROCEDURAL GUIDELINE 19.1 **EYE CARE FOR COMATOSE PATIENTS**

	S	U	NP	Comments
PROCEDURAL STEPS				
1. Performed hand hygiene.	___	___	___	_____
2. Observed patient's eyes for drainage, irritation, redness, and lesions; applied clean gloves if drainage is present.	___	___	___	_____
3. Explained each step of the procedure continually, even if patient is comatose.	___	___	___	_____
4. Assessed for blink reflex.	___	___	___	_____
5. Performed papillary examination.	___	___	___	_____
6. Observed patient's eye movements, noted symmetry of eye movement.	___	___	___	_____
7. Explained procedure to patient and caregivers.	___	___	___	_____
8. Positioned patient properly.	___	___	___	_____
9. Used clean washcloth or cotton balls moistened with water or saline, wiped each eye properly, used separate cotton ball or corner of washcloth for each eye.	___	___	___	_____
10. Used eyedropper to instill prescribed lubricant, wiped away any excess lubricant.	___	___	___	_____
11. Closed patient's eyes and applied patches or a moisture chamber if blink reflex is absent, secured patch without taping eyes.	___	___	___	_____
12. Disposed of excess material, removed gloves, performed hand hygiene.	___	___	___	_____
13. Removed eye patches every 4 hours; observed condition of patient's eyes for drainage, irritation, redness, and lesions.	___	___	___	_____
14. Asked caregiver to explain why eyedrops are important.	___	___	___	_____
15. Documented examination findings, administration of lubricant, and caregiver learning in the appropriate log.	___	___	___	_____
16. Notified health care provider if signs of irritation or infection were present.	___	___	___	_____

Copyright © 2018 by Elsevier Inc. All rights reserved.

Student _____ Date _____

Instructor _____ Date _____

PERFORMANCE CHECKLIST PROCEDURAL GUIDELINE 19.2 **TAKING CARE OF CONTACT LENSES**

	S	U	NP	Comments
PROCEDURAL STEPS				
1. Identified patient using at least two identifiers.	——	——	——	_____
2. Inspected patient's eyes or asked if contact lens is in place.	——	——	——	_____
3. Determined if patient was able to manipulate and hold contact lens and if glasses were available, determined patient's usual contact lens routine.	——	——	——	_____
4. Assessed patient for any unusual visual signs or symptoms.	——	——	——	_____
5. Reviewed types of medication prescribed for patient, especially medications that decrease blink reflexes or lubrication of corneas.	——	——	——	_____
6. Explained procedure to patient.	——	——	——	_____
7. Performed hand hygiene.	——	——	——	_____
8. Verified expiration dates of all solutions, assembled equipment at bedside.	——	——	——	_____
9. Ensured fingernails were short and smooth.	——	——	——	_____
10. Positioned patient appropriately.	——	——	——	_____
11. Applied clean gloves, placed towel just below patient's face.	——	——	——	_____
12. Removed lenses:				
a. Removed soft lenses, completed for each eye.				
(1) Shined a penlight sideways onto eye to locate lens if necessary.	——	——	——	_____
(2) Added two to three drops of sterile saline to patient's eye.	——	——	——	_____
(3) Asked patient to look straight ahead, retracted lower eyelid to expose lower edge of lens.	——	——	——	_____
(4) Used pad of index finger to slide lens down off cornea.	——	——	——	_____
(5) Pulled upper eyelid down with thumb of other hand, compressed lens slightly between thumb and index finger.	——	——	——	_____

Copyright © 2018 by Elsevier Inc. All rights reserved.

	S	U	NP	Comments

(6) Pinched lens and lifted out without allowing edges to stick together, placed lens in storage case. ___ ___ ___ _____

b. Removed hard lenses, completed for each eye.

(1) Inspected eye to ensure lens was positioned directly over cornea, shined penlight sideways to locate lens if necessary. ___ ___ ___ _____

(2) Placed index finger on outer corner of patient's eye, drew skin back toward ear. ___ ___ ___ _____

(3) Asked patient to blink, did not release pressure until blink was completed. ___ ___ ___ _____

(4) Retracted eyelid beyond edge of lens if necessary, pressed lower eyelid against lens to dislodge. ___ ___ ___ _____

(5) Allowed both eyelids to close slightly, grasped lens as it rose, cupped lens in hand. ___ ___ ___ _____

(6) Inspected lens to ensure it was intact, placed lens in storage container. ___ ___ ___ _____

c. Inspected eye after lens removal for redness, pain, swelling, discharge, or tearing. ___ ___ ___ _____

13. Cleaned and disinfected contact lenses:

a. Applied one or two drops of cleaning solution to lens in palm of hand. ___ ___ ___ _____

b. Held lens over emesis basin, rinsed using recommended solution. ___ ___ ___ _____

c. Placed lens in proper storage compartment, placed lenses inside up. ___ ___ ___ _____

d. Filled with disinfectant or storage solution. ___ ___ ___ _____

e. Secured cover(s) over storage case, labeled case properly. ___ ___ ___ _____

14. Inserted lenses:

a. Inserted soft lens, repeated for each eye.

(1) Removed lens from storage case, rinsed with recommended solution, inspected for foreign materials, tears, and other damage. ___ ___ ___ _____

(2) Held lens on tip of index finger concave side up. ___ ___ ___ _____

(3) Inspected lens properly to ensure lens is not inverted. ___ ___ ___ _____

Copyright © 2018 by Elsevier Inc. All rights reserved.

	S	U	NP	Comments
(4) Retracted upper lid properly, pulled lower lid down properly.	___	___	___	_____
(5) Instructed patient to look straight, placed lens on cornea, released lids slowly.	___	___	___	_____
b. Inserted rigid lens, repeated for each eye.				
(1) Removed lens from storage case properly.	___	___	___	_____
(2) Held lens on tip of index finger with concave side up.	___	___	___	_____
(3) Inspected lens to ensure it was moist, clean, clear, and free of cracks.	___	___	___	_____
(4) Wet lens surfaces using solution.	___	___	___	_____
(5) Pulled lower lid down properly.	___	___	___	_____
(6) Instructed patient to look straight, placed lens on cornea, released lids slowly.	___	___	___	_____
c. Asked patient to close eyes briefly and avoid blinking.	___	___	___	_____
15. Inspected eye to ensure lens is on cornea.	___	___	___	_____
16. Asked patient to cover other eye with hand and report if vision was clear and lens was comfortable.	___	___	___	_____
17. Repeated procedure to insert lens in other eye.	___	___	___	_____
18. Discarded solution from case, rinsed case with sterile solution, sterilized or replaced case, allowed case to air dry, disposed of towel, removed gloves, performed hand hygiene.	___	___	___	_____
19. Asked patient if lens felt comfortable.	___	___	___	_____
20. Asked patient if there is blurred vision, pain, and foreign body sensation.	___	___	___	_____
21. Observed eye for drainage or redness.	___	___	___	_____
22. Asked patient to describe how to clean contact lenses.	___	___	___	_____

Copyright © 2018 by Elsevier Inc. All rights reserved.

Student _____ Date _____

Instructor _____ Date _____

PERFORMANCE CHECKLIST SKILL 19.1 **EYE IRRIGATION**

	S	U	NP	Comments

ASSESSMENT

1. In acute emergent situation, flushed eyes with water or lactated Ringer's for at least 15 minutes, used pH testing to determine irrigating volumes.   ___ ___ ___ _____

2. If not an emergency, identified patient using at least two identifiers.   ___ ___ ___ _____

3. Reviewed medication order, including solution and affected eye(s).   ___ ___ ___ _____

4. Obtained history about injury to assess reason for irrigation.   ___ ___ ___ _____

5. Determined patient's ability to open affected eye.   ___ ___ ___ _____

6. Performed a complete eye examination if time allowed.   ___ ___ ___ _____

7. Assessed eye for redness, excessive tearing, discharge, and swelling; asked patient about symptoms of itching, burning, pain, blurred vision, or photophobia.   ___ ___ ___ _____

8. Asked patient to rate level of pain.   ___ ___ ___ _____

9. Assessed patient's ability to cooperate.   ___ ___ ___ _____

PLANNING

1. Identified expected outcomes.   ___ ___ ___ _____

2. Discussed procedure with patient.   ___ ___ ___ _____

3. Checked accuracy and completeness of MAR with written orders.   ___ ___ ___ _____

4. Assembled supplies at bedside.   ___ ___ ___ _____

5. Assisted patient to appropriate position.   ___ ___ ___ _____

IMPLEMENTATION

1. Performed hand hygiene, applied clean gloves.   ___ ___ ___ _____

2. Removed any contact lens if possible, removed gloves, reapplied new gloves.   ___ ___ ___ _____

3. Explained to patient that eye could be closed and no object would touch it.   ___ ___ ___ _____

4. Placed towel or waterproof pad under patient's face and emesis basin below patient's cheek on side of affected eye.   ___ ___ ___ _____

Copyright © 2018 by Elsevier Inc. All rights reserved.

	S	U	NP	Comments

5. Cleaned visible secretions and foreign material from eyelid margins and lashes using moistened gauze; wiped from inner to outer canthus. ___ ___ ___ _____

6. Explained next steps to patient, encouraged relaxation:

   a. Retracted upper and lower eyelids to expose conjunctival sacs. ___ ___ ___ _____

   b. Held lids open properly, did not apply pressure over eye. ___ ___ ___ _____

7. Held irrigating syringe, dropper, or IV tubing in appropriate position. ___ ___ ___ _____

8. Asked patient to look toward brow, irrigated with steady stream toward conjunctival sac, moved from inner to outer canthus. ___ ___ ___ _____

9. Reinforced importance of procedure, encouraged patient appropriately. ___ ___ ___ _____

10. Allowed patient to blink periodically. ___ ___ ___ _____

11. Continued irrigation with prescribed volume or time until secretions were clear. ___ ___ ___ _____

12. Blotted excess moisture from eyelids and face with gauze or towel. ___ ___ ___ _____

13. Disposed of soiled supplies, removed gloves, performed hand hygiene. ___ ___ ___ _____

EVALUATION

1. Observed for verbal and nonverbal signs of anxiety during irrigation. ___ ___ ___ _____

2. Assessed patient's comfort level after irrigation. ___ ___ ___ _____

3. Inspected eye for movement and PERRLA. ___ ___ ___ _____

4. Asked patient about improved visual acuity, had patient read written material. ___ ___ ___ _____

5. Asked patient to explain purpose of drops and when to use them. ___ ___ ___ _____

6. Identified unexpected outcomes. ___ ___ ___ _____

RECORDING AND REPORTING

1. Recorded condition of eye and patient's report of pain and visual symptoms, recorded amount and type of irrigation on MAR. ___ ___ ___ _____

2. Documented evaluation of patient learning. ___ ___ ___ _____

3. Reported continuing symptoms of pain or blurred vision. ___ ___ ___ _____

Copyright © 2018 by Elsevier Inc. All rights reserved.

Student _____ Date _____

Instructor _____ Date _____

PERFORMANCE CHECKLIST SKILL 19.2 **EAR IRRIGATION**

	S	U	NP	Comments

ASSESSMENT

1. Identified patient using two identifiers, compared identifiers with information on MAR. ___ ___ ___ _____

2. Reviewed medication order including solution and affected ear. ___ ___ ___ _____

3. Reviewed medical record for history of ruptured tympanic membrane, placement of myringotomy tubes, or surgery of the auditory canal. ___ ___ ___ _____

4. Inspected pinna and external auditory meatus for redness, swelling, drainage, abrasions, and presence of cerumen or foreign objects; attempted to remove objects by first straightening the ear canal. ___ ___ ___ _____

5. Used otoscope to inspect deeper portions of auditory canal and tympanic membrane. ___ ___ ___ _____

6. Asked if patient is experiencing discomfort. ___ ___ ___ _____

7. Noted patient's ability to hear clearly. ___ ___ ___ _____

8. Reviewed patient's knowledge of purpose for irrigation and normal care of ear. ___ ___ ___ _____

PLANNING

1. Identified expected outcomes. ___ ___ ___ _____

2. Checked accuracy and completeness of each MAR. ___ ___ ___ _____

3. Instilled softener into ear for 2 to 3 days before irrigation if patient had impacted cerumen. ___ ___ ___ _____

4. Explained procedure, warned that irrigation may cause sensation of dizziness, ear fullness, and warmth. ___ ___ ___ _____

IMPLEMENTATION

1. Performed hand hygiene, arranged supplies at bedside. ___ ___ ___ _____

2. Provided privacy. ___ ___ ___ _____

3. Assisted patient to appropriate position, placed towel under patient's head and shoulder, had patient hold emesis basin under ear if able. ___ ___ ___ _____

4. Poured irrigating solution into basin, checked temperature properly. ___ ___ ___ _____

Copyright © 2018 by Elsevier Inc. All rights reserved.

	S	U	NP	Comments

5. Applied gloves, cleaned auricle and outer ear canal with gauze or cotton ball, did not force drainage or cerumen into ear canal.   ___ ___ ___ _____

6. Filled irrigating syringe with solution.   ___ ___ ___ _____

7. Pulled pinna back appropriately based on patient's age, placed tip of device just inside external meatus, left space around irrigating tip and canal.   ___ ___ ___ _____

8. Instilled solution properly, allowed fluid to drain out into basin during instillation, continued until canal was cleaned or solution was used.   ___ ___ ___ _____

9. Maintained flow of irrigation in steady stream until pieces of cerumen flowed from canal.   ___ ___ ___ _____

10. Asked if patient was experiencing pain, nausea, or vertigo.   ___ ___ ___ _____

11. Drained excessive fluid from ear by having patient tilt head.   ___ ___ ___ _____

12. Dried outer ear canal gently with cotton ball, left in place for 5 to 10 minutes.   ___ ___ ___ _____

13. Assisted patient to a sitting position.   ___ ___ ___ _____

14. Removed gloves, disposed of supplies, performed hand hygiene.   ___ ___ ___ _____

EVALUATION

1. Asked patient if discomfort was noted during instillation.   ___ ___ ___ _____

2. Asked patient about sensations of lightheadedness or dizziness.   ___ ___ ___ _____

3. Reinspected condition of meatus and canal.   ___ ___ ___ _____

4. Assessed patient's hearing acuity.   ___ ___ ___ _____

5. Asked patient and family to describe how to use syringe for ear irrigation.   ___ ___ ___ _____

6. Identified unexpected outcomes.   ___ ___ ___ _____

RECORDING AND REPORTING

1. Recorded procedure, amount of solution instilled, time of administration, and irrigated ear in appropriate log.   ___ ___ ___ _____

2. Documented evaluation of patient learning.   ___ ___ ___ _____

3. Reported appearance of external ear and patient's hearing acuity in appropriate log.   ___ ___ ___ _____

Copyright © 2018 by Elsevier Inc. All rights reserved.

Student _____ Date _____

Instructor _____ Date _____

PERFORMANCE CHECKLIST SKILL 19.3 **CARE OF HEARING AIDS**

	S	U	NP	Comments

ASSESSMENT

1. Identified patient using at least two identifiers.

2. Determined whether patient could hear clearly with hearing aid.

3. Asked if patient was able to manipulate and hold hearing aid, observed patient insert aid independently.

4. Assessed if hearing aid was working by removing from ear, turning volume up, and observing for squealing tone.

5. Determined patient's usual hearing aid care practices.

6. Assessed patient for unusual physical or auditory signs/symptoms.

7. Inspected earmold for cracked or rough edges.

8. Inspected for accumulation of cerumen around aid and plugging of opening in aid.

9. Assessed patient's knowledge of and routines for cleansing and caring for hearing aid.

PLANNING

1. Identified expected outcomes.

2. Discussed procedure with patient, explained all steps before removing aid.

3. Assembled supplies at bedside, placed towel over work area.

4. Had patient assume appropriate position.

IMPLEMENTATION

1. Performed hand hygiene, applied clean gloves if necessary.

2. Removed and cleaned hearing aids:

   a. Turned hearing aid off, grasped aid securely, removed device following natural ear contour.

   b. Held aid over towel, wiped exterior with tissue to remove cerumen.

Copyright © 2018 by Elsevier Inc. All rights reserved.

	S	U	NP	Comments

c. Inspected all openings in aid for cerumen, removed cerumen with wax loop or device supplied with aid.

____ ____ ____ _____

d. Inspected earmold for rough edges or frays in cords.

____ ____ ____ _____

e. Opened battery door, placed hearing aid in labeled case, allowed it to air dry.

____ ____ ____ _____

f. Assessed ear for redness, tenderness, discharge, or odor.

____ ____ ____ _____

g. Repeated steps for other hearing aid if bilateral.

____ ____ ____ _____

h. Placed towel beneath patient's ear(s); washed canal(s) with washcloth, soap, and water; rinsed and dried.

____ ____ ____ _____

i. Disposed of towels, removed gloves, performed hand hygiene.

____ ____ ____ _____

j. Placed in storage container with desiccant material if stored, labeled case appropriately, indicated in records where aid was stored.

____ ____ ____ _____

3. Inserted hearing aid(s):

a. Removed hearing aid from storage case, checked battery, ensured volume was off.

____ ____ ____ _____

b. Identified hearing aid as right or left.

____ ____ ____ _____

c. Allowed patient to insert aid when possible, or held hearing aid properly with canal at the bottom, inserted following natural contours to guide into place.

____ ____ ____ _____

d. Anchored any separate pieces.

____ ____ ____ _____

e. Adjusted or had patient adjust volume to comfortable level.

____ ____ ____ _____

f. Repeated insertion for other hearing aid if bilateral.

____ ____ ____ _____

g. Closed and stored case, removed and disposed of gloves, performed hand hygiene.

____ ____ ____ _____

EVALUATION

1. Asked patient to rate comfort after removal or insertion.

____ ____ ____ _____

2. Observed patient during normal conversation and in response to environmental sounds.

____ ____ ____ _____

3. Asked patient and family to show how to care for hearing aids.

____ ____ ____ _____

4. Identified unexpected outcomes.

____ ____ ____ _____

Copyright © 2018 by Elsevier Inc. All rights reserved.

	S	U	NP	Comments

RECORDING AND REPORTING

1. Recorded removal of aid, storage location, and patient's preferred communication techniques, ensured information was in patient's record. ____ ____ ____ _____

2. Documented evaluation of patient learning. ____ ____ ____ _____

3. Reported any signs of infection, injury, or sudden decrease in hearing. ____ ____ ____ _____

Copyright © 2018 by Elsevier Inc. All rights reserved.

Student _____ Date _____

Instructor _____ Date _____

PERFORMANCE CHECKLIST SKILL 21.1 **ADMINISTERING ORAL MEDICATIONS**

	S	U	NP	Comments

ASSESSMENT

1. Checked accuracy and completeness of MAR, clarified incomplete or unclear orders. ___ ___ ___ _____

2. Reviewed pertinent information related to medication. ___ ___ ___ _____

3. Assessed for any contraindications to receiving oral medication, notified health care provider if contraindications were present. ___ ___ ___ _____

4. Assessed risk for aspiration, protected patient by assessing swallowing ability. ___ ___ ___ _____

5. Assessed patient's medical history, history of allergies, medication history, and diet history; listed drug allergies on MAR and medical record, advised patient to wear allergy brace-let if necessary. ___ ___ ___ _____

6. Gathered and reviewed physical assessment findings and laboratory data that influence drug administration. ___ ___ ___ _____

7. Assessed patient's knowledge regarding health and medication use. ___ ___ ___ _____

8. Assessed patient's preference for fluids, deter-mined if medication could be given with these fluids, maintained fluid restrictions. ___ ___ ___ _____

PLANNING

1. Identified expected outcomes. ___ ___ ___ _____

2. Explained procedure to patient, explained specifically if patient wanted to self-administer. ___ ___ ___ _____

3. Collected appropriate equipment and MAR. ___ ___ ___ _____

4. Planned preparation of medication to avoid interruptions and distractions. ___ ___ ___ _____

IMPLEMENTATION

1. Prepared medications:

   a. Performed hand hygiene. ___ ___ ___ _____

   b. Arranged medication tray and cups in prepa-ration area or on cart outside of room. ___ ___ ___ _____

   c. Logged on to ADS or unlocked medicine drawer or cart. ___ ___ ___ _____

238

Copyright © 2018 by Elsevier Inc. All rights reserved.

	S	U	NP	Comments

d. Prepared medication for *one patient at a time,* followed the six rights of medication administration, kept all pages of MARs for one patient together.   _____ _____ _____ _____

e. Selected correct drug, compared name of medication on label with MAR, exited ADS after removing drug(s).   _____ _____ _____ _____

f. Checked or calculated drug dose as necessary, double-checked calculation, checked expiration date on all medications, returned outdated medication to pharmacy.   _____ _____ _____ _____

g. Checked record for medication count and compared current count with supply available if preparing a controlled substance.   _____ _____ _____ _____

h. Prepared solid forms of oral medications.

  (1) Placed unit-dose medication directly into cup without removing wrapper.   _____ _____ _____ _____

  (2) "Popped" medications through foil or paper backing into a medication cup when using a blister pack.   _____ _____ _____ _____

  (3) Had pharmacy split dosage if necessary.   _____ _____ _____ _____

  (4) Placed all medication in one cup, placed medication requiring preadministration assessments in separate cups.   _____ _____ _____ _____

  (5) Crushed medications separately if patient has difficulty swallowing, used pill-crushing device properly, mixed medication with soft food.   _____ _____ _____ _____

i. Prepared liquids.

  (1) Used unit-dose container with correct amount of medication, shook container, administered medication packaged in single-dose cup directly from cup.   _____ _____ _____ _____

  (2) Held bottle with label against palm of hand while pouring.   _____ _____ _____ _____

  (3) Placed medication cap at eye level, filled to desired level on the scale, ensured scale was even with fluid level at surface or base of meniscus.   _____ _____ _____ _____

  (4) Discarded excess liquid appropriately, wiped lip of bottle with paper towel and recapped.   _____ _____ _____ _____

  (5) Prepared medication in oral syringe if appropriate.   _____ _____ _____ _____

Copyright © 2018 by Elsevier Inc. All rights reserved.

	S	U	NP	Comments

j. Returned stock containers or unused medication to shelf or drawer, labeled cups and poured medications before leaving preparation area, did not leave drugs unattended.

k. Compared MAR with labels on prepared drugs before going into patient's room.

2. Administered medications:

a. Took medication to patient at correct time, applied the six rights of medication administration.

b. Identified patient using two identifiers, compared identifiers with information in patient's MAR.

c. Compared MAR with medication labels at bedside, asked patient if he or she has allergies.

d. Explained purpose of each medication, action, and possible side effects; allowed patient to ask any questions.

e. Performed necessary preadministration assessment, asked patient if he or she has any allergies.

f. Assisted patient to appropriate position.

g. Allowed patient to hold cup or tablets if desired, offered preferred liquid.

h. Removed tablets or strips from packet just before use, did not push tablet through foil, placed medication on top of patient's tongue, cautioned against chewing medication.

i. Had patient place sublingually administered medication under tongue and allowed it to dissolve completely.

j. Had patient place buccal-administered medication against mucous membranes of the cheek and gums until medication dissolved.

k. Mixed powdered medication with liquids at bedside, gave mixture to patient to drink.

l. Gave each crushed medication separately with a teaspoon of food.

m. Cautioned patient against chewing or swallowing lozenges.

n. Gave effervescent powders and tablets immediately after dissolving.

Copyright © 2018 by Elsevier Inc. All rights reserved.

	S	U	NP	Comments

o. Placed medication cup to patient's lips if unable to hold cup, introduced each drug to mouth, did not rush or force medication.

p. Stayed until patient completely took all medication by the prescribed route, asked patient to open mouth if necessary.

q. Offered patient nonfat snack if appropriate.

3. Assisted patient to comfortable position.

4. Disposed of soiled supplies, performed hand hygiene.

5. Replenished stock, returned cart to medication room, cleaned work area.

EVALUATION

1. Returned within appropriate time, evaluated patient's response to medications.

2. Asked patient or caregiver to identify drug and explain purpose, action, schedule, and side effects.

3. Asked patient to show where sublingual medication should be placed in mouth.

4. Identified unexpected outcomes.

RECORDING AND REPORTING

1. Recorded pertinent information on MAR immediately after administration, included initials and signature.

2. Recorded patient response to medication, patient teaching, and validation of understanding in appropriate log.

3. Recorded reason for withholding doses in appropriate log.

4. Reported adverse effects/patient response/ withheld drugs to nurse in charge or health care provider.

Copyright © 2018 by Elsevier Inc. All rights reserved.

Student _____ Date _____

Instructor _____ Date _____

PERFORMANCE CHECKLIST SKILL 21.2 **ADMINISTERING MEDICATIONS THROUGH A FEEDING TUBE**

	S	U	NP	Comments

ASSESSMENT

1. Checked accuracy and completeness of each MAR against medication order, clarified incomplete or unclear orders with health care provider. ____ ____ ____ _____

2. Reviewed pertinent information related to medication. ____ ____ ____ _____

3. Assessed for contraindications to receiving medications enterally. ____ ____ ____ _____

4. Assessed patient's medical history, history of allergies, medication history, and diet history; withheld medication and informed health care provider if contraindicated. ____ ____ ____ _____

5. Reviewed postoperative orders for type of enteral tube care if necessary. ____ ____ ____ _____

6. Gathered and reviewed physical assessment data and laboratory data that may influence drug administration. ____ ____ ____ _____

7. Checked with pharmacy for availability of liquid preparation. ____ ____ ____ _____

8. Verified placement of feeding tube before administration. ____ ____ ____ _____

PLANNING

1. Identified expected outcomes. ____ ____ ____ _____

2. Collected appropriate equipment and MAR. ____ ____ ____ _____

IMPLEMENTATION

1. Performed hand hygiene, prepared medications for instillation, checked label against MAR twice, filled graduated container with water, used sterile water if necessary:

   a. Crushed tablets into a fine powder, dissolved each tablet in separate cup of water. ____ ____ ____ _____

   b. Ensured contents of capsule could be expressed from covering, applied gloves, opened capsule and emptied contents into water, dissolved gel caps. ____ ____ ____ _____

   c. Prepared liquid medication appropriately. ____ ____ ____ _____

242

Copyright © 2018 by Elsevier Inc. All rights reserved.

2. Took medication to patient at correct time, applied the six rights of medication administration, performed hand hygiene.

    ____ ____ ____ _____

3. Identified patient using at least two identifiers, compared identifiers with information in MAR.

    ____ ____ ____ _____

4. Compared MAR with medication labels at patient's bedside, asked patient if he or she has allergies.

    ____ ____ ____ _____

5. Explained purpose of each medication, action, and possible adverse effects, allowed patient to ask any questions.

    ____ ____ ____ _____

6. Positioned patient appropriately.

    ____ ____ ____ _____

7. Adjusted infusion pump to hold the tube feeding if continuous enteric tube feeding is infusing.

    ____ ____ ____ _____

8. Applied clean gloves, checked placement of feeding tube.

    ____ ____ ____ _____

9. Check for GRV, returned aspirated contents to stomach if appropriate, held medication and contacted health care provider when GRV was excessive.

    ____ ____ ____ _____

10. Irrigated tubing:

   a. Pinched enteral tube and removed syringe, drew water into syringe, reinserted tip of syringe into tube, released clamp, flushed tubing, clamped tube again, removed syringe.

    ____ ____ ____ _____

   b. Attached syringe using appropriate enteral connector to enteral tube.

    ____ ____ ____ _____

11. Removed bulb or plunger of syringe and reinserted syringe into tip of feeding tube.

    ____ ____ ____ _____

12. Administered first dose by pouring into syringe, allowed to flow by gravity:

   a. Flushed with water if giving only one dose.

    ____ ____ ____ _____

   b. Gave each medication separately, flushed with water between each dose.

    ____ ____ ____ _____

   c. Followed last dose with appropriate amount of water.

    ____ ____ ____ _____

13. Clamped proximal end of feeding tube if feeding was not being administered, capped end of tube.

    ____ ____ ____ _____

14. Followed medication administration if tube feeding was administered by an infusion pump, held feeding if medications were not compatible with feeding solution.

    ____ ____ ____ _____

Copyright © 2018 by Elsevier Inc. All rights reserved.

	S	U	NP	Comments

15. Assisted patient to comfortable position, kept head of bed elevated.   _____ _____ _____ _____

16. Disposed of soiled supplies, rinsed graduated container and syringe, removed and disposed of gloves, performed hand hygiene.   _____ _____ _____ _____

EVALUATION

1. Observed patient for signs of aspiration.   _____ _____ _____ _____

2. Returned within 30 minutes to evaluate patient's response to medications.   _____ _____ _____ _____

3. Asked patient and family to explain why medications are being given through feeding tube.   _____ _____ _____ _____

4. Identified unexpected outcomes.   _____ _____ _____ _____

RECORDING AND REPORTING

1. Recorded method used to check tube placement, GRV, and pH of stomach aspirate in appropriate log.   _____ _____ _____ _____

2. Recorded actual time each drug was administered.   _____ _____ _____ _____

3. Recorded patient's response to medication, patient teaching, and validation of patient understanding in appropriate log.   _____ _____ _____ _____

4. Recorded total amount of water used on proper I&O form.   _____ _____ _____ _____

5. Reported adverse effects, patient response, and withheld drugs to nurse in charge or health care provider.   _____ _____ _____ _____

Copyright © 2018 by Elsevier Inc. All rights reserved.

Student _____ Date _____

Instructor _____ Date _____

PERFORMANCE CHECKLIST SKILL 21.3   **APPLYING TOPICAL MEDICATIONS TO THE SKIN**

	S	U	NP	Comments
ASSESSMENT				
1. Checked accuracy and completeness of MAR with medication order, clarified incomplete or unclear orders with health care provider before administration.	____	____	____	_____
2. Reviewed pertinent information related to medication.	____	____	____	_____
3. Assessed condition of skin or membrane where medication was to be applied; applied clean gloves if necessary; washed, rinsed, and dried site; ensured to remove previously applied medication, debris, or fluids; assessed for symptoms of skin irritation, removed gloves and performed hand hygiene.	____	____	____	_____
4. Assessed patient's medical history, history of allergies, and medication history; asked if patient has had reaction to cream or lotion, listed drug allergies on MAR, patient's medical record, and ID bracelet.	____	____	____	_____
5. Determined amount of topical agent required, assessed skin site, reviewed health care provider's order, read application directions carefully.	____	____	____	_____
6. Assessed patient's knowledge of action and purpose of medication and willingness to adhere to drug regimen.	____	____	____	_____
7. Determined if patient or caregiver was physically able to apply medication.	____	____	____	_____
PLANNING				
1. Identified expected outcomes.	____	____	____	_____
2. Collected appropriate equipment and MAR.	____	____	____	_____
IMPLEMENTATION				
1. Performed hand hygiene, prepared medications for application, checked label against MAR twice, checked expiration date.	____	____	____	_____
2. Took medication to patient at correct time, applied the six rights of medication administration.	____	____	____	_____
3. Assisted patient to comfortable position, arranged supplies at bedside.	____	____	____	_____

Copyright © 2018 by Elsevier Inc. All rights reserved.

4. Identified patient using at least two identifiers, compared identifiers with information in patient's MAR. ____ ____ ____ _____

5. Compared MAR with medication labels at patient's bedside, asked patient if he or she had allergies. ____ ____ ____ _____

6. Explained procedure and discussed the purpose of each medication, action, and possible adverse effects; allowed patient to ask any questions. ____ ____ ____ _____

7. Applied sterile gloves if skin is broken or clean gloves. ____ ____ ____ _____

8. Applied topical creams, ointments, and oil-based lotion:

    a. Exposed affected area, kept unaffected areas covered. ____ ____ ____ _____

    b. Washed, rinsed, and dried affected area before applying medication. ____ ____ ____ _____

    c. Applied topical agent to dry and flaking skin if necessary. ____ ____ ____ _____

    d. Removed gloves, performed hand hygiene, applied new gloves. ____ ____ ____ _____

    e. Placed required amount of medication in hand, softened medication. ____ ____ ____ _____

    f. Told patient initial application of agent may feel cold, spread properly over skin surface, applied to appropriate thickness. ____ ____ ____ _____

    g. Explained to patient that skin may feel greasy after application. ____ ____ ____ _____

9. Applied antianginal ointment:

    a. Removed previous dose paper, folded used paper, and disposed in biohazard container, wiped off residual medication with tissue. ____ ____ ____ _____

    b. Wrote date, time, and nurse's initials on new application paper. ____ ____ ____ _____

    c. Applied desired number of inches of ointment to paper-measuring guide. ____ ____ ____ _____

    d. Selected application site, did not apply to nonintact or hairy surfaces or over scar tissue. ____ ____ ____ _____

    e. Applied ointment to skin surface by placing wrapper directly on skin, did not rub ointment into skin. ____ ____ ____ _____

    f. Secured ointment and paper with tape or dressing, used plastic wrap if necessary. ____ ____ ____ _____

Copyright © 2018 by Elsevier Inc. All rights reserved.

10. Applied transdermal patches:

    a. Removed old patch if necessary, cleansed area, checked between skinfolds for patch.   ____ ____ ____ _____

    b. Disposed of old patch in biohazard trash bag.   ____ ____ ____ _____

    c. Dated and initialed outer side of new patch, noted time of administration.   ____ ____ ____ _____

    d. Chose appropriate new site, did not apply to irritated or oily skin.   ____ ____ ____ _____

    e. Removed the patch from covering, held patch without touching adhesive edges.   ____ ____ ____ _____

    f. Applied patch, ensured edges stick well, applied overlay if provided.   ____ ____ ____ _____

    g. Did not apply patch to previously used sites for at least a week.   ____ ____ ____ _____

    h. Instructed patient not to cut patches.   ____ ____ ____ _____

    i. Instructed patient to always remove old patch before applying new one and not to mix with other therapies.   ____ ____ ____ _____

11. Administered aerosol sprays:

    a. Shook container vigorously, read label for recommended spray distance.   ____ ____ ____ _____

    b. Asked patient to turn face away from spray.   ____ ____ ____ _____

    c. Sprayed medication evenly over affected site.   ____ ____ ____ _____

12. Applied suspension-based lotion:

    a. Shook container vigorously.   ____ ____ ____ _____

    b. Applied lotion to gauze dressing, applied to skin properly.   ____ ____ ____ _____

    c. Explained to patient that area would feel cool and dry.   ____ ____ ____ _____

13. Applied a powder:

    a. Ensured skin was thoroughly dry, dried between skinfolds.   ____ ____ ____ _____

    b. Asked patient to turn face away from powder.   ____ ____ ____ _____

    c. Dusted skin site with fine, thin layer of powder.   ____ ____ ____ _____

Copyright © 2018 by Elsevier Inc. All rights reserved.

14. Assisted patient to comfortable position, reapplied gown, covered with bed linen as desired.

   ___   ___   ___   _____

15. Disposed of soiled supplies properly, removed and disposed of gloves, performed hand hygiene.

   ___   ___   ___   _____

EVALUATION

1. Inspected condition of skin between applications.

   ___   ___   ___   _____

2. Had patient keep a diary of doses taken.

   ___   ___   ___   _____

3. Observed patient or caregiver applying topical medication.

   ___   ___   ___   _____

4. Asked patient to explain how drug works, correct dose, and side effects.

   ___   ___   ___   _____

5. Identified unexpected outcomes.

   ___   ___   ___   _____

RECORDING AND REPORTING

1. Recorded actual time of drugs administered, type of agent, strength, and site of application in the appropriate log.

   ___   ___   ___   _____

2. Recorded patient's response to medication, patient teaching, and validation of patient's understanding in appropriate log.

   ___   ___   ___   _____

3. Described condition of skin before each application in nurse's notes.

   ___   ___   ___   _____

4. Reported adverse effects/patient response/ withheld drugs to nurse in charge or health care provider.

   ___   ___   ___   _____

Copyright © 2018 by Elsevier Inc. All rights reserved.

Student _____ Date _____

Instructor _____ Date _____

PERFORMANCE CHECKLIST SKILL 21.4 **ADMINISTERING OPHTHALMIC MEDICATIONS**

	S	U	NP	Comments
ASSESSMENT				
1. Checked accuracy and completeness of MAR with medication order, clarified incomplete or unclear orders with health care provider.	___	___	___	_____
2. Reviewed pertinent information related to medication.	___	___	___	_____
3. Assessed condition of external eye or ear structures.	___	___	___	_____
4. Determined whether patient had any symptoms of eye discomfort or visual or hearing impairment.	___	___	___	_____
5. Assessed patient's medical history, history of allergies, and medication history, listed drug allergies on MAR and provided allergy bracelet if necessary.	___	___	___	_____
6. Assessed patient's LOC and ability to follow directions.	___	___	___	_____
7. Assessed patient's knowledge regarding drug therapy and desire to self-administer medication.	___	___	___	_____
8. Assessed patient's ability to manipulate and hold dropper or disk.	___	___	___	_____
PLANNING				
1. Identified expected outcomes.	___	___	___	_____
2. Collected appropriate equipment and MAR.	___	___	___	_____
IMPLEMENTATION				
1. Performed hand hygiene, prepared medications for instillation, checked label of medication against MAR twice, checked expiration date on container.	___	___	___	_____
2. Took medication(s) to patient at correct time, applied the six rights of medication administration, performed hand hygiene.	___	___	___	_____
3. Assisted patient to an appropriate position, arranged supplies at bedside.	___	___	___	_____
4. Identified patient using at least two identifiers.	___	___	___	_____

Copyright © 2018 by Elsevier Inc. All rights reserved.

	S	U	NP	Comments

5. Compared MAR with medication labels at bedside, asked patient if he or she had allergies.
____ ____ ____ _____

6. Explained procedure to patient and sensations to expect, discussed purpose of each medication, action, and possible adverse side effects; allowed patient to ask any questions; told patients receiving eyedrops that vision would be blurred and light sensitivity may occur.
____ ____ ____ _____

7. Instilled eye medications:

a. Applied clean gloves, asked patient to assume appropriate position.
____ ____ ____ _____

b. Washed away drainage or crusting along margins, soaked dried crusts, wiped clean from inner to outer canthus, removed gloves, performed hand hygiene.
____ ____ ____ _____

c. Explained there may be burning sensation from the drops.
____ ____ ____ _____

d. Instilled eyedrops.

(1) Applied clean gloves, held cotton ball or tissue below lower eyelid if drainage is present.
____ ____ ____ _____

(2) Exposed conjunctival sac, did not press directly against patient's eyeball.
____ ____ ____ _____

(3) Asked patient to look at ceiling, held eyedropper appropriately above conjunctival sac.
____ ____ ____ _____

(4) Dropped prescribed number of drops into conjunctival sac.
____ ____ ____ _____

(5) Repeated procedure if patient blinked or closed eyes during administration.
____ ____ ____ _____

(6) Applied gentle pressure with tissue to nasolacrimal duct over each eye when administering drops that may cause systemic effects, avoided pressure against patient's eyeball.
____ ____ ____ _____

(7) Asked patient to close eyes gently after instilling drops.
____ ____ ____ _____

e. Instilled ophthalmic ointment.

(1) Applied clean gloves if drainage is present, held applicator above lower lid margin, applied ointment evenly along lower eyelid on conjunctiva.
____ ____ ____ _____

Copyright © 2018 by Elsevier Inc. All rights reserved.

	S	U	NP	Comments
(2) Had patient close eye and rub lid lightly if not contraindicated.	___	___	___	_____
(3) Wiped excess medication from eyelid.	___	___	___	_____
(4) Applied clean eye patch if needed, completely covered affected eye, taped without applying pressure to eye.	___	___	___	_____
f. Inserted intraocular disk.	___	___		_____
(1) Applied clean gloves, opened disk package, positioned convex side of disk on fingertip.	___	___	___	_____
(2) Pulled patient's lower eyelid away from eye, asked patient to look up.	___	___	___	_____
(3) Placed disk properly in the conjunctival sac.	___	___	___	_____
(4) Pulled patient's lower eyelid out and over disk, repeated if disk can still be seen.	___	___	___	_____
8. Removed and disposed of gloves and soiled supplies after administering eye medications, performed hand hygiene.	___	___	___	_____
9. Removed intraocular disk:				
a. Performed hand hygiene, applied clean gloves, pulled eyelid downward on the lower eyelid.	___	___	___	_____
b. Pinched disk and lifted it out of patient's eye.	___	___	___	_____
10. Disposed of soiled supplies appropriately, performed hand hygiene.	___	___	___	_____

EVALUATION

	S	U	NP	Comments
1. Observed response to medication by assessing vision changes, asked if symptoms were relieved, noted side effects or discomfort.	___	___	___	_____
2. Asked patient to discuss drug's purpose, action, side effects, and technique of administration.	___	___	___	_____
3. Asked patient and family to demonstrate inserting the intraocular disk.	___	___	___	_____
4. Identified unexpected outcomes.	___	___	___	_____

RECORDING AND REPORTING

	S	U	NP	Comments
1. Recorded drug, concentration, dose, drop, site, and time on MAR.	___	___	___	_____
2. Recorded patient teaching and validation of understanding in appropriate log.	___	___	___	_____

Copyright © 2018 by Elsevier Inc. All rights reserved.

	S	U	NP	Comments

3. Recorded objective data related to tissues involved, patient's response to medications, and side effects.

4. Reported adverse effects/patient's response/ withheld drugs to nurse in charge or health care provider.

Copyright © 2018 by Elsevier Inc. All rights reserved.

Student _____ Date _____

Instructor _____ Date _____

PERFORMANCE CHECKLIST SKILL 21.5   **ADMINISTERING EAR MEDICATIONS**

	S	U	NP	Comments
ASSESSMENT				
1. Checked accuracy and completeness of MAR with medication order, clarified incomplete or unclear orders with health care provider.	___	___	___	_____
2. Reviewed pertinent information related to medication.	___	___	___	_____
3. Assessed condition of external ear structures.	___	___	___	_____
4. Determined whether patient had any symptoms of ear discomfort or hearing impairment.	___	___	___	_____
5. Assessed patient's medical history, history of allergies, and medication history, listed drug allergies in MAR and provided allergy bracelet if necessary.	___	___	___	_____
6. Assessed patient's LOC and ability to follow directions.	___	___	___	_____
7. Assessed patient's knowledge regarding drug therapy and desire to self-administer medication.	___	___	___	_____
8. Assessed patient's ability to manipulate and hold dropper.	___	___	___	_____
PLANNING				
1. Identified expected outcomes.	___	___	___	_____
2. Collected appropriate equipment and MAR.	___	___	___	_____
IMPLEMENTATION				
1. Performed hand hygiene, prepared medications for instillation, checked label of medication against MAR twice, checked expiration date on container.	___	___	___	_____
2. Took medication(s) to patient at correct time, applied the six rights of medication administration, performed hand hygiene.	___	___	___	_____
3. Arranged supplies at bedside.	___	___	___	_____
4. Identified patient using at least two identifiers.	___	___	___	_____
5. Compared MAR with medication labels at bedside, asked patient if he or she has allergies.	___	___	___	_____

Copyright © 2018 by Elsevier Inc. All rights reserved.

	S	U	NP	Comments

6. Explained procedure to patient and sensations to expect, discussed purpose of each medication, action, and possible adverse side effects; allowed patient to ask any questions. ____ ____ ____ _____

7. Positioned patient appropriately, applied clean gloves if necessary. ____ ____ ____ _____

8. Straightened ear canal by pulling pinna appropriately. ____ ____ ____ _____

9. Wiped away any cerumen or drainage occluding outmost portion of ear canal, did not force cerumen into canal. ____ ____ ____ _____

10. Instilled prescribed drops holding dropper appropriately above ear canal. ____ ____ ____ _____

11. Asked patient to remain side-lying for a few minutes, applied gentle pressure to tragus with finger. ____ ____ ____ _____

12. Inserted portion of cotton ball into outermost part of canal if ordered, did not press cotton into canal. ____ ____ ____ _____

13. Removed cotton after 15 minutes, assisted patient to comfortable position. ____ ____ ____ _____

14. Disposed of soiled supplies properly, performed hand hygiene. ____ ____ ____ _____

EVALUATION

1. Reviewed laboratory results for evidence of pathogens. ____ ____ ____ _____

2. Asked patient to discuss drug's purpose, action, side effects, and technique of administration. ____ ____ ____ _____

3. Asked patient to demonstrate self-administration of eardrops. ____ ____ ____ _____

4. Identified unexpected outcomes. ____ ____ ____ _____

RECORDING AND REPORTING

1. Recorded drug, concentration, dose, drop, site, and time on MAR. ____ ____ ____ _____

2. Recorded patient teaching and validation of understanding in appropriate log. ____ ____ ____ _____

3. Recorded objective data related to tissues involved, patient's response to medications, and side effects in appropriate log. ____ ____ ____ _____

4. Reported adverse effects/patient's response/withheld drugs to nurse in charge or health care provider. ____ ____ ____ _____

Copyright © 2018 by Elsevier Inc. All rights reserved.

Student _____ Date _____

Instructor _____ Date _____

PERFORMANCE CHECKLIST SKILL 21.6 **ADMINISTERING NASAL INSTILLATIONS**

	S	U	NP	Comments

ASSESSMENT

1. Checked accuracy and completeness of each MAR with medication order, clarified incomplete or unclear orders with health care provider.

2. Reviewed pertinent information related to medication.

3. Assessed patient's history and history of allergies, listed drug allergies on MAR, and provided allergy bracelet if needed.

4. Performed hand hygiene, used penlight to inspect condition of nose and sinuses, palpated sinuses for tenderness, noted type of any drainage.

5. Assessed patient's knowledge regarding use of nasal instillations, technique for instillation, and willingness to learn self-administration.

PLANNING

1. Identified expected outcomes.

2. Collected appropriate equipment and MAR.

IMPLEMENTATION

1. Performed hand hygiene, prepared medications for instillation, checked label of medication against MAR twice, checked expiration date on container.

2. Took medication(s) to patient at the proper time, applied the six rights of medication, performed hand hygiene.

3. Identified patient using at least two identifiers, compared with information on MAR.

4. Compared MAR with medication labels at patient's bedside, asked patient if he or she has allergies.

5. Explained procedure to patient and sensations to expect, discussed purpose of each medication, action, and possible adverse effects; allowed patient to ask any questions; told patient that he or she may experience burning, stinging, or a choking sensation.

Copyright © 2018 by Elsevier Inc. All rights reserved.

	S	U	NP	Comments

6. Arranged supplies and medications at bedside, applied clean gloves if necessary.
   ____ ____ ____ _____

7. Shook container, instructed patient to clear or blow nose unless contraindicated.
   ____ ____ ____ _____

8. Administered nose drops:

   a. Assisted patient to proper position depending on affected nasal passage.
   ____ ____ ____ _____

   b. Supported patient's head with nondominant hand.
   ____ ____ ____ _____

   c. Instructed patient to breathe through mouth.
   ____ ____ ____ _____

   d. Held dropper above nares, instilled prescribed number of drops properly.
   ____ ____ ____ _____

   e. Had patient remain in supine position for 5 minutes.
   ____ ____ ____ _____

   f. Offered facial tissue, cautioned patient against blowing nose for several minutes.
   ____ ____ ____ _____

9. Administered nasal spray:

   a. Helped patient into appropriate position.
   ____ ____ ____ _____

   b. Helped patient insert tip of spray into nares, occluded other nostril with finger, pointed spray tip properly.
   ____ ____ ____ _____

   c. Had patient spray medication into nose while inhaling, helped patient remove nozzle, instructed patient to breathe out through mouth.
   ____ ____ ____ _____

   d. Offered facial tissue, cautioned patient against blowing nose for several minutes.
   ____ ____ ____ _____

10. Helped patient to comfortable position until medicine was absorbed.
   ____ ____ ____ _____

11. Disposed of soiled supplies, performed hand hygiene.
   ____ ____ ____ _____

EVALUATION

1. Observed patient for onset of side effects 15 to 30 minutes after administration.
   ____ ____ ____ _____

2. Asked if patient was able to breathe through nose, had patient occlude one nostril at a time and breathe deeply if necessary.
   ____ ____ ____ _____

3. Reinspected condition of nasal passages between instillations.
   ____ ____ ____ _____

4. Asked patient to describe risks of overuse and methods for administration.
   ____ ____ ____ _____

5. Had patient demonstrate self-medication.
   ____ ____ ____ _____

Copyright © 2018 by Elsevier Inc. All rights reserved.

		S	U	NP	Comments

6. Asked patient and family to explain importance of not overusing nasal sprays.
   ___ ___ ___ _____

7. Identified unexpected outcomes.
   ___ ___ ___ _____

RECORDING AND REPORTING

1. Recorded drug, concentration, number of drops, nares, and time on MAR.
   ___ ___ ___ _____

2. Recorded patient teaching and validation of understanding in appropriate log.
   ___ ___ ___ _____

3. Reported any unusual systemic effects/adverse effects/patient response/withheld drugs to nurse in charge or health care provider.
   ___ ___ ___ _____

Copyright © 2018 by Elsevier Inc. All rights reserved.

Student _____ Date _____

Instructor _____ Date _____

PERFORMANCE CHECKLIST SKILL 21.7 **USING METERED-DOSE INHALERS**

	S	U	NP	Comments

ASSESSMENT

1. Checked accuracy and completeness of each MAR against medication order, clarified incomplete or unclear orders with health care provider.

2. Reviewed pertinent information related to medication.

3. Assessed patient's medical history, history of allergies, and medication history, listed drug allergies on MAR and provided allergy bracelet if necessary.

4. Assessed respiratory pattern, auscultated breath sounds, assessed exercise tolerance.

5. Assessed patient's ability to hold, manipulate, and depress canister and inhaler.

6. Asked patient to demonstrate use of device if previously instructed in self-administration.

7. Assessed patient's readiness and ability to learn.

8. Assessed patient's knowledge and understanding of disease and purpose and action of medications.

PLANNING

1. Identified expected outcomes.

2. Collected appropriate equipment and MAR.

IMPLEMENTATION

1. Performed hand hygiene, prepared medications for inhalation, checked label of medication against MAR twice, checked expiration date.

2. Took medication(s) to patient at correct time, applied the six rights of medication administration, performed hand hygiene.

3. Identified patient using at least two identifiers, compared with information on MAR.

4. Compared MAR with medication labels at patient's bedside, asked patient if he or she had allergies.

258

Copyright © 2018 by Elsevier Inc. All rights reserved.

	S	U	NP	Comments

5. Explained procedure to patient, discussed purpose of each medication, action, and possible adverse effects; allowed patient to ask any questions; explained what a metered dose is and how to administer it, warned about overuse and side effects.   ___ ___ ___ _____

6. Allowed adequate time for patient to manipulate equipment, explained and demonstrated how canister fits into inhaler.   ___ ___ ___ _____

7. Explained and demonstrated steps for administering MDI without spacer:

   a. Removed mouthpiece cover from inhaler after inserting MDI canister into holder.   ___ ___ ___ _____

   b. Shook inhaler well for 2 to 5 seconds.   ___ ___ ___ _____

   c. Held inhaler in dominant hand.   ___ ___ ___ _____

   d. Instructed patient to position inhaler properly.   ___ ___ ___ _____

   e. Had patient take deep breath and exhale completely.   ___ ___ ___ _____

   f. Had patient hold inhaler in three-point or bilateral hand position.   ___ ___ ___ _____

   g. Instructed patient to tilt head back and inhale slowly and deeply through mouth for 3 to 5 seconds while depressing canister fully.   ___ ___ ___ _____

   h. Had patient hold breath for about 10 seconds.   ___ ___ ___ _____

   i. Removed MDI from mouth before exhaling.   ___ ___ ___ _____

8. Explained and demonstrated steps to administer MDI using spacer device:

   a. Removed mouthpiece cover from MDI and mouthpiece of spacer device.   ___ ___ ___ _____

   b. Shook inhaler well for 2 to 5 seconds.   ___ ___ ___ _____

   c. Inserted MDI into end of spacer device.   ___ ___ ___ _____

   d. Instructed patient to place spacer mouthpiece in mouth and close lips, avoided covering exhalation slots with lips.   ___ ___ ___ _____

   e. Had patient breathe normally through mouthpiece.   ___ ___ ___ _____

   f. Instructed patient to spray one puff into spacer device.   ___ ___ ___ _____

   g. Had patient breathe in slowly and fully.   ___ ___ ___ _____

   h. Instructed patient to hold breath for 10 seconds.   ___ ___ ___ _____

Copyright © 2018 by Elsevier Inc. All rights reserved.

	S	U	NP	Comments

9. Instructed patient to wait appropriate length of time between inhalations.

10. Instructed patient to not repeat inhalation before next scheduled time.

11. Warned patient he or she may feel gagging sensation.

12. Instructed patient to rinse and spit with warm water 2 minutes after dose.

13. Instructed patient in daily cleaning of inhaler.

14. Assisted patient to comfortable position, performed hand hygiene.

EVALUATION

1. Auscultated patient lungs, listened for abnormal breath sounds, obtained peak flow measures if ordered.

2. Had patient explain and demonstrate steps in use and cleaning of inhaler.

3. Asked patient to explain drug schedule and dose or medication.

4. Asked patient to describe side effects of medication and criteria for calling health care provider.

5. Asked patient to demonstrate inhaler use.

6. Identified unexpected outcomes.

RECORDING AND REPORTING

1. Recorded drug, dose, route, number of inhalations, and time on MAR.

2. Recorded patient teaching and validation of understanding in appropriate log.

3. Recorded patient's response to MDI, side effects, and patient's ability to use MDI.

4. Reported adverse effects/patient response/withheld drugs to nurse in charge or health care provider.

Copyright © 2018 by Elsevier Inc. All rights reserved.

Student _____ Date _____

Instructor _____ Date _____

PERFORMANCE CHECKLIST PROCEDURAL GUIDELINE 21.1 **USING DRY POWDER-INHALED MEDICATIONS**

	S	U	NP	Comments

PROCEDURAL STEPS

1. Checked accuracy and completeness of each MAR with medication order, clarified incomplete or unclear orders with health care provider. ___ ___ ___ _____

2. Reviewed pertinent information related to medication. ___ ___ ___ _____

3. Assessed patient's medical history, history of allergies, and medication history, listed drug allergies on MAR and provided allergy bracelet if necessary. ___ ___ ___ _____

4. Assessed respiratory pattern, auscultated breath sounds. ___ ___ ___ _____

5. Assessed patient's knowledge of medication and readiness to learn. ___ ___ ___ _____

6. Assessed patient's ability to learn. ___ ___ ___ _____

7. Determined patient's ability to hold, manipulate, and activate DPI. ___ ___ ___ _____

8. Assessed patient's technique in using a DPI if previously instructed in self-administration. ___ ___ ___ _____

9. Performed hand hygiene, prepared medication for inhalation, checked label on inhaler against MAR twice, checked expiration date on container. ___ ___ ___ _____

10. Took medication to patient at correct time, applied the six rights of medication administration, performed hand hygiene. ___ ___ ___ _____

11. Identified patient using two identifiers. ___ ___ ___ _____

12. Compared MAR with medication labels at patient's bedside, asked patient if he or she had allergies. ___ ___ ___ _____

13. Explained procedure, discussed purpose of each medication, action, and possible adverse effects; allowed patient to ask any questions; explained about a DPI; warned about overuse and side effects. ___ ___ ___ _____

14. Noted number of doses remaining if external counter was present. ___ ___ ___ _____

Copyright © 2018 by Elsevier Inc. All rights reserved.

	S	U	NP	Comments

15. Prepared DPI for administration, performed hand hygiene.
    ____ ____ ____ _____

16. Had patient place lips over mouthpiece and inhale quickly and deeply, removed inhaler before exhalation.
    ____ ____ ____ _____

17. Had patient hold breath as long as possible and then exhale.
    ____ ____ ____ _____

18. Instructed patient that he or she may not taste the powdered medication.
    ____ ____ ____ _____

19. Had patient rinse and spit with warm water after using DPI.
    ____ ____ ____ _____

20. Returned DPI to closed position or removed loaded capsule, noted number if external counter was present.
    ____ ____ ____ _____

21. Had patient demonstrate use of DPI at next scheduled dose, asked patient to discuss purpose, action, and side effects.
    ____ ____ ____ _____

22. Auscultated breath sounds, evaluated respiratory rate, asked patient about his or her breathing.
    ____ ____ ____ _____

23. Recorded drug, dose, route, inhalations, and time on MAR.
    ____ ____ ____ _____

24. Recorded patient teaching and validation of understanding in appropriate log.
    ____ ____ ____ _____

25. Asked patient to explain when to use medication.
    ____ ____ ____ _____

Copyright © 2018 by Elsevier Inc. All rights reserved.

Student _____ Date _____

Instructor _____ Date _____

PERFORMANCE CHECKLIST SKILL 21.8 **USING SMALL-VOLUME NEBULIZERS**

	S	U	NP	Comments

ASSESSMENT

1. Checked accuracy and completeness of each MAR against medication order, clarified incomplete or unclear orders with health care provider. ___ ___ ___ _____

2. Reviewed pertinent information related to medication. ___ ___ ___ _____

3. Assessed patient's medical history, history of allergies, and medication history, listed drug allergies on MAR and provided allergy bracelet if necessary. ___ ___ ___ _____

4. Assessed patient's ability to grasp and ability to assemble, hold, and manipulate nebulizer equipment. ___ ___ ___ _____

5. Assessed pulse, respirations, breath sounds, pulse oximetry, and peak flow measurement if ordered. ___ ___ ___ _____

6. Assessed patient's knowledge of medication and readiness to learn. ___ ___ ___ _____

7. Assessed patient's ability to learn. ___ ___ ___ _____

8. Assessed patient's ability to manipulate nebulizer mouthpiece and tubing. ___ ___ ___ _____

PLANNING

1. Identified expected outcomes. ___ ___ ___ _____

2. Collected appropriate equipment and MAR. ___ ___ ___ _____

IMPLEMENTATION

1. Performed hand hygiene, prepared medications for inhalation, checked label of medication against MAR twice, checked expiration date. ___ ___ ___ _____

2. Took medication(s) to patient at correct time, applied the six rights of medication administration, performed hand hygiene. ___ ___ ___ _____

3. Identified patient using at least two identifiers, compared with information on MAR. ___ ___ ___ _____

4. Compared MAR with medication labels at patient's bedside, asked patient if he or she had allergies. ___ ___ ___ _____

Copyright © 2018 by Elsevier Inc. All rights reserved.

	S	U	NP	Comments

5. Explained procedure, discussed purpose of each medication, action, and possible adverse effects; allowed patient to ask any questions; explained how to manipulate nebulizer.   ___ ___ ___ _____

6. Assembled nebulizer equipment properly.   ___ ___ ___ _____

7. Added prescribed medication by pouring medicine into nebulizer cup or using dropper or syringe and diluent to instill medication.   ___ ___ ___ _____

8. Attached top securely to nebulizer cup, connected cup to mouthpiece or mask.   ___ ___ ___ _____

9. Connected tubing to aerosol compressor and nebulizer cup.   ___ ___ ___ _____

10. Had patient hold mouthpiece between lips or used mask or adapter.   ___ ___ ___ _____

11. Turned on machine, ensured a sufficient mist was formed.   ___ ___ ___ _____

12. Had patient take a deep breath; encouraged brief, end-inspiratory pause; had patient exhale passively:

   a. Encouraged dyspneic patient to hold every fourth or fifth breath for 5 to 10 seconds.   ___ ___ ___ _____

   b. Reminded patient to repeat breathing pattern until drug was completely nebulized.   ___ ___ ___ _____

   c. Tapped nebulizer cup occasionally.   ___ ___ ___ _____

   d. Monitored patient's pulse during procedure.   ___ ___ ___ _____

13. Turned machine off when medication was completely nebulized, rinsed nebulizer cup per agency policy, dried completely, stored tubing assembly per policy.   ___ ___ ___ _____

14. Instructed patient to rinse and gargle with warm water if steroids were nebulized.   ___ ___ ___ _____

15. Had patient take several breaths and cough after treatment was complete.   ___ ___ ___ _____

16. Assisted patient to comfortable position, performed hand hygiene.   ___ ___ ___ _____

EVALUATION

1. Assessed patient's respirations, breath sounds, cough effort, sputum production, pulse oximetry, and peak flow measures if ordered.   ___ ___ ___ _____

2. Asked patient to explain drug schedule.   ___ ___ ___ _____

Copyright © 2018 by Elsevier Inc. All rights reserved.

	S	U	NP	Comments

3. Asked patient to describe side effects of medication and criteria for calling health care provider. ___ ___ ___ _____

4. Asked patient to explain steps in putting together nebulizer and adding medication. ___ ___ ___ _____

5. Identified unexpected outcomes. ___ ___ ___ _____

RECORDING AND REPORTING

1. Recorded drug, dose, route, length of treatment, and time on MAR. ___ ___ ___ _____

2. Recorded patient teaching and validation of understanding in appropriate log. ___ ___ ___ _____

3. Recorded patient's response to treatment in appropriate log. ___ ___ ___ _____

4. Reported adverse effects/patient response/ withheld drugs to nurse in charge or health care provider. ___ ___ ___ _____

Copyright © 2018 by Elsevier Inc. All rights reserved.

Student _____ Date _____

Instructor _____ Date _____

PERFORMANCE CHECKLIST SKILL 21.9 **ADMINISTERING VAGINAL INSTILLATIONS**

	S	U	NP	Comments
ASSESSMENT				
1. Checked accuracy and completeness of each MAR against medication order, clarified incomplete and unclear orders with health care provider.	___	___	___	_____
2. Reviewed pertinent information related to medication.	___	___	___	_____
3. Assessed patient's medical history, history of allergies, and medication history, listed drug allergies on MAR and provided allergy bracelet if necessary.	___	___	___	_____
4. Performed hand hygiene, applied clean gloves, inspected condition of vaginal tissues during perineal care, noted if drainage was present, removed gloves, performed hand hygiene.	___	___	___	_____
5. Asked if patient was experiencing any symptoms of pruritus, burning, or discomfort.	___	___	___	_____
6. Assessed patient's knowledge of medication and readiness to learn.	___	___	___	_____
7. Assessed patient's ability to manipulate applicator, suppository, or irrigation equipment and to properly position self to insert medication.	___	___	___	_____
PLANNING				
1. Identified expected outcomes.	___	___	___	_____
2. Collected appropriate equipment and MAR.	___	___	___	_____
IMPLEMENTATION				
1. Performed hand hygiene, prepared suppository for administration, checked label of medication against MAR twice, checked expiration date.	___	___	___	_____
2. Took medication(s) to patient at correct time, applied the six rights of medication administration, performed hand hygiene.	___	___	___	_____
3. Identified patient using at least two identifiers, compared with information on MAR.	___	___	___	_____
4. Compared MAR with medication labels at patient's bedside, asked patient if he or she had allergies.	___	___	___	_____

266

Copyright © 2018 by Elsevier Inc. All rights reserved.

	S	U	NP	Comments

5. Explained procedure, discussed purpose of each medication, action, and possible adverse effects; allowed patient to ask any questions; explained procedure if patient planned to self-administer medication.

6. Arranged supplies at bedside, applied clean gloves, provided privacy.

7. Had patient void, assisted patient to proper position.

8. Kept abdomen and lower extremities draped.

9. Ensured vaginal orifice was well illuminated, positioned lamp if necessary.

10. Inserted vaginal suppository:

   a. Removed suppository from wrapper, applied lubricant to rounded end and gloved index finger, ensured suppository was room temperature.

   b. Separated labial folds in front-to-back direction.

   c. Inserted rounded end of suppository along posterior wall of vaginal canal.

   d. Withdrew finger and wiped remaining lubricant from around labia with tissue.

11. Applied cream or foam:

   a. Filled cream or foam applicator following package directions.

   b. Separated labial folds with nondominant-gloved hand.

   c. Inserted applicator properly with dominant gloved hand, pushed applicator plunger to deposit medication into vagina.

   d. Withdrew applicator and placed on paper towel, wiped off residual cream from labia or vaginal orifice with tissue.

12. Administered irrigation and douche:

   a. Placed patient on bedpan with absorbent pad underneath.

   b. Ensured irrigation or douche fluid was at body temperature, ran fluid through container nozzle.

   c. Separated labial folds, directed nozzle toward sacrum.

Copyright © 2018 by Elsevier Inc. All rights reserved.

	S	U	NP	Comments

d. Raised container appropriately above level of vagina, inserted nozzle appropriately, allowed solution to flow while rotating nozzle, administered all irrigating solution.

e. Withdrew nozzle, assisted patient to comfortable position.

f. Allowed patient to remain on bedpan for a few minutes, cleansed perineum with soap and water.

g. Assisted patient off bedpan, dried perineal area.

13. Instructed patient who received suppository, cream, or tablet to remain on back for at least 10 minutes.

14. Washed applicator with soap and water, rinsed, and stored for future use.

15. Offered perineal pad when patient resumes ambulation.

16. Discarded gloves and soiled equipment appropriately, performed hand hygiene.

EVALUATION

1. Performed hand hygiene, applied clean gloves, inspected condition of vaginal canal and external genitalia between applications, assessed vaginal discharge if present, removed gloves, performed hand hygiene.

2. Questioned patient regarding continued pruritus, burning, discomfort, or discharge.

3. Asked patient to discuss purpose, action, and side effects of medication.

4. Asked patient to explain how to draw cream into applicator.

5. Identified unexpected outcomes.

RECORDING AND REPORTING

1. Recorded drug, dose, type of instillation, and time on MAR.

2. Recorded patient teaching, validation of understanding, and ability to self-administer medication in appropriate log.

3. Reported to health care provider if patient stated symptoms persisted or got worse.

4. Reported adverse effects/patient response/withheld drugs to nurse in charge or health care provider.

Copyright © 2018 by Elsevier Inc. All rights reserved.

Student _____   Date _____

Instructor _____   Date _____

PERFORMANCE CHECKLIST SKILL 21.10   **ADMINISTERING RECTAL SUPPOSITORIES**

	S	U	NP	Comments

ASSESSMENT

1. Checked accuracy and completeness of each MAR against medication order, clarified incomplete and unclear orders with health care provider.

2. Reviewed pertinent information related to medication.

3. Assessed patient's medical history for rectal surgeries or cardiac or bleeding problems, history of allergies, and medication history, listed drug allergies on MAR and provided allergy bracelet if necessary.

4. Reviewed any presenting signs of GI alterations.

5. Assessed patient's ability to hold suppository and position self to insert medication.

6. Reviewed patient's knowledge of purpose of drug therapy and interest in self-administering suppository.

PLANNING

1. Identified expected outcomes.

2. Collected appropriate equipment and MAR.

IMPLEMENTATION

1. Performed hand hygiene, prepared suppository for administration, checked label of medication against MAR twice, checked expiration date.

2. Took medication(s) to patient at correct time, applied the six rights of medication administration, performed hand hygiene.

3. Identified patient using at least two identifiers, compared with information on MAR.

4. Compared MAR with medication labels at patient's bedside, asked patient if he or she had allergies.

Copyright © 2018 by Elsevier Inc. All rights reserved.

5. Explained procedure, discussed purpose of each medication, action, and possible adverse effects; allowed patient to ask any questions; explained procedure if patient planned to self-administer medication.

   —   —   —   ————————

6. Arranged supplies at bedside, applied clean gloves, provided privacy.

   —   —   —   ————————

7. Assisted patient to proper position.

   —   —   —   ————————

8. Kept patient draped with only anal area exposed.

   —   —   —   ————————

9. Examined condition of anus externally, palpated rectal walls as needed, disposed of gloves properly if necessary.

   —   —   —   ————————

10. Performed hand hygiene, applied clean gloves if necessary.

   —   —   —   ————————

11. Removed suppository from wrapper, lubricated round end of suppository and index finger, handled area gently if patient had hemorrhoids.

   —   —   —   ————————

12. Asked patient to take slow, deep breaths through mouth and relax anal sphincter.

   —   —   —   ————————

13. Retracted patient's buttocks with nondominant hand, inserted suppository properly.

   —   —   —   ————————

14. Gave suppository through colostomy if ordered.

   —   —   —   ————————

15. Withdrew finger, wiped patient's anal area.

   —   —   —   ————————

16. Asked patient to remain flat for 5 minutes.

   —   —   —   ————————

17. Discarded gloves and supplies in appropriate receptacle, performed hand hygiene.

   —   —   —   ————————

18. Placed call light within reach if suppository contained laxative or fecal softener.

   —   —   —   ————————

19. Reminded patient *not* to flush commode after bowel movement if suppository was given for constipation.

   —   —   —   ————————

EVALUATION

1. Returned to bedside within 5 minutes to determine if suppository was expelled.

   —   —   —   ————————

2. Asked if patient experienced localized anal or rectal discomfort during insertion.

   —   —   —   ————————

3. Evaluated patient for relief of symptoms at appropriate time.

   —   —   —   ————————

4. Asked patient to explain steps to insert suppository.

   —   —   —   ————————

5. Identified unexpected outcomes.

   —   —   —   ————————

Copyright © 2018 by Elsevier Inc. All rights reserved.

	S	U	NP	Comments

RECORDING AND REPORTING

1. Recorded drug, dose, route, and time on MAR. ___ ___ ___ _____

2. Recorded patient response, teaching, and validation of understanding and ability to self-administer medication in appropriate log. ___ ___ ___ _____

3. Reported adverse effects/patient response/ withheld drugs to nurse in charge or health care provider. ___ ___ ___ _____

Copyright © 2018 by Elsevier Inc. All rights reserved.

Student _____ Date _____

Instructor _____ Date _____

PERFORMANCE CHECKLIST SKILL 22.1   **PREPARING INJECTIONS: AMPULES AND VIALS**

	S	U	NP	Comments
ASSESSMENT				
1. Checked accuracy and completeness of each MAR with medication order, reprinted any portion of MAR that was difficult to read.	___	___	___	_____
2. Assessed patient's medical and medication history.	___	___	___	_____
3. Assessed patient's history of allergies, knew types of allergies and normal response.	___	___	___	_____
4. Reviewed medication reference information.	___	___	___	_____
5. Assessed patient's body build, muscle size, and weight if giving subcutaneous or IM medication.	___	___	___	_____
PLANNING				
1. Identify expected outcomes.	___	___	___	_____
IMPLEMENTATION				
1. Performed hand hygiene, prepared supplies.	___	___	___	_____
2. Prepared medications:				
a. Moved medication cart outside patient's room if being used.	___	___	___	_____
b. Unlocked medication cart or logged onto computerized dispensing system.	___	___	___	_____
c. Followed "No-Interruption Zone" policy, prepared medication for one patient at a time, kept all pages of MARs for one patient together, looked at only one patient's electronic MAR at a time.	___	___	___	_____
d. Selected correct drug, compared label with MAR.	___	___	___	_____
e. Checked expiration date on each medication.	___	___	___	_____
f. Calculated drug dose as necessary, double-checked calculations, asked another nurse if needed.	___	___	___	_____
g. Checked record for previous drug count and compared with supply if preparing a controlled substance.	___	___	___	_____
h. Did not leave drugs unattended.	___	___	___	_____

   Copyright © 2018 by Elsevier Inc. All rights reserved.

	S	U	NP	Comments

3. Prepared ampule:

a. Tapped top of ampule until fluid moved from neck of ampule. ____ ____ ____ _____

b. Placed gauze pad around neck of ampule. ____ ____ ____ _____

c. Snapped neck of ampule properly. ____ ____ ____ _____

d. Drew up medication quickly, used a long enough filter needle. ____ ____ ____ _____

e. Held ampule properly, inserted filter needle, did not allow needle to touch rim of ampule. ____ ____ ____ _____

f. Aspirated medication into syringe. ____ ____ ____ _____

g. Kept needle tip under surface of liquid, tipped ampule if needed. ____ ____ ____ _____

h. Did not expel air if air bubbles were aspirated. ____ ____ ____ _____

i. Expelled air bubble properly outside of ampule, did not eject fluid. ____ ____ ____ _____

j. Used sink for disposal of excess fluid, rechecked fluid level in syringe properly. ____ ____ ____ _____

k. Covered needle with safety sheath, replaced filter needle with regular SESIP needle. ____ ____ ____ _____

4. Prepared vial containing solution:

a. Removed cap covering top of unused vial, wiped surface of rubber seal with alcohol, allowed it to dry. ____ ____ ____ _____

b. Picked up syringe, removed cap, drew amount of air into syringe equivalent to volume of medication to be aspirated. ____ ____ ____ _____

c. Inserted needle or needleless device through center of rubber seal, applied pressure to tip of needle during insertion. ____ ____ ____ _____

d. Injected air into air space of vial, held plunger firmly. ____ ____ ____ _____

e. Inverted vial, kept hold on syringe and plunger, grasped so as to counteract pressure in vial. ____ ____ ____ _____

f. Kept tip of needle below fluid level. ____ ____ ____ _____

g. Allowed air pressure to fill syringe gradually with medication, pulled back on plunger if necessary. ____ ____ ____ _____

h. Positioned needle into air space of vial when desired volume is obtained, dislodged air bubbles, ejected air in top of syringe. ____ ____ ____ _____

Copyright © 2018 by Elsevier Inc. All rights reserved.

	S	U	NP	Comments

i. Removed needle or needleless access device from vial. ___ ___ ___ _____

j. Held syringe properly, ensured correct volume and absence of air bubbles, dislodged any remaining air bubbles, ejected any air, rechecked volume of medication. ___ ___ ___ _____

k. Changed needle to appropriate gauge and length if necessary. ___ ___ ___ _____

l. Covered needle with safety sheath or cap. ___ ___ ___ _____

m. Labeled vial properly if using multi-dose vial. ___ ___ ___ _____

5. Prepared vial containing a powder:

a. Removed cap covering vials of medication and diluent, swabbed both seals with alcohol, allowed to dry. ___ ___ ___ _____

b. Drew appropriate volume of diluent into syringe. ___ ___ ___ _____

c. Inserted needle or needleless device through rubber seal of vial of powdered medication, injected diluent, removed needle. ___ ___ ___ _____

d. Mixed medication thoroughly, rolled in palms, did not shake. ___ ___ ___ _____

e. Determined appropriate dose after reconstitution. ___ ___ ___ _____

f. Drew medication into syringe, did not add additional air, followed steps 4e–4l. ___ ___ ___ _____

6. Compared level of medication with MAR. ___ ___ ___ _____

7. Disposed of soiled supplies, placed broken ampule/used vials and used needle or needleless device in puncture- and leak-proof container, cleaned work area, performed hand hygiene. ___ ___ ___ _____

EVALUATION

1. Compared MAR with label of prepared drug, compared dose in syringe with desired dose. ___ ___ ___ _____

2. Identified unexpected outcomes. ___ ___ ___ _____

Copyright © 2018 by Elsevier Inc. All rights reserved.

Student _____ Date _____

Instructor _____ Date _____

PERFORMANCE CHECKLIST PROCEDURAL GUIDELINE 22.1 **MIXING PARENTERAL MEDICATIONS IN ONE SYRINGE**

	S	U	NP	Comments

ASSESSMENT

1. Checked accuracy and completeness of MAR with medication order, reprinted/recopied any portion of MAR that was difficult to read. ⎯⎯ ⎯⎯ ⎯⎯ _____

2. Reviewed pertinent information related to medication. ⎯⎯ ⎯⎯ ⎯⎯ _____

3. Assessed patient's body build, muscle size, and weight if giving subcutaneous or IM medication. ⎯⎯ ⎯⎯ ⎯⎯ _____

4. Considered compatibility of medications to be mixed and type of injection. ⎯⎯ ⎯⎯ ⎯⎯ _____

5. Checked medication's expiration date printed on vial. ⎯⎯ ⎯⎯ ⎯⎯ _____

6. Performed hand hygiene. ⎯⎯ ⎯⎯ ⎯⎯ _____

7. Prepared medication for one patient at a time, followed the six rights of medication administration, selected ampule or vial from drawer or system, compared label of each medication with MAR, ensured correct types of insulin were prepared if necessary. ⎯⎯ ⎯⎯ ⎯⎯ _____

8. Mixed medication from two vials:

   a. Aspirated volume of air equivalent to first medication dose using syringe with needleless device or filter needle. ⎯⎯ ⎯⎯ ⎯⎯ _____

   b. Injected air into vial A, ensured needle or needleless device did not touch solution. ⎯⎯ ⎯⎯ ⎯⎯ _____

   c. Held plunger, withdrew needle and syringe from vial A, aspirated air equivalent to second medication dose into syringe. ⎯⎯ ⎯⎯ ⎯⎯ _____

   d. Inserted needle or device into vial B, injected volume of air into vial B, withdrew medication into syringe. ⎯⎯ ⎯⎯ ⎯⎯ _____

   e. Withdrew needle and syringe from vial B, ensured proper volume had been obtained. ⎯⎯ ⎯⎯ ⎯⎯ _____

   f. Determined what combined value of medications should measure. ⎯⎯ ⎯⎯ ⎯⎯ _____

Copyright © 2018 by Elsevier Inc. All rights reserved.

	S	U	NP	Comments

g. Inserted needle or device into vial A, ensured no medication was expelled into vial, inverted vial, withdrew desired amount of medication into syringe. ____ ____ ____ _____

h. Withdrew needle or device, expelled excess air, checked fluid level in syringe. ____ ____ ____ _____

i. Changed needle or device for appropriate-sized needle if medication was being injected, kept device capped until administration time. ____ ____ ____ _____

9. Mixed insulin:

a. Rolled bottle to resuspend insulin preparation if necessary. ____ ____ ____ _____

b. Wiped off tops of both insulin vials with alcohol. ____ ____ ____ _____

c. Verified insulin dose against MAR. ____ ____ ____ _____

d. Prepared insulin in the proper order if relevant. ____ ____ ____ _____

e. Inserted needle, injected air into first vial, did not let tip of needle touch solution. ____ ____ ____ _____

f. Removed syringe from vial of insulin without aspirating medication. ____ ____ ____ _____

g. Injected air equal to dose of second medication into vial, withdrew correct dose into syringe. ____ ____ ____ _____

h. Removed syringe from vial of insulin without aspirating medication. ____ ____ ____ _____

i. Verified second dosage with MAR, verified with another nurse, determined and verified combined dosage. ____ ____ ____ _____

j. Placed needle back in first vial, ensured no insulin was pushed into vial. ____ ____ ____ _____

k. Inverted vial, withdrew desired amount of insulin into syringe. ____ ____ ____ _____

l. Withdrew needle, checked fluid level in syringe, kept needle sheathed or capped until administration. ____ ____ ____ _____

10. Mixed medications from a vial and an ampule:

a. Prepared medication from vial first as in Skill 22.1. ____ ____ ____ _____

b. Determined what combined volume of medications should measure. ____ ____ ____ _____

c. Used same syringe to prepare medication from ampule as in Skill 22.1. ____ ____ ____ _____

276

Copyright © 2018 by Elsevier Inc. All rights reserved.

	S	U	NP	Comments
d. Withdrew filter needle from ampule, verified fluid level in syringe, changed needle to appropriate SESIP needle, kept device or needle sheathed or capped until administration.	——	——	——	_____
e. Checked syringe for total combined dose of medications.	——	——	——	_____
11. Compared MAR and labels on vials/ampules.	——	——	——	_____
12. Disposed of soiled supplies, placed used ampules/vials and needle or needleless device in puncture- and leak-proof container.	——	——	——	_____
13. Cleaned work area, performed hand hygiene.	——	——	——	_____
14. Checked syringe again for total combined dose.	——	——	——	_____
15. Performed third check for accuracy at patient's bedside.	——	——	——	_____

Copyright © 2018 by Elsevier Inc. All rights reserved.

Student _____   Date _____

Instructor _____   Date _____

PERFORMANCE CHECKLIST SKILL 22.2   **ADMINISTERING INTRADERMAL INJECTIONS**

	S	U	NP	Comments

ASSESSMENT

1. Checked accuracy and completeness of MAR with medication order, recopied any portion of MAR that was difficult to read.   ___ ___ ___ _____

2. Reviewed medication reference information about expected reaction when testing skin with allergen.   ___ ___ ___ _____

3. Assessed patient's history of allergies, known type of allergens, and normal allergic reaction.   ___ ___ ___ _____

4. Assessed for contraindications to ID injections and history of severe adverse reactions to ID injections.   ___ ___ ___ _____

5. Assessed patient's knowledge of purpose and response to skin testing.   ___ ___ ___ _____

6. Checked expiration date for medication.   ___ ___ ___ _____

PLANNING

1. Identified expected outcomes.   ___ ___ ___ _____

IMPLEMENTATION

1. Prepared medications for one patient at a time, checked label of medication with MAR twice.   ___ ___ ___ _____

2. Took medication to patient at correct time, applied the six rights of medication administration.   ___ ___ ___ _____

3. Provided privacy.   ___ ___ ___ _____

4. Identified patient using at least two identifiers, compared identifiers with information in patient's MAR.   ___ ___ ___ _____

5. Compared MAR with medication labels at patient's bedside, asked patient if he or she had allergies.   ___ ___ ___ _____

6. Discussed the purpose of each medication, action, and possible adverse effects; allowed patient to ask any questions, told patient injection will cause burning.   ___ ___ ___ _____

7. Performed hand hygiene, applied clean gloves, kept sheet draped over body parts not requiring exposure.   ___ ___ ___ _____

Copyright © 2018 by Elsevier Inc. All rights reserved.

	S	U	NP	Comments

8. Selected appropriate site, noted lesions or discoloration of skin. ___ ___ ___ _____

9. Assisted patient to comfortable position, had patient extend elbow and support forearm on flat surface. ___ ___ ___ _____

10. Cleansed site with antiseptic swab. ___ ___ ___ _____

11. Held swab or gauze properly. ___ ___ ___ _____

12. Removed needle cap. ___ ___ ___ _____

13. Held syringe properly with bevel of needle pointing up. ___ ___ ___ _____

14. Administered injection:

   a. Stretched skin over site with nondominant hand. ___ ___ ___ _____

   b. Inserted needle properly into skin, advanced to appropriate depth. ___ ___ ___ _____

   c. Injected medication slowly, reinserted needle if necessary. ___ ___ ___ _____

   d. Noted that small bleb appeared on skin surface. ___ ___ ___ _____

   e. Withdrew needle, applied alcohol swab or gauze over site. ___ ___ ___ _____

15. Assisted patient to comfortable position. ___ ___ ___ _____

16. Discarded needle in puncture- and leak-proof container. ___ ___ ___ _____

17. Removed gloves, performed hand hygiene. ___ ___ ___ _____

18. Stayed with patient, observed for allergic reactions. ___ ___ ___ _____

EVALUATION

1. Returned to room in 15 to 30 minutes; asked if patient felt pain, burning, numbness, or tingling at injection site. ___ ___ ___ _____

2. Asked patient to discuss implications of skin testing and signs of hypersensitivity. ___ ___ ___ _____

3. Inspected bleb, drew circle around injection site with skin pencil if necessary, read TB test at appropriate time. ___ ___ ___ _____

4. Asked patient to explain what TB test site might look like in a few days. ___ ___ ___ _____

5. Identified unexpected outcomes. ___ ___ ___ _____

Copyright © 2018 by Elsevier Inc. All rights reserved.

	S	U	NP	Comments

RECORDING AND REPORTING

1. Recorded drug, dose, route, site, and time on MAR; signed MAR. ____ ____ ____ _____

2. Recorded area of ID injection and appearance of skin. ____ ____ ____ _____

3. Reported undesirable effects to health care provider, documented adverse effects properly. ____ ____ ____ _____

4. Recorded patient teaching, validation of understanding, and patient's response to medication. ____ ____ ____ _____

Copyright © 2018 by Elsevier Inc. All rights reserved.

Student _____ Date _____

Instructor _____ Date _____

PERFORMANCE CHECKLIST SKILL 22.3 **ADMINISTERING SUBCUTANEOUS INJECTIONS**

	S	U	NP	Comments
ASSESSMENT				
1. Checked accuracy and completeness of MAR with medication order, reprinted/recopied any portion of MAR that was difficult to read.	___	___	___	_____
2. Assessed patient's medical and medication history.	___	___	___	_____
3. Assessed patient's history of allergies.	___	___	___	_____
4. Reviewed all relevant medication information.	___	___	___	_____
5. Checked expiration date for medication.	___	___	___	_____
6. Observed patient's previous verbal and nonverbal responses to injection.	___	___	___	_____
7. Assessed for contraindication to subcutaneous injections.	___	___	___	_____
8. Assessed patient's symptoms before initiating therapy.	___	___	___	_____
9. Assessed adequacy of patient's adipose tissue.	___	___	___	_____
10. Assessed relevant laboratory results.	___	___	___	_____
11. Assessed patient's knowledge of medication.	___	___	___	_____
PLANNING				
1. Identified expected outcomes.	___	___	___	_____
IMPLEMENTATION				
1. Performed hand hygiene, prepared medication using aseptic technique, checked label of medication with MAR twice.	___	___	___	_____
2. Took medication(s) to patient at correct time, applied the six rights of medication administration, performed hand hygiene.	___	___	___	_____
3. Provided privacy.	___	___	___	_____
4. Identified patient using at least two identifiers.	___	___	___	_____
5. Compared MAR with medication labels at bedside, asked patient if he or she had allergies.	___	___	___	_____
6. Discussed purpose of each medication, action, and possible adverse effects; allowed patient to ask questions; told patient injection would cause a slight burning or stinging sensation.	___	___	___	_____

Copyright © 2018 by Elsevier Inc. All rights reserved.

	S	U	NP	Comments

7. Performed hand hygiene, applied clean gloves, kept sheet draped over body parts not requiring exposure.

8. Selected appropriate injection site, inspected skin over site.

9. Palpated sites, avoided those with masses or tenderness, ensured needle was correct size by measuring skinfold:

   a. Used abdominal or thigh injection sites when administering insulin or heparin.

   b. Chose side abdominal site when administering LMWH.

   c. Rotated insulin site appropriately.

10. Assisted patient to comfortable position, had patient relax site.

11. Relocated site using anatomical landmarks.

12. Cleansed site properly with antiseptic swab.

13. Held swab in nondominant hand.

14. Removed needle cap or sheath.

15. Held syringe properly in dominant hand.

16. Administered injection:

   a. Held skin across injection site.

   b. Injected needle at appropriate angle quickly and firmly, released skin if pinched.

   c. Adjusted injection technique for obese patient if necessary.

   d. Stabilized lower end of syringe barrel with nondominant hand, injected medication slowly, avoided moving syringe.

   e. Withdrew needle quickly while placing swab or gauze over site.

17. Applied pressure to site, did not massage site.

18. Assisted patient to comfortable position.

19. Discarded uncapped needle or needle enclosed in safety shield and attached syringe into puncture- and leak-proof receptacle.

20. Removed gloves, performed hand hygiene.

21. Stayed with patient for several minutes, observed for any allergic reactions.

Copyright © 2018 by Elsevier Inc. All rights reserved.

	S	U	NP	Comments

EVALUATION

1. Returned to room in 15 to 30 minutes; asked if patient felt pain, burning, numbness, or tingling at injection site.

2. Inspected site, noted bruising or induration, provided warm compress to site.

3. Observed patient's response to medication at time correlating with medication's onset, peak, and duration, reviewed laboratory results.

4. Asked patient to explain reason for injection.

5. Identified unexpected outcomes.

RECORDING AND REPORTING

1. Recorded medication, dose, route, site, and time on MAR immediately after administration; signed MAR properly.

2. Recorded patient teaching, validation of understanding, and patient's response to medication in appropriate log.

3. Reported any undesirable effects to health care provider, documented adverse effects in record.

Copyright © 2018 by Elsevier Inc. All rights reserved.

Student _____ Date _____

Instructor _____ Date _____

PERFORMANCE CHECKLIST SKILL 22.4 ADMINISTERING INTRAMUSCULAR INJECTIONS

	S	U	NP	Comments

ASSESSMENT

1. Checked accuracy and completeness of each MAR with medication order, reprinted/recopied any portion of MAR that was difficult to read.

2. Assessed patient's medical and medication history.

3. Assessed patient's history of allergies.

4. Reviewed medication reference information.

5. Checked expiration date for medication.

6. Observed patient's previous verbal and nonverbal responses toward injection.

7. Assessed for contraindications to IM injections.

8. Assessed patient's symptoms before initiating therapy.

9. Assessed patient's knowledge regarding medication to be received.

PLANNING

1. Identified expected outcomes.

IMPLEMENTATION

1. Prepared medication for one patient at a time, kept all pages of MAR for one patient together, checked label of medication with MAR twice.

2. Took medication(s) to patient at correct time, applied the six rights of medication administration, performed hand hygiene.

3. Provided privacy.

4. Identified patient using at least two identifiers, compared identifiers with information on patient's MAR.

5. Compared MAR with medication labels at bedside, asked patient if he or she has allergies.

6. Discussed purpose of each medication, action, and possible adverse effects, told patient injection would cause burning.

Copyright © 2018 by Elsevier Inc. All rights reserved.

	S	U	NP	Comments

7. Performed hand hygiene, applied clean gloves, kept sheet over body parts not requiring exposure.

8. Selected appropriate site, noted integrity and size of muscle, palpated for and avoided areas of tenderness or hardness, rotated sites if necessary.

9. Assisted patient to comfortable position.

10. Relocated site using anatomical landmarks.

11. Cleansed site with antiseptic swab.

12. Held swab in nondominant hand.

13. Removed needle cap or sheath.

14. Held syringe properly in dominant hand.

15. Administered injection:

   a. Positioned nondominant hand below site and pulled skin, injected needle appropriately into muscle.

   b. Grasped body of muscle if necessary.

   c. Stabilized end of syringe barrel, moved dominant hand to plunger, avoided moving syringe.

   d. Pulled back on plunger, injected medication slowly if no blood appeared.

   e. Waited 10 seconds, withdrew needle, released skin, applied gauze over site.

16. Applied pressure to site, did not massage site, applied bandage if needed.

17. Helped patient to comfortable position.

18. Discarded needle and syringe into a puncture- and leak-proof receptacle.

19. Removed gloves, performed hand hygiene.

20. Stayed with patient, observed for allergic reactions.

EVALUATION

1. Returned to room in 15 to 30 minutes; asked if patient felt any pain, numbness, or tingling at injection site.

2. Inspected site, noted bruising or induration, applied warm compress to site.

3. Observed patient's response to medication at times that correlate with medication's onset, peak, and duration.

Copyright © 2018 by Elsevier Inc. All rights reserved.

	S	U	NP	Comments

4. Asked patient to explain the need for the injections and what to expect. ___ ___ ___ _____

5. Identified unexpected outcomes. ___ ___ ___ _____

RECORDING AND REPORTING

1. Recorded medication, dose, route, site, and time given on MAR immediately after administration; signed MAR properly. ___ ___ ___ _____

2. Recorded patient's teaching, validation of understanding, and patient's response to medication in appropriate log. ___ ___ ___ _____

3. Reported any undesirable effects to health care provider, documented adverse effects in record. ___ ___ ___ _____

286

Copyright © 2018 by Elsevier Inc. All rights reserved.

Student _____ Date _____

Instructor _____ Date _____

PERFORMANCE CHECKLIST SKILL 22.5 **ADMINISTERING MEDICATIONS BY INTRAVENOUS BOLUS**

	S	U	NP	Comments
ASSESSMENT				
1. Checked accuracy and completeness of each MAR with medication order, reprinted/recopied any portion of MAR that was difficult to read.	___	___	___	_____
2. Assessed patient's medical and medication history.	___	___	___	_____
3. Reviewed medication reference information.	___	___	___	_____
4. Determined compatibility with IV fluids and additives if necessary.	___	___	___	_____
5. Performed hand hygiene, assessed condition of insertion site for signs of infiltration of phlebitis.	___	___	___	_____
6. Assessed patency of patient's existing IV infusion line or saline lock.	___	___	___	_____
7. Checked patient's history of medication allergies.	___	___	___	_____
8. Assessed patient's symptoms before initiating medication therapy.	___	___	___	_____
9. Assessed patient's understanding of purpose of drug therapy.	___	___	___	_____
PLANNING				
1. Identified expected outcomes.	___	___	___	_____
IMPLEMENTATION				
1. Prepared medications for one patient at a time, kept all pages of MAR for one patient together, checked label of medication with MAR twice.	___	___	___	_____
2. Took medication(s) to patient at the proper time, applied the six rights of medication.	___	___	___	_____
3. Provided privacy.	___	___	___	_____
4. Identified patient using at least two identifiers, compared identifiers with information on MAR.	___	___	___	_____
5. Compared MAR with medication labels at bedside, asked patient if he or she had allergies.	___	___	___	_____

Copyright © 2018 by Elsevier Inc. All rights reserved.

	S	U	NP	Comments

6. Discussed purpose of each medication, action, and possible adverse effects; allowed patient to ask any questions; explained that medication would be given through existing IV line; encouraged patient to report symptoms of discomfort at IV site. ____ ____ ____ _____

7. Performed hand hygiene, applied clean gloves. ____ ____ ____ _____

8. Performed IV push using existing line:

   a. Selected injection port of IV closest to patient, used needleless injection port. ____ ____ ____ _____

   b. Cleaned injection port with antiseptic swab, allowed to dry. ____ ____ ____ _____

   c. Connected needleless tip of syringe to IV line. ____ ____ ____ _____

   d. Occluded IV line by pinching tubing, aspirated for blood return. ____ ____ ____ _____

   e. Released tubing, injected medication, timed administration, allowed IV to infuse when not pushing medication. ____ ____ ____ _____

   f. Withdrew syringe, rechecked IV fluid infusion rate. ____ ____ ____ _____

   g. Stopped IV fluids, clamped line, and flushed line if medication was incompatible with fluids; flushed again after administration at *same rate* as medication. ____ ____ ____ _____

   h. Verified agency policy for stopping IV fluids and medications, disconnected IV line and administered IV push or started a new IV site as appropriate. ____ ____ ____ _____

9. Performed IV push using IV lock:

   a. Prepared flush solutions according to agency policy. ____ ____ ____ _____

   b. Administered medication.

     (1) Cleaned injection port with antiseptic swab. ____ ____ ____ _____

     (2) Inserted syringe with normal saline 0.9% through injection port of IV lock. ____ ____ ____ _____

     (3) Pulled back on plunger, checked for blood return. ____ ____ ____ _____

     (4) Flushed IV site. ____ ____ ____ _____

     (5) Removed saline-filled syringe. ____ ____ ____ _____

     (6) Cleaned injection port with antiseptic swab. ____ ____ ____ _____

Copyright © 2018 by Elsevier Inc. All rights reserved.

	S	U	NP	Comments
(7) Inserted syringe containing prepared medication through injection port.	——	——	——	_____
(8) Injected medication, used a watch to time administration.	——	——	——	_____
(9) Withdrew syringe.	——	——	——	_____
(10) Cleaned injection port with antiseptic swab.	——	——	——	_____
(11) Flushed injection port, injected flush at the same rate medication was delivered.	——	——	——	_____
10. Disposed of uncapped needles and syringes in puncture- and leak-proof container.	——	——	——	_____
11. Stayed with patient for several minutes, observed for allergic reactions.	——	——	——	_____
12. Removed gloves, performed hand hygiene.	——	——	——	_____

EVALUATION

	S	U	NP	Comments
1. Observed patient for adverse reactions during and after administration.	——	——	——	_____
2. Observed IV site during and after injection for sudden swelling.	——	——	——	_____
3. Assessed patient's status after giving medication to evaluate effectiveness.	——	——	——	_____
4. Asked patient to explain what medication is for and when to call the nurse.	——	——	——	_____
5. Identified unexpected outcomes.	——	——	——	_____

RECORDING AND REPORTING

	S	U	NP	Comments
1. Recorded drug, dose, route, and time on MAR immediately after administration; included initials or signature.	——	——	——	_____
2. Recorded patient teaching, validation of understanding, and response to medication in appropriate log.	——	——	——	_____
3. Reported any adverse reactions to health care provider.	——	——	——	_____
4. Recorded patient's medication response in nurses' notes.	——	——	——	_____

Copyright © 2018 by Elsevier Inc. All rights reserved.

Student _____ Date _____

Instructor _____ Date _____

PERFORMANCE CHECKLIST SKILL 22.6   **ADMINISTERING INTRAVENOUS MEDICATIONS BY PIGGYBACK, INTERMITTENT INFUSION SETS, AND MINI-INFUSION PUMPS**

	S	U	NP	Comments
ASSESSMENT				
1. Checked accuracy and completeness of each MAR with medication order, reprinted/recopied any portion of MAR that was difficult to read.	___	___	___	_____
2. Assessed patient's medical and medication history.	___	___	___	_____
3. Assessed patient's history of allergies.	___	___	___	_____
4. Reviewed medication reference information.	___	___	___	_____
5. Determined compatibility of medication with IV fluids if giving medication through existing IV line.	___	___	___	_____
6. Assessed patency of patient's existing IV infusion line or saline lock.	___	___	___	_____
7. Assessed patient's symptoms before initiating therapy.	___	___	___	_____
8. Assessed patient's knowledge of medication.	___	___	___	_____
PLANNING				
1. Identified expected outcomes.	___	___	___	_____
IMPLEMENTATION				
1. Performed hand hygiene, prepared medications for one patient at a time, kept all pages of MAR for one patient together, checked label of medication with MAR twice.	___	___	___	_____
2. Took medication(s) to patient at correct time, applied the six rights of medication administration.	___	___	___	_____
3. Provided privacy, performed hand hygiene, applied clean gloves.	___	___	___	_____
4. Identified patient using at least two identifiers, compared with information on MAR.	___	___	___	_____
5. Compared MAR with medication labels at patient's bedside, asked patient if he or she had allergies.	___	___	___	_____

Copyright © 2018 by Elsevier Inc. All rights reserved.

	S	U	NP	Comments

6. Discussed purpose of each medication, action, and possible adverse effects; allowed patient to ask questions; explained you would give medication through existing IV line; encouraged patient to report discomfort at the site. ___ ___ ___ _____

7. Administered infusion:

   a. Piggyback infusion.

     (1) Connected infusion tubing to medication bag, filled tubing, closed clamp, capped end of tubing. ___ ___ ___ _____

     (2) Hung piggyback medication bag above level of primary fluid bag. ___ ___ ___ _____

     (3) Connected infusion tubing to appropriate connector on upper Y-port of primary infusion line. ___ ___ ___ _____

     (4) Flushed and prepared saline lock if necessary, wiped port with alcohol, let dry, inserted tip of infusion tubing via needleless access. ___ ___ ___ _____

     (5) Regulated flow rate of medication, referred to medication reference for safe flow rate. ___ ___ ___ _____

     (6) Checked flow rate of primary infusion or disconnected tubing, cleansed port, and flushed IV line after infusion. ___ ___ ___ _____

     (7) Regulated continuous main infusion line to ordered rate. ___ ___ ___ _____

     (8) Left IV piggyback and tubing in place or discarded in puncture- and leak-proof container. ___ ___ ___ _____

   b. Volume-control administration set.

     (1) Filled Volutrol with desired amount of IV fluid. ___ ___ ___ _____

     (2) Closed clamp, ensured clamp on air vent Volutrol chamber was open. ___ ___ ___ _____

     (3) Cleaned injection port with antiseptic swab. ___ ___ ___ _____

     (4) Removed needle cap, inserted needleless syringe or needle through port, injected medication, rotated Volutrol between hands. ___ ___ ___ _____

     (5) Regulated IV infusion rate. ___ ___ ___ _____

     (6) Labeled Volutrol with all pertinent information following ISMP safe medication label format. ___ ___ ___ _____

Copyright © 2018 by Elsevier Inc. All rights reserved.

	S	U	NP	Comments
(7) Checked continuous infusion after completion of Volutrol infusion.	——	——	——	————————
(8) Disposed of uncapped needle or needle enclosed in safety shield and syringe in puncture- and leak-proof-container, discarded supplies in appropriate container, performed hand hygiene.	——	——	——	————————
c. Volume-control administration set.				
(1) Connected prefilled syringe to mini-infusion tubing, removed end cap.	——	——	——	————————
(2) Applied pressure to plunger, allowed tubing to fill with medication.	——	——	——	————————
(3) Placed syringe into mini-infusion pump and hung on IV pole, ensured syringe was secured.	——	——	——	————————
(4) Connected end of mini-infusion tubing properly to main IV line or saline lock.	——	——	——	————————
(5) Set pump to deliver medication within time recommended, began infusion.	——	——	——	————————
(6) Checked flow rate or disconnected tubing, cleansed port with alcohol, and flushed IV line after infusion, OR				
(7) Regulated flow rate of main IV infusion.	——	——	——	————————
8. Disposed of supplies in puncture- and leak-proof container.	——	——	——	————————
9. Removed gloves, performed hand hygiene.	——	——	——	————————

EVALUATION

	S	U	NP	Comments
1. Observed patient for signs or symptoms of adverse reaction.	——	——	——	————————
2. Checked infusion rate and condition of IV site periodically during infusion.	——	——	——	————————
3. Asked patient to explain purpose and side effects of medication.	——	——	——	————————
4. Asked patient to explain why medication is received and what to report to the nurse.	——	——	——	————————
5. Identified unexpected outcomes.	——	——	——	————————

RECORDING AND REPORTING

	S	U	NP	Comments
1. Recorded medication, dose, route, rate, and time on MAR immediately; included initials or signature.	——	——	——	————————
2. Recorded volume of fluid in bag or Volutrol on I&O form.	——	——	——	————————

Copyright © 2018 by Elsevier Inc. All rights reserved.

	S	U	NP	Comments
3. Recorded patient teaching, validation of understanding, and patient's response to medication in appropriate log.	___	___	___	_____
4. Reported any adverse reaction to health care provider.	___	___	___	_____

Copyright © 2018 by Elsevier Inc. All rights reserved.

Student _____ Date _____

Instructor _____ Date _____

	S	U	NP	Comments

ASSESSMENT

1. Checked accuracy and completeness of each MAR with medication order, reprinted/recopied any portion of MAR that was difficult to read. ___ ___ ___ _____

2. Assessed patient's medical and medication history. ___ ___ ___ _____

3. Assessed patient's history of allergies. ___ ___ ___ _____

4. Collected drug reference information. ___ ___ ___ _____

5. Assessed patient's previous verbal and nonverbal response to needle insertion. ___ ___ ___ _____

6. Assessed patient pain if analgesic is being administered. ___ ___ ___ _____

7. Assessed for contraindications to CSQI. ___ ___ ___ _____

8. Assessed adequacy of patient's adipose tissue to determine appropriate site. ___ ___ ___ _____

9. Assessed patient's knowledge of medication and use of medication pump. ___ ___ ___ _____

10. Assessed patient's symptoms before initiating therapy, measured blood glucose level if necessary. ___ ___ ___ _____

PLANNING

1. Identified expected outcomes. ___ ___ ___ _____

IMPLEMENTATION

1. Reviewed manufacturer's directions for pump. ___ ___ ___ _____

2. Performed hand hygiene, prepared medication or checked dose on prefilled syringe, connected syringe and prime tubing, compared label of medication with MAR twice. ___ ___ ___ _____

3. Obtained and programmed medication administration pump, placed syringe in pump. ___ ___ ___ _____

4. Compared label on prefilled syringe with MAR. ___ ___ ___ _____

Copyright © 2018 by Elsevier Inc. All rights reserved.

	S	U	NP	Comments

5. Identified patient using at least two identifiers, compared identifiers with information in MAR. ____ ____ ____ _____

6. Compared MAR with medication labels at bedside, asked if patient had any allergies. ____ ____ ____ _____

7. Discussed purpose of each medication, action, and possible adverse effects; allowed patient to ask questions; told patient needle insertion would cause slight burning or stinging. ____ ____ ____ _____

8. Positioned patient, draped, and provided privacy. ____ ____ ____ _____

9. Initiated CSQI:

   a. Assisted patient to comfortable position. ____ ____ ____ _____

   b. Selected appropriate injection site. ____ ____ ____ _____

   c. Performed hand hygiene, applied clean gloves, cleansed injection site with alcohol and antiseptic, allowed both to dry. ____ ____ ____ _____

   d. Held needle in dominant hand, removed needle guard. ____ ____ ____ _____

   e. Pinched or lifted up skin with nondominant hand. ____ ____ ____ _____

   f. Inserted needle per manufacturer's directions. ____ ____ ____ _____

   g. Released skinfold, applied tape over "wings" of needle. ____ ____ ____ _____

   h. Placed occlusive, transparent dressing over insertion site. ____ ____ ____ _____

   i. Attached needle tubing to pump tubing, turned pump on. ____ ____ ____ _____

   j. Disposed of sharps in puncture- and leak-proof container, discarded used supplies, removed gloves, performed hand hygiene. ____ ____ ____ _____

   k. Inspected site before leaving, instructed patient to inform you if site became red or leaked. ____ ____ ____ _____

   l. Stayed with patient, observed for allergic reactions. ____ ____ ____ _____

10. Initiated CSQI:

   a. Verified order, established alternative method for administration if applicable. ____ ____ ____ _____

   b. Stopped infusion pump. ____ ____ ____ _____

   c. Performed hand hygiene. Applied clean gloves. ____ ____ ____ _____

Copyright © 2018 by Elsevier Inc. All rights reserved.

	S	U	NP	Comments
d. Removed dressing without dislodging or removing needle, discarded properly.	___	___	___	_____
e. Removed tape from wings of needle, pulled needle out at same angle it was inserted.	___	___	___	_____
f. Applied pressure at site until no fluid leaked out of skin.	___	___	___	_____
g. Applied sterile gauze or adhesive bandage to site.	___	___	___	_____
11. Disposed of uncapped needles and syringes in puncture-poof and leak-proof container.	___	___	___	_____
12. Removed and disposed of gloves, performed hand hygiene.	___	___	___	_____

EVALUATION

	S	U	NP	Comments
1. Evaluated patient's response to medication.	___	___	___	_____
2. Assessed site every 4 hours for redness, pain, drainage, or swelling.	___	___	___	_____
3. Asked patient to explain purpose of continuous infusion.	___	___	___	_____
4. Identified unexpected outcomes.	___	___	___	_____

RECORDING AND REPORTING

	S	U	NP	Comments
1. Recorded drug, dose, route, site, time, and type of pump in patient's medical record immediately after initiating CSQI; used initials or signature.	___	___	___	_____
2. Followed policy for documentation of opioid waste.	___	___	___	_____
3. Recorded patient's response to medication and appearance of site every 4 hours in appropriate log.	___	___	___	_____
4. Recorded patient teaching, validation of understanding, and patient's response to medication in appropriate log.	___	___	___	_____
5. Reported adverse side effects from medication or infection at insertion site to patient's health care provider.	___	___	___	_____

Copyright © 2018 by Elsevier Inc. All rights reserved.

Student _____ Date _____

Instructor _____ Date _____

PERFORMANCE CHECKLIST SKILL 23.1 **APPLYING AN OXYGEN DELIVERY DEVICE**

	S	U	NP	Comments
ASSESSMENT				
1. Identified patient using at least two identifiers.	___	___	___	_____
2. Performed respiratory assessment.	___	___	___	_____
3. Observed for behavioral changes.	___	___	___	_____
4. Observed for patent airway, removed airway secretions by having patient cough or by suctioning.	___	___	___	_____
5. Noted patient's most recent ABG results or SpO$_2$ value.	___	___	___	_____
6. Reviewed patient's medical record for order for oxygen.	___	___	___	_____
PLANNING				
1. Identified expected outcomes.	___	___	___	_____
2. Explained procedure to patient and family.	___	___	___	_____
3. Gathered equipment and completed necessary charges.	___	___	___	_____
IMPLEMENTATION				
1. Performed hand hygiene, applied face shield and gloves if indicated.	___	___	___	_____
2. Adjusted bed to appropriate height, lowered side rails, checked locks on bed wheel.	___	___	___	_____
3. Attached oxygen delivery device to oxygen tubing, attached to humidified oxygen source adjusted to prescribed flow rate.	___	___	___	_____
4. Applied oxygen device:				
a. Placed tips of cannula into patient's nares, looped tubing over patient's ears, adjusted lanyard.	___	___	___	_____
b. Applied mask over patient's mouth and nose, brought straps over head.	___	___	___	_____
5. Maintained sufficient slack on oxygen tubing, secured to patient's clothes.	___	___	___	_____
6. Observed for proper function of oxygen delivery device.	___	___	___	_____

Copyright © 2018 by Elsevier Inc. All rights reserved.

	S	U	NP	Comments

7. Verified setting on flowmeter and oxygen source for proper setup and prescribed flow rate. ____ ____ ____ _____

8. Checked cannula/mask every 8 hours, kept humidification container filled at all times. ____ ____ ____ _____

9. Posted "Oxygen in Use" signs as needed. ____ ____ ____ _____

10. Disposed of gloves properly, performed hand hygiene. ____ ____ ____ _____

EVALUATION

1. Monitored patient's response to changes in flow rate with SpO$_2$. ____ ____ ____ _____

2. Observed for improvement in physical signs and symptoms. ____ ____ ____ _____

3. Assessed adequacy of oxygen flow each shift. ____ ____ ____ _____

4. Observed patient's ears, nose, nares, and nasal mucous membranes for evidence of skin breakdown. ____ ____ ____ _____

5. Asked patient to explain why oxygen is beneficial. ____ ____ ____ _____

6. Identified unexpected outcomes. ____ ____ ____ _____

RECORDING AND REPORTING

1. Recorded all pertinent information in the appropriate log. ____ ____ ____ _____

2. Documented evaluation of patient learning. ____ ____ ____ _____

3. Reported unexpected outcomes to health care provider or nurse in charge. ____ ____ ____ _____

Copyright © 2018 by Elsevier Inc. All rights reserved.

Student _____ Date _____

Instructor _____ Date _____

PERFORMANCE CHECKLIST SKILL 23.2 **ADMINISTERING OXYGEN THERAPY TO A PATIENT WITH AN ARTIFICIAL AIRWAY**

	S	U	NP	Comments
ASSESSMENT				
1. Identified patient using at least two identifiers.	___	___	___	_____
2. Assessed patient's respiratory status.	___	___	___	_____
3. Observed for patent airway, removed airway secretions by having patient cough and by suctioning.	___	___	___	_____
4. Monitored SpO_2, noted patient's most recent ABG levels.	___	___	___	_____
5. Reviewed patient's medical record for order for oxygen; noted delivery method, flow rate, and duration of oxygen therapy.	___	___	___	_____
PLANNING				
1. Identified expected outcomes.	___	___	___	_____
2. Explained purpose of T tube or tracheostomy collar to patient and family.	___	___	___	_____
IMPLEMENTATION				
1. Gathered equipment, completed necessary charges.	___	___	___	_____
2. Performed hand hygiene, applied clean gloves and other appropriate PPE.	___	___	___	_____
3. Attached T tube or tracheostomy collar to oxygen tubing and to humidified air or oxygen source if indicated.	___	___	___	_____
4. Adjusted flow rate properly if oxygen was ordered, adjusted nebulizer to proper FiO_2 setting, attached T tube to artificial airway, placed tracheostomy collar over tracheostomy tube.	___	___	___	_____
5. Observed that T tube does not pull on artificial airway or cause pressure on skin, suctioned secretions as necessary.	___	___	___	_____
6. Observed oxygen tubing for accumulation of fluid, drained tube away from patient if necessary, disconnected from collar or T tube, discarded fluid in proper receptacle.	___	___	___	_____
7. Set up suction equipment at patient's bedside.	___	___	___	_____
8. Removed gloves and goggles, performed hand hygiene.	___	___	___	_____

Copyright © 2018 by Elsevier Inc. All rights reserved.

	S	U	NP	Comments

EVALUATION

1. Monitored patient's ABG levels or measured SpO$_2$. ___ ___ ___ _____

2. Performed respiratory assessment. ___ ___ ___ _____

3. Observed position of oxygen delivery device, ensured it was not pulling on the artificial airway. ___ ___ ___ _____

4. Asked patient and family to explain why oxygen is attached to tracheostomy tube. ___ ___ ___ _____

5. Identified unexpected outcomes. ___ ___ ___ _____

RECORDING AND REPORTING

1. Recorded respiratory findings and all pertinent information in the appropriate log. ___ ___ ___ _____

2. Documented evaluation of patient learning. ___ ___ ___ _____

3. Reported unexpected outcomes to health care provider or nurse in charge. ___ ___ ___ _____

Copyright © 2018 by Elsevier Inc. All rights reserved.

Student _____ Date _____

Instructor _____ Date _____

PERFORMANCE CHECKLIST SKILL 23.3 **USING INCENTIVE SPIROMETRY**

	S	U	NP	Comments

ASSESSMENT

1. Identified patient using at least two identifiers. ___ ___ ___ _____

2. Identified patients who would benefit from incentive spirometry. ___ ___ ___ _____

3. Assessed patient for confusion, malnutrition, cognitive impairment, and decreased necessary motor skills. ___ ___ ___ _____

4. Assessed patient's respiratory status. ___ ___ ___ _____

5. Assessed level of pain. ___ ___ ___ _____

6. Reviewed health care provider's order for incentive spirometry. ___ ___ ___ _____

PLANNING

1. Identified expected outcomes. ___ ___ ___ _____

2. Explained procedure to patient and family. ___ ___ ___ _____

3. Indicated to patient where the target volume is on the IS, demonstrated use if possible. ___ ___ ___ _____

IMPLEMENTATION

1. Gathered equipment, completed necessary charges. ___ ___ ___ _____

2. Performed hand hygiene. ___ ___ ___ _____

3. Positioned patient in appropriate position. ___ ___ ___ _____

4. Instructed patient to hold IS upright, exhale completely, and place lips tightly around mouthpiece. ___ ___ ___ _____

5. Instructed patient to take slow, deep breath and maintain a constant flow, removed mouthpiece at point of maximal inhalation, had patient hold breath for 3 seconds and exhale normally. ___ ___ ___ _____

6. Had patient repeat maneuver, encouraged patient to reach prescribed goal. ___ ___ ___ _____

7. Encouraged patient to independently use IS at prescribed frequency. ___ ___ ___ _____

8. Performed hand hygiene. ___ ___ ___ _____

Copyright © 2018 by Elsevier Inc. All rights reserved.

EVALUATION

1. Observed patient's ability to use incentive spirometer by return demonstration. ____ ____ ____ _____

2. Assessed if patient was able to achieve target volume or frequency. ____ ____ ____ _____

3. Auscultated chest during respiratory cycle, obtained pulse oximeter reading. ____ ____ ____ _____

4. Asked patient to show how to use IS and how frequently to use it. ____ ____ ____ _____

5. Identified unexpected outcomes. ____ ____ ____ _____

RECORDING AND REPORTING

1. Recorded lung sounds before and after incentive spirometry, frequency of use, volumes achieved, and adverse effects in appropriate log. ____ ____ ____ _____

2. Documented evaluation of learning. ____ ____ ____ _____

Copyright © 2018 by Elsevier Inc. All rights reserved.

Student _____ Date _____

Instructor _____ Date _____

PERFORMANCE CHECKLIST SKILL 23.4 **CARE OF A PATIENT RECEIVING NONINVASIVE POSITIVE-PRESSURE VENTILATION**

	S	U	NP	Comments
ASSESSMENT				
1. Identified patient using at least two identifiers.	___	___	___	_____
2. Assessed patient safety, asked patient about dyspnea, observed for signs associated with hypoxia.	___	___	___	_____
3. Observed patient's skin over bridge of nose, around ears, and back of head.	___	___	___	_____
4. Observed patient's ability to clear and remove airway secretions by coughing.	___	___	___	_____
5. Monitored patient's vital signs and pulse oximetry, obtained most recent ABG results.	___	___	___	_____
6. Assessed patient's LOC, behaviors, and ability to maintain and protect airway.	___	___	___	_____
7. Reviewed patient's medical record for medical order for CPAP/BiPAP and appropriate settings.	___	___	___	_____
PLANNING				
1. Identified expected outcomes.	___	___	___	_____
2. Explained to patient and family purpose and reasons for CPAP/BiPAP.	___	___	___	_____
IMPLEMENTATION				
1. Collaborated with respiratory therapist to gather equipment and complete necessary charges.	___	___	___	_____
2. Performed hand hygiene, applied clean gloves and any necessary PPE.	___	___	___	_____
3. Adjusted bed to appropriate height, lowered side rail nearest you, checked locks on wheels.	___	___	___	_____
4. Determined correct mask size.	___	___	___	_____
5. Connected CPAP/BiPAP device delivery tubing to pressure generator.	___	___	___	_____
6. Connected patient to pulse oximetry.	___	___	___	_____
7. Set CPAP/BiPAP initial settings properly.	___	___	___	_____
8. Selected FiO_2 level as indicated.	___	___	___	_____
9. Ensured humidification and heating devices are on.	___	___	___	_____

Copyright © 2018 by Elsevier Inc. All rights reserved.

	S	U	NP	Comments

10. Ensured mask is tight fitting with no air leaks or pressure points.

11. Disposed of supplies appropriately, removed gloves and PPE, performed hand hygiene.

12. Provided continuous care:

  a. Ensured all alarms are active and ventilator circuit is properly functioning.

  b. Ensured that emergency resuscitation equipment is at bedside.

  c. Investigated any alarms that come with ventilator or patient monitor.

  d. Repositioned patient every 2 hours.

EVALUATION

1. Observed for decreased anxiety, improved LOC and cognitive abilities, and other indicators of response to therapy.

2. Monitored pulse oximetry.

3. Observed skin integrity over bridge of nose, asked patient about level of comfort.

4. Observed and monitored patient's and family's ability to manipulate device and face mask if NIPPV is planned for use in the home.

5. Asked patient to explain why NIPPV therapy is necessary.

6. Identified unexpected outcomes.

RECORDING AND REPORTING

1. Recorded respiratory findings, CPAP/BiPAP settings, vital signs, pulse oximetry, patient response, and patient teaching outcomes, and skin assessment in appropriate log.

2. Documented evaluation of patient learning.

3. Reported sudden change in respiratory status and decline in ABG levels or pulse oximetry values to nurse in charge or health care provider.

Copyright © 2018 by Elsevier Inc. All rights reserved.

Student _____ Date _____

Instructor _____ Date _____

PERFORMANCE CHECKLIST PROCEDURAL GUIDELINE 23.1 **USE OF A PEAK FLOWMETER**

	S	U	NP	Comments

PROCEDURAL STEPS

1. Reviewed medical record for patient's baseline PEFR. ___ ___ ___ _____

2. Assessed previous PEFR readings and target set by patient's health care provider. ___ ___ ___ _____

3. Helped patient to appropriate position. ___ ___ ___ _____

4. Assessed patient's baseline knowledge of when and how to use PEFR. ___ ___ ___ _____

5. Slid mouthpiece into base of numbered scale. ___ ___ ___ _____

6. Instructed patient to take deep breath. ___ ___ ___ _____

7. Had patient place meter mouthpiece in mouth and close lips firmly. ___ ___ ___ _____

8. Had patient blow out hard and fast in one breath through mouth. ___ ___ ___ _____

9. Monitored PEFR results, assessed if patient is in expected range. ___ ___ ___ _____

10. Informed patient of his or her acceptable range. ___ ___ ___ _____

11. Asked patient to demonstrate recording PEFR using traffic light pattern if patient is to record at home. ___ ___ ___ _____

12. Asked patient to demonstrate how to use PEFR device. ___ ___ ___ _____

13. Compared patient's PEFR with personal best. ___ ___ ___ _____

14. Recorded PEFR measurement before and after therapy and patient's ability to perform PEFR. ___ ___ ___ _____

15. Instructed patient to clean unit weekly following manufacturer's instructions. ___ ___ ___ _____

Copyright © 2018 by Elsevier Inc. All rights reserved.

Student _____ Date _____

Instructor _____ Date _____

PERFORMANCE CHECKLIST SKILL 23.5   **CARE OF A PATIENT ON A MECHANICAL VENTILATOR**

	S	U	NP	Comments
ASSESSMENT				
1. Identified patient using at least two identifiers.	___	___	___	_____
2. Assessed patient's LOC, ability to cooperate, and need for special positioning.	___	___	___	_____
3. Assessed patient's need for sedation.	___	___	___	_____
4. Assessed patient's respiratory status.	___	___	___	_____
5. Assessed patient's cardiovascular condition.	___	___	___	_____
6. Assessed for signs of inadvertent extubation.	___	___	___	_____
7. Checked ventilator, $EtCO_2$, SpO_2, and ventilator and cardiac alarms at appropriate times; compared with health care provider's orders.	___	___	___	_____
8. Applied gloves, verified placement of artificial airway, determined that tube was securely placed:				
a. Auscultated over trachea for presence of air leak.	___	___	___	_____
b. Used cuff pressure monitoring device.	___	___	___	_____
9. Ensured suctioning system is functioning properly.	___	___	___	_____
10. Observed for patent airway, removed secretions by suctioning if necessary, removed and disposed of gloves, performed hand hygiene.	___	___	___	_____
11. Assessed integrity of patient's oral mucous membrane and skin around stabilization device.	___	___	___	_____
12. Noted patient's most recent ABG results or SpO_2, determined if any factors changed during mechanical ventilation.	___	___	___	_____
13. Determined method for communication with patient, reviewed previous communication techniques if possible.	___	___	___	_____
14. Reviewed patient's medical record for order for mechanical ventilation; noted mode, rate, oxygen settings, and tidal volume.	___	___	___	_____

306

Copyright © 2018 by Elsevier Inc. All rights reserved.

	S	U	NP	Comments

PLANNING

1. Identified expected outcomes.

2. Explained ventilator system to patient and family, included purpose and reasons for initiation of mechanical ventilation.

3. Positioned patient properly.

IMPLEMENTATION

1. Performed hand hygiene, applied clean gloves and other PPE.

2. Attached mechanical ventilator to ET or tracheostomy tube, observed for proper functioning of mechanical ventilator.

3. Verified that ET or tracheostomy tube was properly positioned during an inspiratory and expiratory cycle.

4. Observed patient for synchronization with mechanical ventilation and response to therapy.

5. Monitored heart rate, blood pressure, respiratory rate, and cardiac rhythm.

6. Reassessed and marked level of ET tube at the lips or nares.

7. Ensured suction equipment is set up and functioning.

8. Repositioned patient to promote best oxygenation and ventilation, monitored SpO_2 levels during and after positioning.

9. Collaborated with health care provider about status of patient, response to therapy, and ongoing monitoring.

10. Performed hourly safety checks on patient and ventilator system:

    a. Ensured patient could reach call light.

    b. Checked security of all ventilator connections, ensured all alarms were turned on.

    c. Verified all settings were correct and corresponded to health care provider's orders.

    d. Checked and refilled humidifier, checked tubing for condensation, drained and appropriately discarded any liquid.

    e. Observed temperature gauges, ensured gas was delivered at correct temperature.

11. Performed mouth care at least four times per 24 hours.

Copyright © 2018 by Elsevier Inc. All rights reserved.

	S	U	NP	Comments

12. Inserted bite block if necessary. _____ _____ _____ _____

13. Administered sedating drugs as indicated. _____ _____ _____ _____

14. Performed daily interruption in sedation, assessed readiness to extubate. _____ _____ _____ _____

15. Administered medication as ordered for PUD prophylaxis. _____ _____ _____ _____

16. Instituted DVT prophylaxis as ordered. _____ _____ _____ _____

17. Performed nursing activities to prevent hazards of immobility. _____ _____ _____ _____

18. Ensured communication method is in place for patient. _____ _____ _____ _____

19. Kept patient informed on progress and plan for weaning from mechanical ventilator. _____ _____ _____ _____

20. Removed PPE, performed hand hygiene. _____ _____ _____ _____

EVALUATION

1. Reassessed and monitored patient's response to mechanical ventilation every 1 to 4 hours. _____ _____ _____ _____

2. Observed SpO_2 and $EtCO_2$, monitored gas exchange. _____ _____ _____ _____

3. Observed integrity of patient ventilator system. _____ _____ _____ _____

4. Observed and evaluated effectiveness of communication methods. _____ _____ _____ _____

5. Asked patient and family to explain why mechanical ventilation is necessary. _____ _____ _____ _____

6. Identified unexpected outcomes. _____ _____ _____ _____

RECORDING AND REPORTING

1. Recorded all pertinent information in appropriate log. _____ _____ _____ _____

2. Recorded any nursing interventions, including oral care, repositioning, ROM exercises, and medications. _____ _____ _____ _____

3. Documented evaluation of patient learning. _____ _____ _____ _____

4. Reported sudden change in patient's respiratory status and ventilator-associated problems to nurse in charge or health care provider. _____ _____ _____ _____

Copyright © 2018 by Elsevier Inc. All rights reserved.

Student _____ Date _____

Instructor _____ Date _____

PERFORMANCE CHECKLIST SKILL 24.1   **PERFORMING POSTURAL DRAINAGE**

	S	U	NP	Comments
ASSESSMENT				
1. Identified patient using at least two identifiers.	___	___	___	_____
2. Assessed patient for history of decreased LOC and muscle weakness or disease processes.	___	___	___	_____
3. Reviewed medical record; assessed for signs and symptoms consistent with atelectasis, lobar collapse pneumonia, or bronchiectasis; ineffective coughing; thick, sticky, tenacious, and discolored secretions that are difficult to cough up.	___	___	___	_____
4. Auscultated all lung fields for decreased breath sounds and adventitious lung sounds.	___	___	___	_____
5. Assessed vital signs and pulse oximetry before postural drainage treatment.	___	___	___	_____
6. Determined patient's and caregiver's understanding of and ability to perform home postural drainage.	___	___	___	_____
7. Determined patient's level of comfort.	___	___	___	_____
PLANNING				
1. Identified expected outcomes.	___	___	___	_____
2. Explained procedure to patient and family:				
a. Administered analgesia 20 minutes before CPT maneuvers if necessary.	___	___	___	_____
b. Explained purpose and rationale for procedure, explained details of procedure.	___	___	___	_____
c. Encouraged high fluid intake program unless contraindicated, maintained record of fluid I&O.	___	___	___	_____
d. Planned treatments so they did not overlap with meals or tube feeding, stopped gastric tube feedings for 30 to 45 minutes before postural drainage, checked for residual feeding in patient's stomach, held treatment if necessary.	___	___	___	_____
e. Scheduled treatments at appropriate times.	___	___	___	_____
f. Had patient remove any restrictive clothing.	___	___	___	_____

Copyright © 2018 by Elsevier Inc. All rights reserved.

	S	U	NP	Comments

IMPLEMENTATION

1. Provided privacy, performed hand hygiene, applied gloves.

2. Used findings from physical assessment and chest x-ray film to select congested areas for drainage.

3. Assisted patient to appropriate position, placed pillows for support and comfort, draped patient appropriately.

4. Had patient maintain position for 10 to 15 minutes.

5. Performed chest percussion and vibration after 15 minutes.

6. Had patient sit up and cough, saved secretions if necessary, suctioned if necessary.

7. Had patient rest briefly if necessary, noted pulse oximeter readings.

8. Had patient take sips of water.

9. Repeated steps 3–8, ensured each treatment did not exceed 30 to 60 minutes.

10. Offered or assisted patient with oral hygiene.

11. Removed gloves and performed hand hygiene.

EVALUATION

1. Auscultated lung fields.

2. Inspected character and amount of sputum.

3. Reviewed diagnostic reports.

4. Obtained vital signs and pulse oximetry.

5. Asked patient to explain importance of positioning.

6. Identified unexpected outcomes.

RECORDING AND REPORTING

1. Recorded all pertinent information in the appropriate log.

2. Documented evaluation of patient learning.

Copyright © 2018 by Elsevier Inc. All rights reserved.

Student _____ Date _____

Instructor _____ Date _____

PERFORMANCE CHECKLIST PROCEDURAL GUIDELINE 24.1 **USING AN ACAPELLA DEVICE**

	S	U	NP	Comments
PROCEDURAL STEPS				
1. Identified patient using at least two identifiers.	____	____	____	_____
2. Verified need for a health care provider's order.	____	____	____	_____
3. Performed respiratory assessment, determined lung segments requiring percussion or vibration.	____	____	____	_____
4. Assessed patient's and family's understanding of the device and procedure, explained and clarified procedure as needed.	____	____	____	_____
5. Prepared Acapella device properly.	____	____	____	_____
6. Instructed patient to:				
a. Sit comfortably.	____	____	____	_____
b. Take in a breath larger than normal but not full capacity.	____	____	____	_____
c. Place mouthpiece into mouth and maintain a tight seal.	____	____	____	_____
d. Hold breath for 2 to 3 seconds.	____	____	____	_____
e. Try not to cough, exhale slowly for 3 to 4 seconds through device.	____	____	____	_____
f. Repeat cycle for 5 to 10 breaths as tolerated.	____	____	____	_____
g. Remove mouthpiece, perform forced exhalations.	____	____	____	_____
h. Repeat steps a–g as ordered.	____	____	____	_____
7. Auscultated lung fields.	____	____	____	_____
8. Obtained vital signs and pulse oximetry.	____	____	____	_____
9. Inspected color, character, and amount of sputum.	____	____	____	_____
10. Assisted patient with oral hygiene.	____	____	____	_____
11. Asked patient to demonstrate use of Acapella device.	____	____	____	_____
12. Reviewed unexpected outcomes for Skill 24.1.	____	____	____	_____
13. Documented procedure and patient's tolerance, documented evaluation of patient learning.	____	____	____	_____

Copyright © 2018 by Elsevier Inc. All rights reserved.

Student _____ Date _____

Instructor _____ Date _____

PERFORMANCE CHECKLIST PROCEDURAL GUIDELINE 24.2 **PERFORMING PERCUSSION AND VIBRATION**

	S	U	NP	Comments

PROCEDURAL STEPS

1. Identified patient using at least two identifiers. ___ ___ ___ _____

2. Assessed patient, reviewed medical record for signs, symptoms, and conditions that indicate need to perform these skills. ___ ___ ___ _____

3. Performed respiratory assessment to assess breathing pattern. ___ ___ ___ _____

4. Auscultated lung sounds over lung segments drained during postural drainage. ___ ___ ___ _____

5. Identified and assessed area of rib cage over affected bronchial segment; determined if percussion or vibration were contraindicated. ___ ___ ___ _____

6. Determined patient's understanding, assessed patient's ability to cooperate with therapy. ___ ___ ___ _____

7. Explained procedure in detail. ___ ___ ___ _____

8. Helped patient to relax during procedure, had patient practice exhaling slowly through pursed lips while relaxing chest wall muscles. ___ ___ ___ _____

9. Performed hand hygiene, applied clean gloves. ___ ___ ___ _____

10. Elevated bed to working height, stood close to bed with arms in front and knees slightly bent. ___ ___ ___ _____

11. Positioned patient based on physical assessment and chest x-ray findings. ___ ___ ___ _____

12. Performed percussion and vibration:

    a. Percussion and vibration with hands.

       (1) Performed percussion for 3 to 5 minutes in each position as tolerated, began percussion on appropriate part of chest wall, asked if patient experienced any discomfort. ___ ___ ___ _____

       (2) Placed hands properly on chest wall. ___ ___ ___ _____

       (3) Clapped with proper motion. ___ ___ ___ _____

       (4) Alternately clapped chest with cupped hands, performed clapping at proper speed. ___ ___ ___ _____

Copyright © 2018 by Elsevier Inc. All rights reserved.

	S	U	NP	Comments

(5) Performed chest wall vibration and shaking over each affected area, performed vibrations in sets of three followed by coughing.

(a) Placed flat portion of hand over area; had patient take slow, deep breath through nose. ___ ___ ___ _____

(b) Resisted chest wall gently as it rose. ___ ___ ___ _____

(c) Had patient hold breath for 2 to 3 seconds and exhale through pursed lips while contracting abdominal muscles and relaxing chest wall muscles. ___ ___ ___ _____

(d) Vibrated chest wall properly while patient was exhaling. ___ ___ ___ _____

(e) Repeated vibration three times, had patient cascade cough, vibrated chest wall as patient coughed, followed natural movement of ribs when applying pressure, allowed patient to sit up and cough as needed. ___ ___ ___ _____

(f) Monitored patient's tolerance of vibration and ability to relax chest wall and breathe properly as instructed. ___ ___ ___ _____

(g) Performed three or four sets of three vibrations each followed by coughing. ___ ___ ___ _____

b. HFCWC device.

(1) Placed vest on patient, assessed for proper fit. ___ ___ ___ _____

(2) Assessed chest wall motion. ___ ___ ___ _____

(3) Connected tubing to generator and vest port, turned on. ___ ___ ___ _____

(4) Adjusted pressure control as ordered. ___ ___ ___ _____

(5) Adjusted frequency. ___ ___ ___ _____

(6) Administered any aerosol therapy as prescribed. ___ ___ ___ _____

(7) Depressed and maintained pressure on control to initiate vest therapy. ___ ___ ___ _____

(8) Released control after 5 to 10 minutes. ___ ___ ___ _____

13. Instructed patient to cough, suctioned if necessary. ___ ___ ___ _____

14. Continued with treatment, usually 15 to 30 minutes. ___ ___ ___ _____

15. Assisted with oral hygiene. ___ ___ ___ _____

Copyright © 2018 by Elsevier Inc. All rights reserved.

	S	U	NP	Comments
16. Removed gloves, performed hand hygiene.	___	___	___	_____
17. Taught patient and significant others procedure for home use of devices; if necessary, referred for outpatient or home care follow-up.	___	___	___	_____
18. Auscultated lung fields.	___	___	___	_____
19. Obtained vital signs and pulse oximetry.	___	___	___	_____
20. Inspected color, character, and amount of sputum.	___	___	___	_____
21. Asked patient to explain importance of keeping airways clear of secretions.	___	___	___	_____
22. Documented procedure, patient's response, and evaluation of patient learning.	___	___	___	_____

Copyright © 2018 by Elsevier Inc. All rights reserved.

Student _____ Date _____

Instructor _____ Date _____

PERFORMANCE CHECKLIST SKILL 25.1   **PERFORMING OROPHARYNGEAL SUCTIONING**

	S	U	NP	Comments
ASSESSMENT				
1. Identified patient using at least two identifiers.	___	___	___	_____
2. Identified risk factors for airway obstruction.	___	___	___	_____
3. Assessed for signs and symptoms of hypoxia.	___	___	___	_____
4. Obtained patient's oxygen saturation level via pulse oximetry, kept oximeter in place.	___	___	___	_____
5. Determined patient's ability to hold or manipulate catheter and knowledge about procedure.	___	___	___	_____
6. Assessed for signs and symptoms of upper airway obstruction.	___	___	___	_____
7. Auscultated for presence of adventitious sounds.	___	___	___	_____
PLANNING				
1. Identified expected outcomes.	___	___	___	_____
2. Performed hand hygiene, gathered equipment, provided privacy.	___	___	___	_____
3. Explained procedure to patient, encouraged patient to cough out secretions, showed how to splint painful areas during procedure, had patient practice coughing if able.	___	___	___	_____
4. Positioned patient properly, draped patient properly.	___	___	___	_____
IMPLEMENTATION				
1. Performed hand hygiene, applied clean gloves and necessary PPE.	___	___	___	_____
2. Filled cup or basin with appropriate amount of water or saline.	___	___	___	_____
3. Checked that suction machine was functioning properly.	___	___	___	_____
4. Removed patient's oxygen mask if present, kept mask near patient's face.	___	___	___	_____
5. Inserted catheter into mouth along gum line to pharynx, moved catheter around until secretions cleared, encouraged patient to cough, replaced oxygen mask.	___	___	___	_____

Copyright © 2018 by Elsevier Inc. All rights reserved.

	S	U	NP	Comments

6. Rinsed catheter with water until tubing was cleared of secretions, turned off suction, placed catheter in clean area. ___ ___ ___ _____

7. Washed patient's face if necessary. ___ ___ ___ _____

8. Observed respiratory status, repeated procedure if indicated, used standard suction catheter if needed. ___ ___ ___ _____

9. Removed towel or drape, placed in trash or laundry if soiled, repositioned patient appropriately. ___ ___ ___ _____

10. Discarded remainder of water into appropriate receptacle, washed and dried basin, discarded cup in appropriate receptacle. ___ ___ ___ _____

11. Removed gloves and PPE, disposed of in appropriate receptacle, performed hand hygiene. ___ ___ ___ _____

12. Positioned patient, provided oral hygiene as needed. ___ ___ ___ _____

EVALUATION

1. Compared assessment findings before and after procedure. ___ ___ ___ _____

2. Auscultated chest and airways for adventitious sounds. ___ ___ ___ _____

3. Inspected mouth for any vomitus. ___ ___ ___ _____

4. Obtained postsuction SpO_2 measure, compared with presuction level. ___ ___ ___ _____

5. Asked patient to demonstrate how suction catheter is used. ___ ___ ___ _____

6. Identified unexpected outcomes. ___ ___ ___ _____

RECORDING AND REPORTING

1. Recorded all pertinent information in the appropriate log. ___ ___ ___ _____

2. Recorded patient's and caregiver's understanding of safe oral suctioning. ___ ___ ___ _____

3. Reported any unresolved outcomes to health care provider. ___ ___ ___ _____

Copyright © 2018 by Elsevier Inc. All rights reserved.

Student _____ Date _____

Instructor _____ Date _____

PERFORMANCE CHECKLIST SKILL 25.2 **AIRWAY SUCTIONING**

	S	U	NP	Comments
ASSESSMENT				
1. Identified patient using at least two identifiers.	___	___	___	_____
2. Performed hand hygiene, applied clean gloves, assessed for signs of upper or lower airway obstruction.	___	___	___	_____
3. Assessed vital signs and symptoms associated with hypoxia and hypercapnia.	___	___	___	_____
4. Assessed for risk factors for upper or lower airway obstruction.	___	___	___	_____
5. Identified patient with increased risk for ineffective airway clearance.	___	___	___	_____
6. Assessed for excessive secretions or coughing, secretions visible in airway, signs of respiratory distress, and other signs of need for suctioning.	___	___	___	_____
7. Assessed patency of ET with capnography/end-tidal carbon dioxide detector.	___	___	___	_____
8. Assessed factors that may affect volume and consistency of secretions, including fluid balance, lack of humidity, and infection.	___	___	___	_____
9. Assessed patient's peak inspiratory pressure or tidal volume for endotracheal suctioning.	___	___	___	_____
10. Identified contraindications of nasotracheal suctioning.	___	___	___	_____
11. Reviewed sputum microbiology data in laboratory report.	___	___	___	_____
12. Determine presence of signs of hypoxia or hypercapnia.	___	___	___	_____
13. Assessed patient's understanding of procedure and presence of any apprehension.	___	___	___	_____
PLANNING				
1. Identified expected outcomes.	___	___	___	_____
2. Assisted patient to appropriate position.	___	___	___	_____
3. Positioned pulse oximeter on patient's finger, took reading and left oximeter in place.	___	___	___	_____

Copyright © 2018 by Elsevier Inc. All rights reserved.

	S	U	NP	Comments

4. Explained how procedure would clear airway and relieve breathing; explained that temporary coughing, sneezing, gagging, or shortness of breath was normal. ____ ____ ____ _____

IMPLEMENTATION

1. Performed hand hygiene, applied PPE if necessary. ____ ____ ____ _____

2. Adjusted bed to appropriate height, lowered side rail nearest self, checked locks on bed wheel. ____ ____ ____ _____

3. Connected one end of tubing to suction machine, placed other end near patient, turned device on, set suction pressure as low as possible, occluded end of tubing to check pressure. ____ ____ ____ _____

4. Prepared suction catheter:

   a. Opened suction kit or catheter using aseptic technique, placed drape across patient's chest or on bedside table, did not allow suction catheter to touch any nonsterile surface. ____ ____ ____ _____

   b. Opened sterile basin, placed on bedside table, did not touch inside of basin, filled properly with sterile saline solution or water. ____ ____ ____ _____

   c. Opened packet of water-soluble lubricant if necessary, applied to catheter. ____ ____ ____ _____

5. Applied sterile gloves properly. ____ ____ ____ _____

6. Picked up suction catheter with dominant hand, picked up connecting tubing with nondominant hand, secured catheter to tubing. ____ ____ ____ _____

7. Placed catheter tip in sterile basin, suctioned small amount of saline by occluding suction vent. ____ ____ ____ _____

8. Suctioned airway:

   a. Performed nasopharyngeal and nasotracheal suctioning.

      (1) Increased oxygen flow rate for face masks as ordered or had patient breathe deeply. ____ ____ ____ _____

      (2) Coated distal end of catheter with lubricant. ____ ____ ____ _____

318

Copyright © 2018 by Elsevier Inc. All rights reserved.

	S	U	NP	Comments

(3) Removed oxygen delivery device if applicable, inserted catheter into nares without applying suction, instructed patient to deep breathe.

    (a) For nasopharyngeal suctioning, inserted catheter properly through naris and advance to back of pharynx, did not force, performed intermittent suction, withdrew catheter while rotating it between fingers. ____ ____ ____ _____

    (b) For nasotracheal suctioning, advanced catheter properly through naris and into trachea, inserted catheter when patient takes deep breath, pulled back when patient begins to cough. Had patient turn head if needed, applied intermittent suctioning, withdrew catheter while rotating it between fingers. ____ ____ ____ _____

(4) Reapplied oxygen-delivery device, encouraged patient to breathe deep if able. ____ ____ ____ _____

(5) Rinsed catheter and connecting tubing with normal saline or water until cleared.

(6) Assessed need to repeat procedure, did not perform more than two passes with the catheter, allowed patient to rest at least 1 minute, asked patient to deep breathe and cough. ____ ____ ____ _____

b. Performed artificial airway suctioning.

(1) Hyperoxygenated patient appropriately before suctioning. ____ ____ ____ _____

(2) Opened swivel adapter or removed delivery device if patient was receiving mechanical ventilation. ____ ____ ____ _____

(3) Advised patient that suctioning will begin, inserted catheter without applying suction until resistance was met or patient coughed, pulled back. ____ ____ ____ _____

(4) Applied intermittent suction by placing thumb over vent and withdrawing catheter while rotating it between thumb and forefinger, encouraged patient to cough, watched for respiratory distress. ____ ____ ____ _____

Copyright © 2018 by Elsevier Inc. All rights reserved.

	S	U	NP	Comments

(5) Closed swivel adapter or replaced oxygen delivery device if patient was receiving mechanical ventilation, hyperoxygenated patient appropriately.

(6) Rinsed catheter and connected rubbing with normal saline until clear, used continuous suction.

(7) Assessed patient's vital signs, cardiopulmonary status, and ventilatory measures for secretion clearance; repeated steps to clear secretions; allowed adequate time between passes.

(8) Performed oropharyngeal suctioning after pharynx and trachea are clear.

9. Disconnected catheter from tubing, rolled catheter in fingers, pulled glove off inside out so catheter remained in glove, pulled off other glove over first in same way, discarded appropriately, turned off suction device.

10. Removed towel, placed in appropriate receptacle, repositioned patient, applied clean gloves to continue personal care.

11. Readjusted oxygen to original level if indicated.

12. Discarded remainder of saline appropriately, discarded basin appropriately or rinsed and placed in soiled utility room.

13. Removed PPE and discarded, performed hand hygiene.

14. Placed unopened suction kit on machine table or at head of bed.

15. Assisted patient to comfortable position, provided oral hygiene as needed.

EVALUATION

1. Compared patient's vital signs, cardiopulmonary assessments, and $EtCO_2$ and SpO_2 values before and after suctioning; compared FiO_2 and tidal volumes if on ventilator.

2. Asked patient if breathing was easier and if congestion had decreased.

3. Auscultated lungs, compared patient's respiratory assessment before and after suctioning.

4. Observed character of airway secretions.

5. Asked patient to explain why suctioning is required.

6. Identified unexpected outcomes.

320

Copyright © 2018 by Elsevier Inc. All rights reserved.

	S	U	NP	Comments

RECORDING AND REPORTING

1. Recorded amount, consistency, color, and odor of secretions, size of catheter, route of suctioning, and patient response in appropriate log. ___ ___ ___ _____

2. Recorded need for and type of hyperoxygenation and percent oxygenation used. ___ ___ ___ _____

3. Recorded patient's and caregiver's understanding. ___ ___ ___ _____

4. Documented vital signs presuctioning and postsuctioning, cardiopulmonary status, and ventilation measured in the appropriate log. ___ ___ ___ _____

5. Reported patient's intolerance or unexpected changes to health care provider. ___ ___ ___ _____

Copyright © 2018 by Elsevier Inc. All rights reserved.

Student _____ Date _____

Instructor _____ Date _____

PERFORMANCE CHECKLIST PROCEDURAL GUIDELINE 25.1   **CLOSED (IN-LINE) SUCTIONING**

	S	U	NP	Comments

PROCEDURAL STEPS

1. Performed assessment as in Skill 25.2.
    ___ ___ ___ _____

2. Performed hand hygiene, gathered equipment, provided privacy.
    ___ ___ ___ _____

3. Identified patient using at least two identifiers.
    ___ ___ ___ _____

4. Explained procedure and importance of coughing during procedure to patient.
    ___ ___ ___ _____

5. Adjusted bed to appropriate height, lowered side rail nearest self, checked locks on bed wheels.
    ___ ___ ___ _____

6. Assisted patient to appropriate position, placed towel across patient's chest.
    ___ ___ ___ _____

7. Applied clean gloves and face shield, attached suction:

    a. Opened catheter package, attached closed suction catheter to ventilator circuit, connected Y on ventilator circuit to catheter with flex tubing.
    ___ ___ ___ _____

    b. Connected tubing to suction machine and end of closed-system or in-line suction catheter, turned device on, set regulator to appropriate negative pressure, checked pressure.
    ___ ___ ___ _____

8. Hyperoxygenated patient, did not manually ventilate.
    ___ ___ ___ _____

9. Unlocked suction control mechanism if required, opened saline port, attached saline syringe or vial.
    ___ ___ ___ _____

10. Picked up suction catheter in plastic sleeve with dominant hand.
    ___ ___ ___ _____

11. Waited until patient inhaled to insert catheter, used repeated maneuver of pushing catheter and sliding plastic sleeve back until resistance was felt or patient coughed, pulled back.
    ___ ___ ___ _____

Copyright © 2018 by Elsevier Inc. All rights reserved.

	S	U	NP	Comments

12. Encouraged patient to cough, applied suction while withdrawing catheter, applied suction for no longer than 15 seconds, withdrew catheter completely.

13. Reassessed cardiopulmonary status, determined need for subsequent suctioning, repeated steps 8–12 one more time to clear secretions, allowed time between suction passes.

14. Withdrew catheter into sheath, ensured colored indicator line was visible in sheath, attached appropriate solution to side port, squeezed vial or pushed syringe while applying suction, rinsed catheter with saline until clear, locked suction mechanism, turned off suction.

15. Hyperoxygenated for at least 1 minute.

16. Performed Skill 25.1 or 25.2 with separate suction catheter if patient requires oral or nasal suctioning.

17. Placed Yankauer catheter on clean, dry surface for either reuse or within patient's reach if appropriate.

18. Positioned patient appropriately, removed gloves and PPE and discarded appropriately, performed hand hygiene.

19. Compared patient's vital signs and SpO$_2$ before and after suctioning.

20. Auscultated lung fields, compared with baseline.

21. Observed airway secretions.

22. Asked patient if breathing is easier and congestion is decreased.

23. Verified patient understanding of suctioning procedure.

Copyright © 2018 by Elsevier Inc. All rights reserved.

Student _____   Date _____

Instructor _____   Date _____

PERFORMANCE CHECKLIST SKILL 25.3   **PERFORMING ENDOTRACHEAL TUBE CARE**

	S	U	NP	Comments
ASSESSMENT				
1. Identified patient using at least two identifiers.	___	___	___	_____
2. Auscultated lungs, observed respiratory rate and depth.	___	___	___	_____
3. Performed hand hygiene, applied clean gloves, observed condition of tissue surrounding ET tube for impaired skin integrity.	___	___	___	_____
4. Observed patency of airway.	___	___	___	_____
5. Observed for signs of cuff overinflation or underinflation.	___	___	___	_____
6. Observed for factors that increase risk of complications from ET tube.	___	___	___	_____
7. Assessed patient's ability to verbalize around ET tube or for presence of audible air leak.	___	___	___	_____
8. Determined proper ET tube depth, marked on tube and in patient's records.	___	___	___	_____
9. Assessed patient's knowledge of procedure.	___	___	___	_____
PLANNING				
1. Identified expected outcomes.	___	___	___	_____
2. Performed hand hygiene, gathered equipment, provided privacy.	___	___	___	_____
3. Obtained assistance from available staff.	___	___	___	_____
4. Assisted patient to appropriate position, elevated head of bed.	___	___	___	_____
5. Explained procedure and patient's need to participate.	___	___	___	_____
IMPLEMENTATION				
1. Performed hand hygiene, applied clean gloves and PPE, ensured assistants did so also.	___	___	___	_____
2. Placed clean towel across patient's chest.	___	___	___	_____
3. Performed endotracheal or oropharyngeal suction if indicated.	___	___	___	_____
4. Connected Yankauer suction catheter to suction source, ensured suction source is on and functioning.	___	___	___	_____
5. Removed oral airway or bite block if present.	___	___	___	_____

Copyright © 2018 by Elsevier Inc. All rights reserved.

	S	U	NP	Comments

6. Brushed teeth, used solution or paste to break down plaque buildup, suctioned secretions as necessary. ____ ____ ____ _____

7. Used chlorhexidine solution and oral swabs to clean mouth, suctioned oropharyngeal secretions as necessary, applied moisturizer to oral mucosa and lips. ____ ____ ____ _____

8. Prepared ET tube securement options:

   a. Prepared tape properly for tape method. ____ ____ ____ _____

   b. Prepared commercial ET tube holder properly. ____ ____ ____ _____

9. Removed old tape or device:

   a. Removed tape while one person stabilizes ET tube, used tape removed if necessary. ____ ____ ____ _____

   b. Removed Velcro strips from ET tube, removed ET tube holder from patient. ____ ____ ____ _____

10. Removed any secretions or adhesive from patient's face, cleaned and dried facial skin, used adhesive remover if necessary. ____ ____ ____ _____

11. Noted level of ET tube, moved oral ET tube to other side of mouth, performed oral care as needed, cleaned oral airway or bite block, reinserted as necessary. ____ ____ ____ _____

12. Secured tube while assistant holds ET tube:

   a. Used tape method.

     (1) Slipped tape properly under patient's head and neck, centered tape. ____ ____ ____ _____

     (2) Secured tape properly on one side of face, tore remaining tape in half, secured each piece properly to face and tube. ____ ____ ____ _____

     (3) Pulled other side of tape, secured to opposite side of face. ____ ____ ____ _____

   b. Used commercially available ET tube securement device.

     (1) Threaded ET tube through opening, ensured pilot balloon was accessible. ____ ____ ____ _____

     (2) Placed strips of ET tube holder under patient at occipital region of the head. ____ ____ ____ _____

     (3) Verified that ET tube was at established depth. ____ ____ ____ _____

     (4) Attached Velcro at base of patient's head, left slack in strips. ____ ____ ____ _____

     (5) Verified that tube was secure and there were no pressure areas. ____ ____ ____ _____

Copyright © 2018 by Elsevier Inc. All rights reserved.

	S	U	NP	Comments

13. Reinserted oral airway and secured with tape for unconscious patient.

14. Cleaned and dried face and neck, shaved male patient as necessary.

15. Discarded soiled items in appropriate receptacle, removed towel, placed in laundry.

16. Repositioned patient, asked what else he or she needs.

17. Removed gloves and PPE, discarded, performed hand hygiene, placed clean items in storage.

EVALUATION

1. Compared respiratory assessments before and after ET tube care.

2. Observed depth and position of ET tube.

3. Assessed security of tape.

4. Assessed skin around mouth and mucous membrane for intactness and pressure sores.

5. Compared $EtCO_2$ values from before and after ET tube care.

6. Observed for signs of inadequate or excessive cuff inflation.

7. Identified unexpected outcomes.

RECORDING AND REPORTING

1. Documented all pertinent information in the appropriate log.

2. Recorded repositioning of ET tube, side of placement, and securement technique used.

3. Reported unequal breath sounds, accidental extubation, cuff leak, or respiratory distress to health care provider.

Copyright © 2018 by Elsevier Inc. All rights reserved.

Student _____ Date _____

Instructor _____ Date _____

PERFORMANCE CHECKLIST SKILL 25.4   **PERFORMING TRACHEOSTOMY CARE**

	S	U	NP	Comments
ASSESSMENT				
1. Identified patient using at least two identifiers.	___	___	___	_____
2. Performed hand hygiene, applied clean gloves, observed for signs of cuff overinflation or underinflation.	___	___	___	_____
3. Observed for need for tracheostomy care due to secretions at stoma site or in tube.	___	___	___	_____
4. Observed skin around tracheal stoma, under TT, and under tracheal ties for skin breakdown.	___	___	___	_____
5. Assessed patient's hydration status, humidity delivered to airway, status of existing infection, patient's nutritional status, and ability to cough.	___	___	___	_____
6. Assessed patient's cardiopulmonary status, SpO_2, $EtCO_2$, vital sins, respiratory effort, lung sounds, and LOC, kept pulse oximeter in place.	___	___	___	_____
7. Assessed patient's and caregiver's understanding of and ability to perform tracheostomy care.	___	___	___	_____
8. Checked when tracheostomy care was last performed.	___	___	___	_____
PLANNING				
1. Identified expected outcomes.	___	___	___	_____
2. Obtained nurse, NAP, or respiratory therapist to assist.	___	___	___	_____
3. Performed hand hygiene, gathered supplies and arranged at bedside, provided privacy.	___	___	___	_____
4. Assisted patient to appropriate position.	___	___	___	_____
5. Explained procedure and patient's participation.	___	___	___	_____
IMPLEMENTATION				
1. Applied PPE as necessary.	___	___	___	_____
2. Adjusted bed to appropriate height, lowered side rail, checked locks on bed wheel.	___	___	___	_____

Copyright © 2018 by Elsevier Inc. All rights reserved.

	S	U	NP	Comments

3. Preoxygenated patient for 30 seconds, asked patient to take 5 to 6 deep breaths, suctioned tracheostomy, removed soiled dressing, discarded in glove with coiled catheter. ____ ____ ____ _____

4. Performed hand hygiene, prepared equipment on bedside table:

   a. Opened sterile kit and two gauze packages, poured saline on one, opened cotton swab packages, poured saline on one, did not re-cap saline. ____ ____ ____ _____

   b. Opened sterile tracheostomy dressing package. ____ ____ ____ _____

   c. Unwrapped sterile basin, poured proper amount of saline into it. ____ ____ ____ _____

   d. Opened sterile brush package, placed in basin. ____ ____ ____ _____

   e. Prepared TT fixation device.

      (1) Prepared length of twill tape, cut ends diagonally, laid aside to dry. ____ ____ ____ _____

      (2) Opened commercially prepared package according to manufacturer's directions. ____ ____ ____ _____

   f. Opened inner cannula package if appropriate. ____ ____ ____ _____

5. Applied sterile glove, kept dominant hand sterile throughout procedure. ____ ____ ____ _____

6. Removed oxygen source if present. ____ ____ ____ _____

7. Provided care of tracheostomy with reusable inner cannula:

   a. Unlocked and removed inner cannula while touching only outer aspect of the tube, dropped inner cannula into normal saline basin. ____ ____ ____ _____

   b. Replaced tracheostomy collar, T tube, or ventilator oxygen source over outer cannula. ____ ____ ____ _____

   c. Used small brush to remove secretions inside and outside inner cannula. ____ ____ ____ _____

   d. Held inner cannula over basin, rinsed with saline, used nondominant hand to pour. ____ ____ ____ _____

   e. Removed oxygen source, replaced inner cannula, secured locking mechanism, reapplied ventilator after hyperoxygenating if needed. ____ ____ ____ _____

Copyright © 2018 by Elsevier Inc. All rights reserved.

	S	U	NP	Comments

8. Provided care of tracheostomy with disposable inner cannula:

   a. Removed new cannula from packaging.   ____ ____ ____ _____

   b. Withdrew inner cannula while touching only the outer aspect of the tube, replaced and locked new cannula.   ____ ____ ____ _____

   c. Disposed of contaminated cannula in appropriate receptacle, reconnected ventilator or oxygen supply.   ____ ____ ____ _____

9. Cleaned exposed outer cannula surfaces and stoma under faceplate properly with wet cotton and gauze.   ____ ____ ____ _____

10. Used dry gauze to pat skin and cannula surfaces dry.   ____ ____ ____ _____

11. Secured tracheostomy:

   a. Used tracheostomy tie method.

     (1) Instructed assistant to apply clean gloves and hold tube in place, cut old ties.   ____ ____ ____ _____

     (2) Inserted one end of tie through faceplate eyelet, pulled ends even.   ____ ____ ____ _____

     (3) Slid ends of tie behind head, inserted ties through proper eyelets.   ____ ____ ____ _____

     (4) Pulled snugly.   ____ ____ ____ _____

     (5) Tied ends properly, allowed proper amount of space within tie.   ____ ____ ____ _____

     (6) Inserted fresh dressing under clean ties and faceplate.   ____ ____ ____ _____

   b. Used tracheostomy tube holder method.

     (1) Instructed assistant to apply clean gloves and hold tube in place, or left TT holder in place until new device is secure.   ____ ____ ____ _____

     (2) Aligned strap under patient's neck, ensured Velcro attachments were properly placed.   ____ ____ ____ _____

     (3) Placed narrow end of tie under and through faceplate eyelets, pulled ends even, secured with Velcro.   ____ ____ ____ _____

     (4) Verified space under neck strap.   ____ ____ ____ _____

12. Performed oral care with toothbrush or oral swabs and chlorhexidine rinse.   ____ ____ ____ _____

Copyright © 2018 by Elsevier Inc. All rights reserved.

	S	U	NP	Comments
13. Positioned patient comfortably, assessed respiratory status.	___	___	___	_____
14. Ensured oxygen or humidification delivery sources were in place and set at correct levels.	___	___	___	_____
15. Removed gloves and PPE, discarded appropriately, performed hand hygiene.	___	___	___	_____
16. Replaced cap on normal saline bottles, stored reusable liquids, dated container, stored unused supplies appropriately.	___	___	___	_____

EVALUATION

	S	U	NP	Comments
1. Compared assessments before and after tracheostomy care.	___	___	___	_____
2. Assessed fit of new tracheostomy ties, asked patient if tube felt comfortable, palpated tube for pulsation for air under the skin.	___	___	___	_____
3. Inspected inner and outer cannulas for secretions.	___	___	___	_____
4. Assessed stoma for inflammation, edema, or discolored secretions.	___	___	___	_____
5. Observed for excessive phonation, presence of gastric secretions in airway, or tracheoesophageal fistula.	___	___	___	_____
6. Asked patient to demonstrate cleaning tube and place new ties.	___	___	___	_____
7. Identified unexpected outcomes.	___	___	___	_____

RECORDING AND REPORTING

	S	U	NP	Comments
1. Recorded all pertinent information in the appropriate log.	___	___	___	_____
2. Recorded condition of stoma and skin around stoma site and under dressing.	___	___	___	_____
3. Recorded interventions that were performed to address patient complications.	___	___	___	_____
4. Recorded patient's and caregiver's understanding.	___	___	___	_____
5. Reported accidental decannulation or respiratory distress to health care provider.	___	___	___	_____

Copyright © 2018 by Elsevier Inc. All rights reserved.

Student _____ Date _____

Instructor _____ Date _____

PERFORMANCE CHECKLIST SKILL 26.1 **OBTAINING A 12-LEAD ELECTROCARDIOGRAM**

	S	U	NP	Comments

ASSESSMENT

1. Identified patient using at least two identifiers. ___ ___ ___ _____

2. Determined indications for obtaining ECG, assessed patient's history and cardiopulmonary status. ___ ___ ___ _____

3. Assessed patient's level of understanding of procedure. ___ ___ ___ _____

4. Assessed patient's ability to follow directions and remain in position. ___ ___ ___ _____

PLANNING

1. Identified expected outcomes. ___ ___ ___ _____

2. Provided privacy. ___ ___ ___ _____

IMPLEMENTATION

1. Prepared patient for procedure:

   a. Removed or repositioned clothing to expose patient's chest and arms. ___ ___ ___ _____

   b. Placed patient in an appropriate position. ___ ___ ___ _____

   c. Instructed patient to lie still without talking and to not cross legs. ___ ___ ___ _____

2. Turned machine on, entered required demographic information. ___ ___ ___ _____

3. Performed hand hygiene. ___ ___ ___ _____

4. Cleaned and prepared isolated electrode area, clipped excess hair from electrode area. ___ ___ ___ _____

5. Applied electrodes in correct positions, applied electrode paste if necessary:

   a. Placed chest leads correctly. ___ ___ ___ _____

   b. Placed leads on extremities correctly. ___ ___ ___ _____

6. Checked 12-lead machine for messages to correct electrode or lead issues, obtained lead if no messages occur. ___ ___ ___ _____

7. Disconnected leads and wiped excess electrode paste from chest if tracing is without artifact. ___ ___ ___ _____

8. Immediately delivered ECG to appropriate health care provider if STAT. ___ ___ ___ _____

Copyright © 2018 by Elsevier Inc. All rights reserved.

	S	U	NP	Comments

EVALUATION

1. Noted and documented if patient is experiencing any chest discomfort.   ____ ____ ____ _____

2. Discussed findings and results of 12-lead ECG with health care provider.   ____ ____ ____ _____

3. Asked patient to explain need for ECG.   ____ ____ ____ _____

4. Identified unexpected outcomes.   ____ ____ ____ _____

RECORDING AND REPORTING

1. Recorded date and time ECG was obtained, reason for ECG, and to whom ECG was given.   ____ ____ ____ _____

2. Reported any unexpected outcomes.   ____ ____ ____ _____

3. Documented evaluation of patient learning.   ____ ____ ____ _____

Copyright © 2018 by Elsevier Inc. All rights reserved.

Student _____ Date _____

Instructor _____ Date _____

PERFORMANCE CHECKLIST SKILL 26.2 **APPLYING A CARDIAC MONITOR**

	S	U	NP	Comments

ASSESSMENT

1. Identified patient using at least two identifiers. _____ _____ _____ _____

2. Determined reason for continuous cardiac monitoring. _____ _____ _____ _____

3. Assessed patient's level of understanding of procedure. _____ _____ _____ _____

4. Checked skin for excess oil or moisture, wiped chest and limbs with clean towel. _____ _____ _____ _____

PLANNING

1. Identified expected outcomes. _____ _____ _____ _____

2. Provided privacy. _____ _____ _____ _____

IMPLEMENTATION

1. Prepared patient for procedure:

   a. Removed or repositioned patient's gown to expose only chest, kept abdomen and thighs covered. _____ _____ _____ _____

   b. Placed patient in appropriate position. _____ _____ _____ _____

2. Performed hand hygiene. _____ _____ _____ _____

3. Cleaned and prepared chest area for electrode placement, clipped excess hair from electrode area. _____ _____ _____ _____

4. Applied electrodes in correct positions for three- or five-electrode system. _____ _____ _____ _____

5. Attached monitor to electrodes. _____ _____ _____ _____

6. Checked bedside monitor or telemetry station for messages. _____ _____ _____ _____

7. Checked that ECG rhythm can be visualized in monitor or viewing station. _____ _____ _____ _____

8. Changed ECG electrode daily or more often if necessary. _____ _____ _____ _____

9. Customized alarm limits within 1 hour of assuming care of patient and on condition changes. _____ _____ _____ _____

EVALUATION

1. Documented distress experienced by patient. _____ _____ _____ _____

2. Ensured all appropriate alarms are on. _____ _____ _____ _____

Copyright © 2018 by Elsevier Inc. All rights reserved.

	S	U	NP	Comments
3. Asked patient to explain why monitoring is important.	___	___	___	_____
4. Identified unexpected outcomes.	___	___	___	_____

RECORDING AND REPORTING

	S	U	NP	Comments
1. Reviewed alarm trends and waveforms once per shift and on report of alarm.	___	___	___	_____
2. Recorded at least one rhythm strip per shift in the appropriate log.	___	___	___	_____
3. Documented evaluation of patient learning.	___	___	___	_____
4. Reported unexpected outcomes immediately to health care provider.	___	___	___	_____

Copyright © 2018 by Elsevier Inc. All rights reserved.

Student _____ Date _____

Instructor _____ Date _____

PERFORMANCE CHECKLIST SKILL 27.1 **MANAGING CLOSED CHEST DRAINAGE SYSTEMS**

	S	U	NP	Comments

ASSESSMENT

1. Identified patient using two identifiers. ___ ___ ___ _____

2. Performed complete respiratory assessment, baseline vital signs, and pulse oximetry:

   a. Assessed for signs of respiratory distress and hypoxia. ___ ___ ___ _____

   b. Assessed for sharp stabbing chest pain, asked patient to rate comfort level. ___ ___ ___ _____

3. Assessed patient for known allergies. ___ ___ ___ _____

4. Reviewed patient's medication record for anti-coagulant therapy. ___ ___ ___ _____

5. Reviewed patient's hemoglobin and hemato-crit levels. ___ ___ ___ _____

6. For patient with chest tubes, observed chest tube dressing and insertion site, tubing for kinks or clots, and proper positioning of drainage system. ___ ___ ___ _____

7. Determined patient's knowledge of procedure. ___ ___ ___ _____

PLANNING

1. Identified expected outcomes. ___ ___ ___ _____

IMPLEMENTATION

1. Determined whether informed consent is needed, completed "time-out" procedure. ___ ___ ___ _____

2. Reviewed health care provider order for chest tube placement. ___ ___ ___ _____

3. Performed hand hygiene. ___ ___ ___ _____

4. Set up water-seal system:

   a. Obtained chest drainage system, removed wrappers. ___ ___ ___ _____

   b. Stood system upright, added water to appropriate compartments, maintained sterility of drainage tubing. ___ ___ ___ _____

5. Set up waterless system:

   a. Removed sterile wrappers. ___ ___ ___ _____

Copyright © 2018 by Elsevier Inc. All rights reserved.

	S	U	NP	Comments

b. Connected tubing between suction-control chamber and suction source for three-chamber system. ___ ___ ___ _____

c. Instilled water or NS into diagnostic indicator injection port. ___ ___ ___ _____

6. Secured all tubing connections properly, turned on suction. ___ ___ ___ _____

7. Turned off suction and unclamped drainage tubing before connecting patient to system. ___ ___ ___ _____

8. Administered ordered premedication. ___ ___ ___ _____

9. Provided psychological support to patient. ___ ___ ___ _____

10. Performed hand hygiene, applied clean gloves, positioned patient properly for tube insertion. ___ ___ ___ _____

11. Assisted health care provider with tube insertion, provided equipment and local analgesic. ___ ___ ___ _____

12. Assisted health care provider to attach drainage system, removed clamp, turned on suction. ___ ___ ___ _____

13. Taped or zip-tied all connections. ___ ___ ___ _____

14. Checked systems for proper function. ___ ___ ___ _____

15. Positioned patient appropriately. ___ ___ ___ _____

16. Checked patency of air vents in system. ___ ___ ___ _____

17. Positioned excess tubing appropriately and secured with clamp. ___ ___ ___ _____

18. Adjusted tubing to hang in a straight line from chest tube to drainage center. ___ ___ ___ _____

19. Placed two rubber-tipped hemostats in easily accessible position. ___ ___ ___ _____

20. Disposed of sharps in proper container, disposed of used supplies, performed hand hygiene. ___ ___ ___ _____

21. Cared for patient after chest tube insertion:

a. Performed hand hygiene, applied clean gloves, assessed vital signs, oxygen saturation, skin color, respiratory status, and insertion site at appropriate intervals. ___ ___ ___ _____

b. Monitored color, consistency, and amount of chest tube drainage at appropriate intervals, indicated level of fluid, date, and time properly. ___ ___ ___ _____

c. Observed chest dressing for drainage. ___ ___ ___ _____

336

Copyright © 2018 by Elsevier Inc. All rights reserved.

	S	U	NP	Comments

d. Applied clean gloves, palpated tube for swelling and crepitus.

___ ___ ___ _____

e. Ensured tubing is free of kinks and dependent loops.

___ ___ ___ _____

f. Observed for fluctuation of drainage and clots or debris in tubing.

___ ___ ___ _____

g. Kept drainage system upright and below level of patient's chest.

___ ___ ___ _____

h. Checked for air leaks by monitoring bubbling in water-seal chamber.

___ ___ ___ _____

i. Removed gloves, disposed of soiled equipment in appropriate biohazard container, performed hand hygiene.

___ ___ ___ _____

EVALUATION

1. Evaluated patient for decreased respiratory distress and chest pain, auscultated patient's lungs and observed chest expansion.

___ ___ ___ _____

2. Monitored vital signs and SpO_2.

___ ___ ___ _____

3. Reassessed patient's level of comfort, compared with level before chest tube insertion.

___ ___ ___ _____

4. Evaluated patient ability to use deep breathing exercises while maintaining comfort.

___ ___ ___ _____

5. Monitored continued functioning of system.

___ ___ ___ _____

6. Asked patient to explain why he or she has a chest tube.

___ ___ ___ _____

7. Identified unexpected outcomes.

___ ___ ___ _____

RECORDING AND REPORTING

1. Recorded pertinent information in the appropriate log.

___ ___ ___ _____

2. Recorded patient comfort and baseline vitals in the appropriate log.

___ ___ ___ _____

3. Reported any unexpected outcomes to nurse in charge or health care provider.

___ ___ ___ _____

Copyright © 2018 by Elsevier Inc. All rights reserved.

Student _____ Date _____

Instructor _____ Date _____

PERFORMANCE CHECKLIST SKILL 27.2   **ASSISTING WITH REMOVAL OF CHEST TUBES**

	S	U	NP	Comments
ASSESSMENT				
1. Identified patient using at least two identifiers.	___	___	___	_____
2. Performed respiratory assessment, assessed for lung reexpansion:				
a. Noted trend in water-seal fluctuation over last 24 hours.	___	___	___	_____
b. Provided results of chest x-ray.	___	___	___	_____
c. Confirmed that drainage has decreased to appropriate volume.	___	___	___	_____
d. Percussed lung for resonance.	___	___	___	_____
e. Auscultated lung sounds.	___	___	___	_____
3. Assessed patient's level of comfort, determined when last analgesic medication was given.	___	___	___	_____
4. Determined patient's understanding of chest tube removal procedure.	___	___	___	_____
5. Did not clamp chest tube before removal; assessed changes in vital signs, oxygen saturation, chest pain, apprehension, and symptoms of tension pneumothorax.	___	___	___	_____
PLANNING				
1. Identified expected outcomes.	___	___	___	_____
2. Explained procedure to patient.	___	___	___	_____
IMPLEMENTATION				
1. Administered prescribed medication for pain relief 30 minutes before procedure.	___	___	___	_____
2. Performed "time-out" procedure with health care provider.	___	___	___	_____
3. Performed hand hygiene, applied PPE if needed.	___	___	___	_____
4. Assisted patient to appropriate position, placed pad under chest tube site.	___	___	___	_____
5. Supported patient physically and emotionally while health care provider removed dressing and clips and sutures.	___	___	___	_____
6. Assisted patient to appropriate position.	___	___	___	_____

338

Copyright © 2018 by Elsevier Inc. All rights reserved.

	S	U	NP	Comments
7. Removed used equipment from bedside, placed in appropriate receptacle.	___	___	___	_____
8. Removed gloves, performed hand hygiene.	___	___	___	_____

EVALUATION

	S	U	NP	Comments
1. Auscultated lung sounds.	___	___	___	_____
2. Palpated over lung, observed patient for subcutaneous emphysema.	___	___	___	_____
3. Evaluated for respiratory distress in the first few hours after removal.	___	___	___	_____
4. Evaluated patient's vital signs, oxygen saturation, pulmonary status, and psychological status.	___	___	___	_____
5. Reviewed chest x-ray film.	___	___	___	_____
6. Asked about patient's level of pain, observed for nonverbal cues.	___	___	___	_____
7. Checked chest dressing for drainage and patency, noted wound for signs of healing.	___	___	___	_____
8. Asked patient to explain chest tube removal.	___	___	___	_____
9. Identified unexpected outcomes.	___	___	___	_____

RECORDING AND REPORTING

	S	U	NP	Comments
1. Recorded removal of tube and all pertinent information in the appropriate log.	___	___	___	_____
2. Recorded vital signs and respiratory assessment in the appropriate log.	___	___	___	_____
3. Reported unexpected outcomes to the nurse in charge or health care providers.	___	___	___	_____

Copyright © 2018 by Elsevier Inc. All rights reserved.

Student _____ Date _____

Instructor _____ Date _____

PERFORMANCE CHECKLIST SKILL 27.3 **AUTOTRANSFUSION OF CHEST TUBE DRAINAGE**

	S	U	NP	Comments
ASSESSMENT				
1. Identified patient using at least two identifiers.	___	___	___	_____
2. Performed assessment outlined in Skill 27.1.	___	___	___	_____
3. Determined presence of active bleeding through chest tube.	___	___	___	_____
4. Assessed IV site, noted size of IV catheter.	___	___	___	_____
5. Obtained baseline laboratory data.	___	___	___	_____
PLANNING				
1. Identified expected outcomes.	___	___	___	_____
2. Explained procedure to patient.	___	___	___	_____
IMPLEMENTATION				
1. Set up system:				
a. Set up ATS according to instructions and to maintain sterility of unit.	___	___	___	_____
b. Ensured all connections were tight and all clamps were open.	___	___	___	_____
2. Performed hand hygiene, applied gloves.	___	___	___	_____
3. Prepared chest drainage for reinfusion:				
a. Opened replacement bag following directions, closed the two white clamps.	___	___	___	_____
b. Used high-negativity relief valve to reduce excessive negativity.	___	___	___	_____
c. Performed bag transfer.				
(1) Closed clamps on chest drainage tubing.	___	___	___	_____
(2) Closed clamps on top of initial ATS collection bag.	___	___	___	_____
(3) Connected chest drainage tube to new bag.	___	___	___	_____
(4) Ensured all connections were tight.	___	___	___	_____
(5) Opened all clamps on chest drainage tube and replacement bag.	___	___	___	_____
d. Connected connectors of initial bag, removed appropriately.	___	___	___	_____
e. Secured replacement bag, secured frame onto the hook.	___	___	___	_____

Copyright © 2018 by Elsevier Inc. All rights reserved.

	S	U	NP	Comments

f. Placed thumbs on metal frame, pushed up to slide bag out, removed replacement bag.   ___ ___ ___ _____

4. Reinfused chest drainage:

   a. Used a new microaggregate filter to reinfuse each autotransfusion bag.   ___ ___ ___ _____

   b. Accessed bag by inverting bag and spiking it and twisting.   ___ ___ ___ _____

   c. Squeezed bag upside down to remove air, primed filler with blood.   ___ ___ ___ _____

   d. Hung bag on IV pole; primed until all air was gone; clamped tubing, attached to patient's IV access, and adjusted clamp to deliver reinfusion at appropriate rate.   ___ ___ ___ _____

   e. Added anticoagulants properly if ordered.   ___ ___ ___ _____

   f. Monitored patient's vital signs and SpO_2 properly.   ___ ___ ___ _____

5. Discontinued autotransfusion:

   a. Clamped chest drainage tube briefly, connected directly to chest drainage unit with red and blue connectors.   ___ ___ ___ _____

   b. Opened chest drainage tube clamp.   ___ ___ ___ _____

6. Discarded used supplies and performed hand hygiene.   ___ ___ ___ _____

EVALUATION

1. Monitored vital signs, hematocrit, and hemoglobin.   ___ ___ ___ _____

2. Monitored chest drainage system and patient's lung sounds.   ___ ___ ___ _____

3. Evaluated IV infusion site for infiltration and phlebitis.   ___ ___ ___ _____

4. Asked patient to explain why he or she needed this procedure.   ___ ___ ___ _____

5. Identified unexpected outcomes.   ___ ___ ___ _____

RECORDING AND REPORTING

1. Recorded drainage and reinfusion with times and amounts, patient response, condition of the IV site, and patient teaching and understanding in the appropriate log.   ___ ___ ___ _____

Copyright © 2018 by Elsevier Inc. All rights reserved.

Student _____ Date _____

Instructor _____ Date _____

PERFORMANCE CHECKLIST SKILL 28.1   **INSERTING AN OROPHARYNGEAL AIRWAY**

	S	U	NP	Comments
ASSESSMENT				
1. Identified need to insert oral airway.	___	___	___	_____
2. Determined factors that may contribute to upper airway obstruction.	___	___	___	_____
3. Ensured patient does not have dentures in.	___	___	___	_____
4. Assessed caregiver's knowledge of procedure.	___	___	___	_____
PLANNING				
1. Identified expected outcomes.	___	___	___	_____
2. Ensured family caregiver understands need for oropharyngeal airway.	___	___	___	_____
IMPLEMENTATION				
1. Positioned unconscious patient appropriately.	___	___	___	_____
2. Performed hand hygiene, applied clean gloves and PPE.	___	___	___	_____
3. Used padded tongue blade to open patient's mouth, used thumb and forefingers as necessary.	___	___	___	_____
4. Inserted oral airway:				
a. Held oral airway properly until back of throat was found, turned airway over and followed natural curve of tongue.	___	___	___	_____
5. Suctioned secretions as needed.	___	___	___	_____
6. Reassessed patient's respiratory status, auscultated lungs.	___	___	___	_____
7. Cleaned patient's face with tissue or washcloth.	___	___	___	_____
8. Discarded tissue into appropriate receptacle, placed washcloth in soiled linen bag, removed and discarded gloves and PPE, performed hand hygiene.	___	___	___	_____
9. Administered mouth care frequently.	___	___	___	_____
EVALUATION				
1. Observed patient's respiratory status and compared respiratory assessments before and after insertion.	___	___	___	_____

Copyright © 2018 by Elsevier Inc. All rights reserved.

	S	U	NP	Comments

2. Assessed that airway was patent and that patient's tongue did not obstruct airway.

3. Observed adjacent and underlying tissue for signs of redness, abrasion, or bruising.

4. Reassessed need for oral airway if patient pushed airway out with tongue or coughed.

5. Asked family to explain why oral airway is important.

6. Identified unexpected outcomes.

RECORDING AND REPORTING

1. Recorded assessment findings, size of airway, other interventions, and patient response in the appropriate log.

Copyright © 2018 by Elsevier Inc. All rights reserved.

Student _____ Date _____

Instructor _____ Date _____

PERFORMANCE CHECKLIST SKILL 28.2   **USING AN AUTOMATED EXTERNAL DEFIBRILLATOR**

	S	U	NP	Comments

ASSESSMENT

1. Established a person's unresponsiveness, called for help. ___ ___ ___ _____

2. Established absence of respirations and lack of circulation. ___ ___ ___ _____

PLANNING

1. Identified expected outcomes. ___ ___ ___ _____

IMPLEMENTATION

1. Assessed patient for unresponsiveness, not breathing or moving, and pulselessness. ___ ___ ___ _____

2. Activated code team in accordance with policy and procedure. ___ ___ ___ _____

3. Started chest compressions, continued until AED was attached to patient and device advised you to not touch the patient. ___ ___ ___ _____

4. Placed AED next to patient near chest or head. ___ ___ ___ _____

5. Turned power on. ___ ___ ___ _____

6. Attached the device properly, ensured cables were connected to the AED. ___ ___ ___ _____

7. Did *not* touch the patient when the AED prompted you, announced "Clear," allowed AED to analyze rhythm, pressed button if required. ___ ___ ___ _____

8. Announced "Clear," performed a visual check to ensure no one was in contact with the victim. ___ ___ ___ _____

9. Began chest compressions after the shock, continued for 2 minutes, did *not* remove the pads. ___ ___ ___ _____

10. Delivered two breaths using mouth-to-mouth with a barrier device or mask, delivered 10 to 12 breaths per minute. ___ ___ ___ _____

11. Cleared patient when AED prompted you, continued until patient regained pulse or a health care provider determined death. ___ ___ ___ _____

EVALUATION

1. Inspected pad adhesion to chest wall, applied new set of pads if necessary. ___ ___ ___ _____

Copyright © 2018 by Elsevier Inc. All rights reserved.

	S	U	NP	Comments

2. Continued efforts until patient regained pulse or health care provider determined death. _____ _____ _____ _____

3. Provided updates to family on patient's status. _____ _____ _____ _____

4. Identified unexpected outcomes. _____ _____ _____ _____

RECORDING AND REPORTING

1. Reported arrest via hospital-wide communication system immediately, included exact location. _____ _____ _____ _____

2. Documented arrest properly. _____ _____ _____ _____

3. Recorded all other pertinent information in the appropriate log. _____ _____ _____ _____

Copyright © 2018 by Elsevier Inc. All rights reserved.

Student _____ Date _____

Instructor _____ Date _____

PERFORMANCE CHECKLIST SKILL 28.3   **CODE MANAGEMENT**

	S	U	NP	Comments
ASSESSMENT				
1. Determined if patient was unconscious by shaking the patient and shouting, assessed patient unresponsiveness.	___	___	___	_____
PLANNING				
1. Identified expected outcomes.	___	___	___	_____
2. Activated hospital's code team or EMS immediately, told co-workers to bring AED and crash cart to bedside.	___	___	___	_____
IMPLEMENTATION: PRIMARY SURVEY				
1. Checked carotid pulse properly.	___	___	___	_____
2. Placed patient on a hard surface, ensured patient was flat, logrolled patient if trauma was suspected.	___	___	___	_____
3. Applied clean gloves and face shield.	___	___	___	_____
4. Opened airway by head tilt–chin lift or jaw thrust.	___	___	___	_____
5. Determined if patient has spontaneous respirations.	___	___	___	_____
6. Attempted to ventilate patient with slow breaths using appropriate method.	___	___	___	_____
7. Inserted oral airway if available.	___	___	___	_____
8. Suctioned secretions if necessary or turned patient's head to one side if appropriate.	___	___	___	_____
9. Applied AED immediately if appropriate and available in absence of patient's pulse.	___	___	___	_____
10. Initiated chest compressions if AED was unavailable, used correct hand position and compression ratio.	___	___	___	_____
IMPLEMENTATION: SECONDARY SURVEY				
1. Gave leader verbal report of events performed before code team's arrival.	___	___	___	_____
2. Delegated tasks appropriately while core group continued resuscitation efforts:				
a. Assisted victim's roommates or visitors away from code scene, assigned others to communicate with family.	___	___	___	_____

346

Copyright © 2018 by Elsevier Inc. All rights reserved.

	S	U	NP	Comments

b. Delegated someone to remove excess equipment from the room.

c. Had someone bring patient's chart or access patient's electronic medical record.

d. Assigned a nurse as recorder of events.

e. Assigned a nurse to get medications and supplies to hand off to code team members.

3. Attached manual defibrillator/monitor to patient appropriately.

4. Continued CPR and defibrillation if cardiac rhythm was "shockable":

   a. Turned on defibrillator, selected proper energy level.

   b. Applied conductive gel or gel pads to patient's chest.

   c. Placed paddles or pads on patient's chest wall.

   d. Verified that everyone had cleared the patient, called, "Clear."

5. Established IV access with large-bore IV needle, began infusion of 0.9% NS.

6. Assisted with procedure as needed.

7. Continued CPR until appropriate point.

8. Assisted code team with ET intubation if respirations were absent, had appropriate equipment available, ensured light source on laryngoscope was functional.

9. Assisted in confirmation of ET tube placement or advanced airway support.

10. Ventilated bag device on intubation.

11. Obtained ordered laboratory and diagnostic studies.

EVALUATION

1. Reassessed the primary and secondary surveys throughout the code event.

2. Palpated carotid pulse at least every 5 minutes after first minute of CPR.

3. Observed for spontaneous return of respirations or heart rate every 2 minutes.

4. Ensured that interruptions in CPR were minimized.

Copyright © 2018 by Elsevier Inc. All rights reserved.

	S	U	NP	Comments
5. Asked patient to explain why CPR was performed.	___	___	___	_____
6. Identified unexpected outcomes.	___	___	___	_____

RECORDING AND REPORTING

	S	U	NP	Comments
1. Reported arrest immediately, included exact location.	___	___	___	_____
2. Recorded all pertinent information in the appropriate log.	___	___	___	_____

Copyright © 2018 by Elsevier Inc. All rights reserved.

Student _____ Date _____

Instructor _____ Date _____

PERFORMANCE CHECKLIST SKILL 29.1 **INSERTION OF A SHORT-PERIPHERAL INTRAVENOUS DEVICE**

	S	U	NP	Comments
ASSESSMENT				
1. Reviewed accuracy of health care provider's order; followed six rights of medication administration, checked resources to ensure safe and correct administration.	___	___	___	_____
2. Performed hand hygiene, identified patient using two identifiers.	___	___	___	_____
3. Assessed patient's knowledge of procedure and reason for prescribed therapy, determined arm placement preference.	___	___	___	_____
4. Determined if patient was going to undergo any surgeries or operations.	___	___	___	_____
5. Assessed laboratory data.	___	___	___	_____
6. Assessed patient's history of allergies, especially to iodine, adhesive, or latex.	___	___	___	_____
PLANNING				
1. Identified expected outcomes.	___	___	___	_____
2. Collected appropriate equipment, ensured infusion set for the EID is correct.	___	___	___	_____
IMPLEMENTATION				
1. Performed hand hygiene.	___	___	___	_____
2. Instructed patient about rationale for infusion, medications ordered, procedure, and signs and symptoms of complications.	___	___	___	_____
3. Assisted patient to comfortable position, provided adequate lighting.	___	___	___	_____
4. Collected and organized equipment on bedside or overbed table.	___	___	___	_____
5. Changed patient's gown to more easily removable gown if available.	___	___	___	_____
6. Selected appropriate-size catheter, opened sterile packages using sterile aseptic technique.	___	___	___	_____
7. Prepared short extension tubing with appropriate connector:				
a. Removed cap from needleless connector, attached syringe with normal saline, primed tubing and connector, removed all air, left syringe attached to tubing.	___	___	___	_____

Copyright © 2018 by Elsevier Inc. All rights reserved.

	S	U	NP	Comments

b. Maintained sterility of end of connector, set aside for attaching to catheter hub after successful venipuncture.

8. Prepared tubing and solution for continuous infusion:

   a. Checked IV solution using six rights of administration, scanned bar codes on patient's wrist and IV fluid container if appropriate, ensured additives had been added, checked solution and bag.

   b. Opened infusion set, maintained sterility.

   c. Placed roller clamp below drip chamber, moved roller clamp to *off* position.

   d. Removed protective sheath over IV tubing port on bag or bottle.

   e. Removed protective cap from IV tubing spike, inserted spike into port of IV bag, cleansed rubber stopper, inserted spike into rubber stopper.

   f. Compressed drip chamber and released, filled drip chamber one-third to one-half full.

   g. Primed infusion tubing by filling with IV solution, removed protective cape on tubing, opened roller clamp, inverted Y connector to displace air, returned roller clamp to *off* position, replaced protective cap on end of tubing, labeled IV tubing.

   h. Ensured tubing was clear of air and bubbles, checked entire length of tubing.

   i. If optional long extension tubing was used, removed protective cap, attached to distal end of IV tubing, primed extension tubing, inserted tubing into EID with power off.

9. Performed hand hygiene.

10. Applied tourniquet around arm above antecubital fossa, checked for presence of radial pulse.

11. Selected appropriate vein for VAD insertion:

    a. Used most distal site in nondominant arm if possible.

    b. Palpated vein; noted resilience, soft feeling while releasing pressure; avoided veins that felt hard.

    c. Selected a well-dilated vein.

Copyright © 2018 by Elsevier Inc. All rights reserved.

	S	U	NP	Comments

d. Avoided areas with tenderness, redness, rash, pain, or infection; extremity affected by previous CVA, paralysis, dialysis shunt, or mastectomy; sites distal to previous venipuncture site; sclerosed or hardened veins; infiltrate site; areas of venous valves or phlebotic vessels; and fragile dorsal veins in older patients. ___ ___ ___ _____

e. Chose site that did not interfere with ADL. ___ ___ ___ _____

12. Released tourniquet temporarily. ___ ___ ___ _____

13. Performed hand hygiene, applied clean gloves and other PPE. ___ ___ ___ _____

14. Placed adapter end of extension set or needless connector for saline lock nearby in the sterile package. ___ ___ ___ _____

15. Cleaned site and dried, performed skin antisepsis with CHG solution and allowed to dry. ___ ___ ___ _____

16. Reapplied tourniquet properly, checked presence of pulse distal to tourniquet. ___ ___ ___ _____

17. Performed venipuncture, anchored vein below site, instructed patient to relax hand, warned patient of a sharp stick, inserted needle appropriately. ___ ___ ___ _____

18. Observed for blood return through flashback chamber, advanced catheter appropriately, loosened stylet over the needle catheter, held skin taught while stabilizing needle, advanced catheter off needle, threaded catheter into vein properly, placed stylet directly into sharps container. ___ ___ ___ _____

19. Stabilized catheter with nondominant hand, released cuff or tourniquet with the other, applied pressure above insertion site, kept catheter stable with index finger. ___ ___ ___ _____

20. Connected Luer-Lok end of tubing to end of catheter hub, secured connection ends, avoided touching sterile connection ends. ___ ___ ___ _____

21. Attached prefilled syringe of saline to set, aspirated to remove air and excess blood return, slowly injected saline into VAD, removed and discarded syringe. ___ ___ ___ _____

22. Observed insertion site for swelling ___ ___ ___ _____

23. Applied sterile dressing over site:

Copyright © 2018 by Elsevier Inc. All rights reserved.

	S	U	NP	Comments

a. Applied TSM dressing.

   (1) Removed adherent backing, applied one edge and smoothed remaining dressing over IV insertion site, left Luer-Lok connection uncovered, pressed dressing and removed outer covering, placed tape over Luer-Lok connection.

b. Applied sterile gauze dressing.

   (1) Placed sterile tape over catheter hub.

   (2) Placed gauze pad over insertion site and catheter hub, secured edges with tape, did not cover connection between IV tubing and catheter hub.

   (3) Folded and taped gauze appropriately, placed under Luer-Lok connection and secured, avoided applying tape or gauze around arm, did not use rolled bandages to secure VAD.

24. Secured IV catheter using engineered stabilization device.

25. Looped set tubing alongside arm, placed tape over tubing and secured.

26. Labeled dressing properly.

27. Disposed of sharps in the appropriate container, discarded supplies, removed gloves, performed hand hygiene.

28. Instructed patient in how to move without dislodging VAD.

EVALUATION

1. Observed patient at established intervals for function, intactness, and patency of IV system and for correct type, amount, and infusion rate.

2. Evaluated patient to determine response to therapy.

3. Evaluated patient at established intervals for signs of IV-related complications.

4. Asked patient to describe symptoms to report.

5. Identified unexpected outcomes.

RECORDING AND REPORTING

1. Recorded all pertinent information in the appropriate log.

2. Documented type and rate of infusion and device ID number if using an EID.

Copyright © 2018 by Elsevier Inc. All rights reserved.

	S	U	NP	Comments

3. Recorded patient's status, IV fluid, amount infused, and integrity and patency of system according to policy.

      ___ ___ ___   _____

4. Recorded level of patient's understanding in appropriate log.

      ___ ___ ___   _____

5. Reported pertinent information to oncoming nursing staff.

      ___ ___ ___   _____

6. Reported signs and symptoms of IV-related complications to health care provider.

      ___ ___ ___   _____

7. Recorded signs and symptoms of IV-related complications, interventions, and patient response to treatments.

      ___ ___ ___   _____

Copyright © 2018 by Elsevier Inc. All rights reserved.

Student _____   Date _____

Instructor _____   Date _____

PERFORMANCE CHECKLIST SKILL 29.2   **REGULATING INTRAVENOUS FLOW RATES**

	S	U	NP	Comments

ASSESSMENT

1. Reviewed accuracy and completeness of health care provider order, followed six rights of drug administration. ___ ___ ___ _____

2. Performed hand hygiene, identified patient using two identifiers. ___ ___ ___ _____

3. Applied clean gloves, inspected and palpated skin around IV site, asked patient how IV site feels, assessed VAD for patency and signs of IV-related complications, disposed of gloves, performed hand hygiene. ___ ___ ___ _____

4. Assessed IV system for patency. ___ ___ ___ _____

5. Identified patient risk for fluid and electrolyte imbalance. ___ ___ ___ _____

6. Assessed patient's knowledge of how positioning of IV site affects flow rate. ___ ___ ___ _____

PLANNING

1. Identified expected outcomes. ___ ___ ___ _____

2. Calculated flow rate with calculator or paper and pencil. ___ ___ ___ _____

3. Prepared patient and caregiver by explaining procedure, its purpose, and expectations of patient. ___ ___ ___ _____

4. Checked order to see how long each liter should infuse, calculated if necessary. ___ ___ ___ _____

5. Checked agency policy regarding KVO flow rate if needed. ___ ___ ___ _____

6. Used hourly rate to program EID or calculate minute flow rate. ___ ___ ___ _____

7. Knew calibration of infusion set. ___ ___ ___ _____

8. Selected appropriate formula to calculate minute flow drops based on drop factor of infusion set. ___ ___ ___ _____

IMPLEMENTATION

1. Regulated gravity infusion:

   a. Ensured IV container is at an appropriate height. ___ ___ ___ _____

Copyright © 2018 by Elsevier Inc. All rights reserved.

	S	U	NP	Comments

b. Opened roller clamp on tubing until there are drops in drip chamber, counted drip rate for 1 minute, adjusted roller clamp if needed.

____ ____ ____ _____

c. Monitored drip rate at least hourly.

____ ____ ____ _____

2. Regulated EID:

a. Closed roller clamp on primed IV infusion tubing.

____ ____ ____ _____

b. Inserted infusion tubing into chamber of control mechanism.

____ ____ ____ _____

c. Secured part of IV tubing through "air in line" alarm system, closed door, turned on power, selected drop rate, closed door, and pressed start. If infusing, accessed EID library and set rate and dose limits.

____ ____ ____ _____

d. Opened infusion tubing drip regulator completely while EID is in use.

____ ____ ____ _____

e. Monitored infusion rate and IV site for complications, used watch to verify rate of infusion.

____ ____ ____ _____

f. Assessed IV system from container to VAD insertion site when alarm signals.

____ ____ ____ _____

3. Attached label to IV solution container with date and time container changed.

____ ____ ____ _____

4. Taught patient purpose of EID, purpose of alarms, to avoid raising hand or arm that affects flow rate, and to avoid touching clamp.

____ ____ ____ _____

5. Removed and disposed of used supplies, performed hand hygiene.

____ ____ ____ _____

EVALUATION

1. Observed patient every 1 to 2 hours, noted volume of IV rate infused and rate of infusion.

____ ____ ____ _____

2. Evaluated patient's response to therapy.

____ ____ ____ _____

3. Evaluated patient at established intervals for signs of IV-related complications.

____ ____ ____ _____

4. Asked patient to explain what causes pump to alarm and what to do when it does.

____ ____ ____ _____

5. Identified unexpected outcomes.

____ ____ ____ _____

Copyright © 2018 by Elsevier Inc. All rights reserved.

	S	U	NP	Comments

RECORDING AND REPORTING

1. Recorded IV solution, rate of infusion, and integrity and patency of system in appropriate log.

2. Recorded use of EID or control device and device ID number.

3. Recorded patient response and unexpected outcomes.

4. Recorded patient's level of understanding and ability to follow instructions.

5. Reported rate of and volume left in infusion to next nurse assigned to care for patient.

Copyright © 2018 by Elsevier Inc. All rights reserved.

Student _____ Date _____

Instructor _____ Date _____

PERFORMANCE CHECKLIST SKILL 29.3 **CHANGING INTRAVENOUS SOLUTIONS**

	S	U	NP	Comments

ASSESSMENT

1. Reviewed accuracy and completeness of health care provider's order, followed six rights of drug administration. ___ ___ ___ _____

2. Noted date and time when IV tubing and solution were last changed. ___ ___ ___ _____

3. Identified patient using at least two identifiers. ___ ___ ___ _____

4. Determined patient's understanding of need for continued IV therapy. ___ ___ ___ _____

5. Performed hand hygiene, applied clean gloves, inspected and palpated skin around IV site, assessed VAD for patency and signs of IV-related complications. ___ ___ ___ _____

6. Checked infusion system from solution container to VAD insertion site for integrity, determined compatibility of all IV solutions and additives, discarded gloves and performed hand hygiene. ___ ___ ___ _____

7. Checked pertinent laboratory values. ___ ___ ___ _____

PLANNING

1. Identified expected outcomes. ___ ___ ___ _____

2. Performed hand hygiene, gathered equipment, had solution prepared at least 1 hour before needed, allowed solution to warm to room temperature, checked that solution is properly labeled, followed any light sensitivity restrictions. ___ ___ ___ _____

3. Prepared patient and caregiver by explaining procedure, its purpose, and what is expected of patient. ___ ___ ___ _____

IMPLEMENTATION

1. Changed solution at an appropriate time. ___ ___ ___ _____

2. Performed hand hygiene. ___ ___ ___ _____

3. Prepared new solution for changing, hung bag on IV pole and removed protective cover from tubing port, OR removed metal cap and rubber disks from glass bottle. ___ ___ ___ _____

Copyright © 2018 by Elsevier Inc. All rights reserved.

	S	U	NP	Comments

4. Closed roller clamp on existing solution, removed tubing from EID, removed old fluid container from IV pole, held container with tubing port pointing upward.

5. Removed spike from old solution container, inserted into new container.

6. Hung new container of solution on IV pole.

7. Checked for air in tubing, removed properly if necessary.

8. Ensured drip chamber is one-third to one-half full.

9. Regulated flow to ordered rate using either roller clamp or EID.

10. Placed time label on side of container, labeled appropriately.

11. Instructed patient on purpose of new IV solution and additives, flow rate, potential side effects, how to avoid occluding tubing, and what to report.

EVALUATION

1. Observed patient every 1 to 2 hours for functioning, intactness, and patency of IV system, infusion rate, and type and amount of IV solution infused.

2. Determined patient's response to therapy.

3. Observed patient for signs of FVD or FVE to determine response to IV therapy.

4. Evaluated patient for signs of IV-related complications.

5. Asked patient to describe what to do if IV is dripping.

6. Identified unexpected outcomes.

RECORDING AND REPORTING

1. Recorded amount and type of solution, flow rate, and integrity and patency of system in the appropriate log.

2. Recorded use of EID or control device and device ID number.

3. Recorded what IV problems patient knows to report.

4. Recorded patient response to therapy and unexpected outcomes.

5. Reported rate of and volume left in infusion to next nurse assigned to care for patient.

Copyright © 2018 by Elsevier Inc. All rights reserved.

Student _____ Date _____

Instructor _____ Date _____

PERFORMANCE CHECKLIST SKILL 29.4 **CHANGING INFUSION TUBING**

	S	U	NP	Comments
ASSESSMENT				
1. Noted date and time when IV tubing was last changed.	___	___	___	_____
2. Identified patient using at least two identifiers, compared with information in MAR.	___	___	___	_____
3. Performed hand hygiene, assessed tubing for puncture, contamination, or occlusion that required immediate change.	___	___	___	_____
4. Determined patient's understanding of need for continued IV therapy.	___	___	___	_____
PLANNING				
1. Identified expected outcomes.	___	___	___	_____
2. Prepared patient by explaining procedure, its purpose, and expectations of patient.	___	___	___	_____
3. Coordinated IV tubing changes with solution changes when possible.	___	___	___	_____
4. Collected equipment.	___	___	___	_____
IMPLEMENTATION				
1. Performed hand hygiene, opened new infusion set and add-on pieces, kept protective coverings in place, placed roller clamp below drip chamber and moved clamp to off position, secured all connections.	___	___	___	_____
2. Applied clean gloves, removed IV dressing if necessary.	___	___	___	_____
3. Prepared IV tubing with new IV container.	___	___	NP	_____
4. Prepared IV tubing with existing continuous IV infusion bag:				
a. Moved roller clamp on new IV tubing to off position.	___	___	___	_____
b. Slowed rate of infusion through old tubing.	___	___	___	_____
c. Compressed and filled drip chamber of old tubing.	___	___	___	_____

Copyright © 2018 by Elsevier Inc. All rights reserved.

	S	U	NP	Comments

d. Inverted container, removed old tubing, kept spike sterile and upright.

   ____   ____   ____   _____

e. Inserted spike of new tubing into solution container, hung solution bag on IV pole, compressed and released drip chamber on new tubing, filled drip chamber appropriately.

f. Removed protective cover on end of tubing, opened roller clamp, primed new tubing with solution, stopped infusion, replaced cap, placed end of adapter near patient's IV site.

g. Stopped EID of turned roller clamp on old tubing to *off* position.

5. Prepared tubing with extension set or saline lock:

   a. Used sterile technique to connect new injection cap to new extension set.

   b. Scrubbed injection cap with antiseptic swab and allowed to dry, attached syringe with saline flush solution, injected into extension set.

6. Reestablished infusion:

   a. Disconnected old tubing from extension set, inserted Luer-Lok of new tubing or saline lock into connection.

   b. Opened roller clamp on new tubing for continuous infusion, regulated drip using roller clamp or EID.

   c. Attached tape or label with date and time of change onto tubing below drip chamber.

   d. Formed a loop of tubing, secured to patient's arm with tape.

7. Removed and discarded old IV tubing, applied new dressing if necessary, removed and disposed of gloves, performed hand hygiene.

8. Taught patient how to move and turn properly with IV tubing.

EVALUATION

1. Observed patient every 1 to 2 hours for function, intactness, and patency of IV system and leaking at connection sites.

2. Evaluated patient for signs of IV-related complications.

Copyright © 2018 by Elsevier Inc. All rights reserved.

	S	U	NP	Comments

3. Asked patient to explain how to prevent tubing from being pinched and what signs should be reported to a nurse. ____ ____ ____ _____

4. Identified unexpected outcomes. ____ ____ ____ _____

RECORDING AND REPORTING

1. Recorded tubing change, type of solution, volume, and rate in appropriate record; recorded parenteral fluids appropriately. ____ ____ ____ _____

2. Recorded what IV problems patient knows to report. ____ ____ ____ _____

Copyright © 2018 by Elsevier Inc. All rights reserved.

Student _____ Date _____

Instructor _____ Date _____

PERFORMANCE CHECKLIST SKILL 29.5 **CHANGING A SHORT-PERIPHERAL INTRAVENOUS DRESSING**

	S	U	NP	Comments
ASSESSMENT				
1. Identified patient using at least two identifiers, compared with information in MAR.	___	___	___	_____
2. Determined when dressing was last changed.	___	___	___	_____
3. Performed hand hygiene, applied new gloves, observed dressing for moisture and intactness, determined source of any moisture.	___	___	___	_____
4. Inspected and palpated skin around IV site, assessed VAD for patency and signs of IV-related complications, removed and discarded gloves.	___	___	___	_____
5. Assessed patient's understanding of need for continued IV infusion.	___	___	___	_____
PLANNING				
1. Identified expected outcomes.	___	___	___	_____
2. Explained procedure and purpose to patient and caregiver, explained that patient will need to hold affected extremity still, explained how long procedure will take.	___	___	___	_____
3. Performed hand hygiene, collected equipment and organized on bedside or overbed table, applied clean gloves.	___	___	___	_____
IMPLEMENTATION				
1. Removed dressing appropriately:				
a. Removed TSM dressing by stabilizing catheter, pulling up corners of dressing properly until dressing is removed.	___	___	___	_____
b. Removed gauze dressing by stabilizing catheter hub while loosening tape and removing old dressing one layer at a time.	___	___	___	_____
2. Assessed VAD insertion site for signs of IV-related complications, determined if VAD requires removal, removed if ordered.	___	___	___	_____

Copyright © 2018 by Elsevier Inc. All rights reserved.

	S	U	NP	Comments

3. Assessed integrity of engineered stabilization advice, assessed for signs of adhesive-related skin injury.

4. Performed skin antisepsis to insertion site with CHG solution and allowed to dry.

5. Applied skin protectant to area if necessary.

6. Applied sterile dressing over site while stabilizing catheter:

   a. Applied TSM dressing appropriately.

   b. Applied sterile gauze dressing appropriately.

7. Secured new engineered catheter stabilization device if necessary.

8. Removed and discarded glove and used equipment, performed hand hygiene.

9. Applied site protection device if appropriate.

10. Anchored extension tubing or IV tubing along arm and secured, avoided placing tape over dressing.

11. Labeled dressing properly.

12. Performed hand hygiene.

EVALUATION

1. Evaluated function, patency of IV system, and flow rate after changing dressing.

2. Evaluated patient for signs of IV-related complications.

3. Asked patient to describe problems to report that would require a dressing change.

4. Identified unexpected outcomes.

RECORDING AND REPORTING

1. Recorded time and reason for change, type of dressing, patency of system, and description of VAD in appropriate log.

2. Recorded what IV problems patient knows to report.

3. Reported that dressing was changed and any significant information to incoming nurse.

4. Reported and documented complication, interventions, and responses.

Copyright © 2018 by Elsevier Inc. All rights reserved.

Student _____ Date _____

Instructor _____ Date _____

PERFORMANCE CHECKLIST PROCEDURAL GUIDELINE 29.1   **DISCONTINUING A SHORT-PERIPHERAL INTRAVENOUS ACCESS**

	S	U	NP	Comments
PROCEDURAL STEPS				
1. Reviewed accuracy and completeness of order for discontinuation of VAD.	___	___	___	_____
2. Performed hand hygiene, collected equipment.	___	___	___	_____
3. Identified patient using at least two identifiers.	___	___	___	_____
4. Applied clean gloves, observed existing IV site for signs of IV-related complications, palpated catheter site through intact dressing.	___	___	___	_____
5. Assessed if patient is receiving anticoagulant or has history of coagulopathy.	___	___	___	_____
6. Assessed patient's understanding of reason for IV infusion to be discontinued.	___	___	___	_____
7. Explained procedure to patient before you removed catheter, explained that patient needs to hold affected extremity still.	___	___	___	_____
8. Turned IV tubing roller clamp to *off* position or turned EID off first.	___	___	___	_____
9. Removed VAD dressing and engineered stabilization device.	___	___	___	_____
10. Stabilized catheter hub properly.	___	___	___	_____
11. Placed clean sterile gauze above site, withdrew catheter properly, kept hub parallel to skin.	___	___	___	_____
12. Applied pressure to site for appropriate length of time.	___	___	___	_____
13. Inspected catheter for intactness after removal, noted tip and integrity length.	___	___	___	_____
14. Observed site for evidence of any complications.	___	___	___	_____
15. Applied clean gauze dressing over insertion site, secured with tape.	___	___	___	_____

Copyright © 2018 by Elsevier Inc. All rights reserved.

	S	U	NP	Comments
16. Discarded used supplies, removed gloves, performed hand hygiene.	____	____	____	_____
17. Documented procedure in patient's medical record.	____	____	____	_____
18. Asked patient to explain why IV is being removed.	____	____	____	_____

Copyright © 2018 by Elsevier Inc. All rights reserved.

Student _____ Date _____

Instructor _____ Date _____

PERFORMANCE CHECKLIST SKILL 29.6   **MANAGING CENTRAL VASCULAR ACCESS DEVICES**

	S	U	NP	Comments

ASSESSMENT

1. Reviewed accuracy and completeness of order for insertion of CVAD for size and type, assessed treatment schedule, followed six rights of medication administration. ___ ___ ___ _____

2. Identified patient using at least two identifiers, compared identifiers with information on MAR. ___ ___ ___ _____

3. Performed hand hygiene, assessed patient's hydration status. ___ ___ ___ _____

4. Assessed patient for any surgical procedures of the upper chest or anatomical irregularities of the proposed insertion site. ___ ___ ___ _____

5. Assessed CVAD placement site for skin integrity and signs of infection, applied gloves if drainage is present. ___ ___ ___ _____

6. Assessed patient for allergy to iodine, lidocaine, latex, or CHG. ___ ___ ___ _____

7. Assessed type of CVAD intended for placement, reviewed manufacturer's directions. ___ ___ ___ _____

8. Assessed for proper function of CVAD before therapy. ___ ___ ___ _____

9. Assessed if lumens require flushing or site needs dressing change. ___ ___ ___ _____

10. Assessed patient's understanding of CVAD and knowledge of purpose, care, and maintenance; asked patient to discuss steps in care and perform procedure. ___ ___ ___ _____

PLANNING

1. Identified expected outcomes. ___ ___ ___ _____

2. Explained procedure and purpose to patient and caregiver, explained that patient must not move during procedure, offered pain medication and opportunity to toilet. ___ ___ ___ _____

3. Performed hand hygiene, collected and organized equipment on bedside or overbed table. ___ ___ ___ _____

Copyright © 2018 by Elsevier Inc. All rights reserved.

	S	U	NP	Comments

IMPLEMENTATION

1. Performed catheter insertion for nontunneled device:

   a. Assisted physician in positioning patient properly. ___ ___ ___ _____

   b. Performed hand hygiene. ___ ___ ___ _____

   c. Used scissors or electric clippers to remove hair around insertion site, explained rationale to patient. ___ ___ ___ _____

   d. Applied PPE. ___ ___ ___ _____

   e. Added sterile equipment to CVA kit as needed. ___ ___ ___ _____

   f. Prepared site with CHG solution, allowed to dry. ___ ___ ___ _____

   g. Removed gloves, performed hand hygiene. ___ ___ ___ _____

   h. Set up IV bag, filled tubing, covered end of tubing with sterile cap. ___ ___ ___ _____

   i. Wiped off top of lidocaine bottle with alcohol, held bottle upside down, applied topical anesthetic agents before insertion if necessary. ___ ___ ___ _____

   j. Once catheter is removed, adjusted IV infusion to prescribed rate, connected to electronic infusion pump once chest x-ray study was obtained. ___ ___ ___ _____

2. Performed insertion site care and dressing change:

   a. Positioned patient properly. ___ ___ ___ _____

   b. Prepared dressing materials. ___ ___ ___ _____

   c. Performed hand hygiene, applied mask, provided mask for patient. ___ ___ ___ _____

   d. Applied clean gloves, removed old dressing properly, discarded appropriately. ___ ___ ___ _____

   e. Removed catheter stabilization device properly if used. ___ ___ ___ _____

   f. Inspected catheter, insertion site, and surrounding skin, compared length measurements if dislodgement is suspected. ___ ___ ___ _____

   g. Removed and discarded gloves, performed hand hygiene, opened CVAD dressing kit using sterile technique, applied sterile gloves. ___ ___ ___ _____

Copyright © 2018 by Elsevier Inc. All rights reserved.

	S	U	NP	Comments
h. Cleaned site appropriately.	___	___	___	_____
i. Applied skin protectant to entire area, allowed to dry completely.	___	___	___	_____
j. Used chlorhexidine-impregnated dressing if appropriate.	___	___	___	_____
k. Applied sterile TSM dressing or gauze over insertion site.	___	___	___	_____
l. Applied new catheter stabilization device appropriately if needed.	___	___	___	_____
m. Applied appropriate label.	___	___	___	_____
n. Disposed of supplies and used equipment appropriately, removed gloves, performed hand hygiene.	___	___	___	_____

3. Took blood sample properly:

	S	U	NP	Comments
a. Applied clean gloves.	___	___	___	_____
b. Turned off all infusions for at least 1 minute before drawing blood, drew blood from a peripheral vein if necessary.	___	___	___	_____
c. Used appropriate lumen of a multilumen catheter.	___	___	___	_____
d. Syringe method.				
(1) Removed end of IV tubing or injection cap from the catheter hub, kept end of tubing sterile.	___	___	___	_____
(2) Disinfected catheter hub with antiseptic solution, allowed to dry.	___	___	___	_____
(3) Attached an empty syringe, unclamped catheter, and withdrew blood for discard sample.	___	___	___	_____
(4) Reclamped catheter, removed syringe with blood, discarded in appropriate biohazard container.	___	___	___	_____
(5) Cleansed hub with another antiseptic solution, allowed to dry completely.	___	___	___	_____
(6) Attached second syringe(s) to obtain required volume of blood for specimen.	___	___	___	_____
(7) Unclamped catheter if necessary to withdraw blood.	___	___	___	_____
(8) Reclamped catheter after obtaining specimen, removed syringe.	___	___	___	_____

Copyright © 2018 by Elsevier Inc. All rights reserved.

	S	U	NP	Comments

(9) Cleansed catheter hub with antiseptic solution, allowed to dry. ___ ___ ___ _____

(10) Attached prefilled injection cap to syringe of sodium chloride to catheter, used appropriate flush/clamp/disconnect sequence, ensured clamp is engaged. ___ ___ ___ _____

(11) Removed syringe, discarded into appropriate container. ___ ___ ___ _____

e. Transferred blood using transfer vacuum device. ___ ___ ___ _____

f. Flushed catheter with heparin solution, ensured clamp is engaged. ___ ___ ___ _____

g. Removed syringe, scrubbed hub with antiseptic and allowed to dry, attached injection cap or IV tubing, resumed infusion as ordered or clamped catheter if needed. ___ ___ ___ _____

h. Disposed of soiled equipment and used supplies, removed gloves, performed hand hygiene. ___ ___ ___ _____

4. Changed injection cap properly:

a. Determined if injection caps should be changed. ___ ___ ___ _____

b. Primed new injection cap(s) properly. ___ ___ ___ _____

c. Clamped catheter lumens one at a time if needed. ___ ___ ___ _____

d. Cleansed catheter hub and injection cap, removed and disposed of old injection cap. ___ ___ ___ _____

e. Cleansed exposed hub with antiseptic, connected new injection caps on catheter hub. ___ ___ ___ _____

f. Flushed catheter with sodium chloride followed by heparin solution, ensured clamp is engaged. ___ ___ ___ _____

g. Disposed of all soiled supplies and used equipment, removed gloves, performed hand hygiene. ___ ___ ___ _____

5. Discontinued nontunneled catheter appropriately:

a. Verified order to discontinue line, checked agency policy for the person who should discontinue CVAD. ___ ___ ___ _____

Copyright © 2018 by Elsevier Inc. All rights reserved.

	S	U	NP	Comments

b. Prepared to convert IV fluids or medications to a short peripheral or middle before CVAD continuation. _____ _____ _____ _____

c. Positioned patient appropriately. _____ _____ _____ _____

d. Performed hand hygiene. _____ _____ _____ _____

e. Turned off IV fluids infusing through central line, converted to alternate VAD. _____ _____ _____ _____

f. Placed moisture-proof pad under site. _____ _____ _____ _____

g. Applied PPE. _____ _____ _____ _____

h. Removed CVAD dressing appropriately. _____ _____ _____ _____

i. Removed catheter securement device with alcohol. _____ _____ _____ _____

j. Removed gloves, performed hand hygiene, opened CVAD dressing change kit and suture removal kit, added additional items to sterile fields, applied sterile gloves. _____ _____ _____ _____

k. Performed skin antisepsis of insertion site with CHG, allowed to dry. _____ _____ _____ _____

l. Applied sterile gauze to site, instructed patient to take a deep breath and perform Valsalva maneuver as catheter is withdrawn. _____ _____ _____ _____

m. Removed catheter smoothly and properly, inspected catheter for intactness, applied pressure to site until bleeding stopped, stopped removal if resistance is met. _____ _____ _____ _____

n. Applied petroleum-based ointment to exit site, applied sterile occlusive dressing to site, changed dressing every 24 hours until healed. _____ _____ _____ _____

o. Labeled dressing properly. _____ _____ _____ _____

p. Inspected catheter integrity, discarded in biohazard container. _____ _____ _____ _____

q. Returned patient to comfortable position, ensured short peripheral IV or midline was infusing at correct rate. _____ _____ _____ _____

r. Disposed of soiled supplies, removed gloves and PPE, performed hand hygiene. _____ _____ _____ _____

Copyright © 2018 by Elsevier Inc. All rights reserved.

	S	U	NP	Comments

EVALUATION

1. Consulted x-ray film examination reports for catheter placement.

2. Determined daily continued need for CVAD.

3. Evaluated for postinsertion complications:

    a. Auscultated breath sounds, evaluated for shortness of breath, chest pain, and absent breath sounds.

    b. Monitored vital signs.

    c. Monitored patient complaints of pain, numbness, tingling, or weakness.

4. Evaluated patient to determine response to infusion therapy.

5. Evaluated patient for signs of CVAD-related complications.

6. Observed all connection points, ensured they are secure.

7. Asked patient to describe problems that might develop and what to report to a nurse.

8. Identified unexpected outcomes.

RECORDING AND REPORTING

1. Notified health care provider of signs and symptoms of any complications.

2. Documented catheter site care in nurses' notes.

3. Documented patient's ability to explain instructions.

4. Documented catheter removal in nurses' notes.

5. Documented blood draw in nurses' notes.

6. Documented in nurses' notes unexpected outcomes, health care provider notification, interventions, and patient response to treatment.

Copyright © 2018 by Elsevier Inc. All rights reserved.

Student _____   Date _____

Instructor _____   Date _____

PERFORMANCE CHECKLIST SKILL 30.1 **INITIATING BLOOD THERAPY**

	S	U	NP	Comments

ASSESSMENT

1. Verified health care provider's order for specific blood or blood product and all pertinent information. ___ ___ ___ _____

2. Obtained patient's transfusion history, noted known allergies and previous transfusion reactions, verified that type and cross-match had been completed appropriately. ___ ___ ___ _____

3. Verified that IV cannula was patent and without complications, administered blood or blood components using appropriate peripheral catheter. ___ ___ ___ _____

4. Assessed laboratory values such as hematocrit, coagulation values, platelet count, and potassium. ___ ___ ___ _____

5. Checked that patient had completed and signed transfusion consent before retrieving blood. ___ ___ ___ _____

6. Knew indications or reasons for a transfusion, packed RBCs if necessary. ___ ___ ___ _____

7. Obtained and recorded pretransfusion baseline vital signs, notified health care provider if patient was febrile. ___ ___ ___ _____

8. Assessed patient's need for IV fluids or medications while transfusion was infusing. ___ ___ ___ _____

9. Assessed patient's understanding of procedure and rationale. ___ ___ ___ _____

PLANNING

1. Identified expected outcomes. ___ ___ ___ _____

IMPLEMENTATION

1. Performed preadministration protocol:

   a. Obtained blood component following agency protocol. ___ ___ ___ _____

   b. Checked blood bag for signs of contamination and presence of leaks. ___ ___ ___ _____

   c. Compared verbally; correctly verified patient, blood product, and type with another qualified person before initiating transfusion. ___ ___ ___ _____

Copyright © 2018 by Elsevier Inc. All rights reserved.

	S	U	NP	Comments
(1) Identified patient using at least two identifiers.	——	——	——	————————
(2) Matched transfusion record number and patient's ID number.	——	——	——	————————
(3) Ensured patient's name is correct on all documents.	——	——	——	————————
(4) Checked unit number on blood bag with blood bank, checked expiration date and time.	——	——	——	————————
(5) Ensured blood type matches transfusion record and blood bag.	——	——	——	————————
(6) Checked that patient's blood type and Rh type are compatible with donor's.	——	——	——	————————
(7) Checked expiration date and time on unit of blood.	——	——	——	————————
(8) Checked patient ID information with blood unit label, did not administer if patient has no ID bracelet.	——	——	——	————————
(9) Verified patient and unit identification record process properly.	——	——	——	————————
d. Reviewed purpose of transfusion, asked patient to report any changes he or she may feel during the transfusion.	——	——	——	————————
e. Had patient empty urine drainage collection container or applied gloves and emptied for him or her.	——	——	——	————————
2. Administered transfusion:				
a. Performed hand hygiene, applied gloves, reinspected blood product for leakage or unusual appearance.	——	——	——	————————
b. Opened Y-tubing blood administration set, used multiset if needed.	——	——	——	————————
c. Set all clamps to *off* position.	——	——	——	————————
d. Spiked normal saline IV bag with spike, hung bag on pole, primed tubing, opened upper clamp on saline side of tubing, squeezed drip chamber until fluid covered filter and appropriate amount of drip chamber.	——	——	——	————————
e. Maintained clamp on blood product side of tubing in *off* position, opened common tubing clamp, closed clamp when tubing was filled with saline, maintained protective sterile cap on tubing connector.	——	——	——	————————

Copyright © 2018 by Elsevier Inc. All rights reserved.

	S	U	NP	Comments

f. Prepared blood component for administration, agitated blood unit bag, removed covering from access port, spiked unit with other Y connection, closed saline clamp, opened blood unit clamp, primed tubing with blood, ensured residual air was removed. ___ ___ ___ _____

g. Maintained asepsis, attached primed tubing to patient's VAD, connected primed blood administration tubing to patient's VAD. ___ ___ ___ _____

h. Opened tubing clamp, regulated blood flow properly. ___ ___ ___ _____

i. Monitored patient's vital signs at the appropriate times. ___ ___ ___ _____

j. Regulated rate appropriately if there was no transfusion reaction, checked drop factor for the blood tubing. ___ ___ ___ _____

k. Cleared IV line with saline, discarded blood bag appropriately, maintained patency when consecutive units were ordered. ___ ___ ___ _____

l. Disposed of all supplies appropriately, removed gloves, performed hand hygiene. ___ ___ ___ _____

EVALUATION

1. Observed IV site and status of infusion each time vitals were taken. ___ ___ ___ _____

2. Observed for change in vital signs and signs of transfusion reactions. ___ ___ ___ _____

3. Observed patient, assessed laboratory values to determine response. ___ ___ ___ _____

4. Asked patient to describe reasons for and risks and benefits of transfusion. ___ ___ ___ _____

5. Identified unexpected outcomes. ___ ___ ___ _____

RECORDING AND REPORTING

1. Recorded pretransfusion medication, vital signs, location and condition of IV site, and patient education. ___ ___ ___ _____

2. Recorded type and volume of blood component; unit/donor/recipient identification, compatibility, and expiration date; and patient's response, documented transfusion notes appropriately. ___ ___ ___ _____

3. Recorded volume of NS a blood component infused. ___ ___ ___ _____

Copyright © 2018 by Elsevier Inc. All rights reserved.

	S	U	NP	Comments
4. Recorded amount of blood received by autotransfusion and patient's response.	——	——	——	_____
5. Recorded vital signs before and after initiation, and after transfusion.	——	——	——	_____
6. Documented evaluation of patient learning.	——	——	——	_____
7. Reported signs of transfusion reaction immediately.	——	——	——	_____
8. Reported any intratransfusion/posttransfusion deterioration in cardiac, pulmonary, or renal status.	——	——	——	_____

Copyright © 2018 by Elsevier Inc. All rights reserved.

Student _____ Date _____

Instructor _____ Date _____

PERFORMANCE CHECKLIST SKILL 30.2 **MONITORING FOR ADVERSE TRANSFUSION REACTIONS**

	S	U	NP	Comments
ASSESSMENT				
1. Identified patient using at least two identifiers.	___	___	___	_____
2. Observed patient for fever with or without chills in conjunction with initiation of transfusion.	___	___	___	_____
3. Assessed patient for tachycardia/tachypnea and dyspnea.	___	___	___	_____
4. Observed patient for drop in blood pressure.	___	___	___	_____
5. Observed patient for hives or skin rash.	___	___	___	_____
6. Observed patient for flushing.	___	___	___	_____
7. Observed patient for gastrointestinal symptoms.	___	___	___	_____
8. Observed patient for wheezing, chest pain, and possible cardiac arrest.	___	___	___	_____
9. Remained alert to patient complaints of headache or muscle pain in presence of a fever.	___	___	___	_____
10. Monitored patient for DIC, renal failure, anemia, and hemoglobinemia/hemoglobinuria by reviewing laboratory test results.	___	___	___	_____
11. Auscultated patient's lungs, monitored CVP if possible.	___	___	___	_____
12. Observed patient for signs of liver damage and bone marrow suppression.	___	___	___	_____
13. Observed for mild hypothermia, cardiac dysrhythmias, hypotension, hypocalcemia, and hemochromatosis in patients receiving massive transfusions.	___	___	___	_____
PLANNING				
1. Identified expected outcomes.	___	___	___	_____
2. Ensured patient can explain signs of a transfusion reaction.	___	___	___	_____
IMPLEMENTATION				
1. Responded to suspected transfusion reaction:				

376

Copyright © 2018 by Elsevier Inc. All rights reserved.

	S	U	NP	Comments

a. Stopped transfusion immediately.   ___ ___ ___ _____

b. Removed blood component and tubing containing blood product, replaced with normal saline and new tubing, connected tubing to hub of VAD, administered antihistamine instead if appropriate.   ___ ___ ___ _____

c. Maintained patent VAD line using normal saline.   ___ ___ ___ _____

d. Obtained vital signs, did not leave patient alone.   ___ ___ ___ _____

e. Notified health care provider.   ___ ___ ___ _____

f. Notified blood bank.   ___ ___ ___ _____

g. Obtained blood samples from extremity not receiving transfusion if needed.   ___ ___ ___ _____

h. Returned remainder of blood component and attached blood tubing to blood bank according to policy.   ___ ___ ___ _____

i. Monitored patient's vital signs as frequently as needed.   ___ ___ ___ _____

j. Administered prescribed medication according to type and severity of transfusion reaction.   ___ ___ ___ _____

k. Initiated cardiac resuscitation if necessary.   ___ ___ ___ _____

l. Obtained first voided urine sample, sent to laboratory, inserted catheter if necessary.   ___ ___ ___ _____

EVALUATION

1. Continued monitoring patient for signs and symptoms of transfusion reactions.   ___ ___ ___ _____

2. Asked patient to explain reactions that can occur and what signs to report.   ___ ___ ___ _____

3. Identified unexpected outcomes.   ___ ___ ___ _____

RECORDING AND REPORTING

1. Documented exact time transfusion reaction was first noted, all vital signs and assessments, treatments, and patient response; completed transfusion reaction report.   ___ ___ ___ _____

2. Documented evaluation of patient learning.   ___ ___ ___ _____

3. Reported presence of transfusion reaction and physical assessment findings to nurse in charge or health care provider.   ___ ___ ___ _____

Copyright © 2018 by Elsevier Inc. All rights reserved.

Student _____ Date _____

Instructor _____ Date _____

PERFORMANCE CHECKLIST SKILL 31.1 **PERFORMING A NUTRITIONAL SCREENING AND PHYSICAL EXAMINATION**

	S	U	NP	Comments
ASSESSMENT				
1. Identify patient using at least two identifiers.	___	___	___	_____
2. Asked patient to report usual body weight, noted recent changes in weight, asked if any weight loss was intentional.	___	___	___	_____
3. Performed hand hygiene, measured actual body weight properly.	___	___	___	_____
4. Measured actual height properly.	___	___	___	_____
5. Calculated ideal body weight properly.	___	___	___	_____
6. Calculated BMI properly.	___	___	___	_____
7. Obtained dietary information, including history, cultural or religious restrictions, and medications and supplements.	___	___	___	_____
8. Performed physical assessment, noted physical changes reflecting nutritional deficiencies.	___	___	___	_____
9. Review results of relevant laboratory tests.	___	___	___	_____
10. Determined patient's ability to manipulate eating utensils and self-feed.	___	___	___	_____
11. Completed a nutritional screening tool if required.	___	___	___	_____
12. Explained to patient that nutritional assessment was complete and how information will be applied to patient care.	___	___	___	_____
IMPLEMENTATION				
1. Provided patient help with feeding based on assessment findings.	___	___	___	_____
2. Instituted aspiration precautions.	___	___	___	_____
EVALUATION				
1. Reviewed history and physical findings, noted abnormal findings or areas of concern.	___	___	___	_____
2. Compared patient's weight for height with IBW, compared BMI with recommended BMI.	___	___	___	_____
3. Compared normal laboratory test levels with patient's levels.	___	___	___	_____

Copyright © 2018 by Elsevier Inc. All rights reserved.

	S	U	NP	Comments

4. Computed any score on nutritional screening tool. ___ ___ ___ _____

5. Asked patient to describe what the screening will determine. ___ ___ ___ _____

6. Identified unexpected outcomes. ___ ___ ___ _____

RECORDING AND REPORTING

1. Documented assessment results in appropriate log. ___ ___ ___ _____

2. Documented evaluation of patient or caregiver learning. ___ ___ ___ _____

3. Notified health care provider of abnormal findings. ___ ___ ___ _____

4. Made referral to the RD. ___ ___ ___ _____

Copyright © 2018 by Elsevier Inc. All rights reserved.

Student _____ Date _____

Instructor _____ Date _____

PERFORMANCE CHECKLIST SKILL 31.2   **ASSISTING AN ADULT PATIENT WITH ORAL NUTRITION**

	S	U	NP	Comments

ASSESSMENT

1. Identified patient using at least two identifiers. ___ ___ ___ _____

2. Reviewed health care provider's diet order for type of diet and supplements. ___ ___ ___ _____

3. Assessed presence and condition of teeth, determined if dentures were poorly fitted, rated any pain severity on a pain scale. ___ ___ ___ _____

4. Assessed neurologic patient's cranial nerve function. ___ ___ ___ _____

5. Determined to what extent patient is able to self-feed; assessed physical motor skills; evaluated LOC, visual acuity, peripheral vision, and mood. ___ ___ ___ _____

6. Assessed patient's appetite, tolerance of foods, recent fluid intake, cultural and religious preferences, and food likes and dislikes. ___ ___ ___ _____

7. Assessed patient for generalized fatigue, pain, or shortness of breath. ___ ___ ___ _____

8. Asked if patient feels nauseated, assessed recent bowel pattern and auscultated for bowel sounds. ___ ___ ___ _____

9. Assessed need for toileting, handwashing, and oral care before feeding. ___ ___ ___ _____

10. Reviewed nursing history for patient's most recent weight and laboratory. ___ ___ ___ _____

PLANNING

1. Identified expected outcomes. ___ ___ ___ _____

2. Allowed patient to rest 30 minutes between assessment and mealtime. ___ ___ ___ _____

3. Administered analgesic if ordered. ___ ___ ___ _____

4. Explained to patient how you plan to set up and help with meal, allowed time for questions. ___ ___ ___ _____

Copyright © 2018 by Elsevier Inc. All rights reserved.

	S	U	NP	Comments

IMPLEMENTATION

1. Prepared patient's room for mealtime:

   a. Performed hand hygiene, cleared over-bed table, arranged needed supplies. ___ ___ ___ _____

   b. Assisted patient to comfortable position. ___ ___ ___ _____

2. Prepared patient for meal:

   a. Assisted patient with elimination needs, performed hand hygiene. ___ ___ ___ _____

   b. Applied clean gloves and offered oral hygiene, rinsed and reinserted dentures if present, removed gloves and performed hand hygiene. ___ ___ ___ _____

   c. Consulted with health care provider on best therapy for patient with oral mucositis. ___ ___ ___ _____

   d. Helped patient put on glasses or insert contact lenses. ___ ___ ___ _____

3. Checked environment for distractions, reduced noise level if possible. ___ ___ ___ _____

4. Obtained special assistive devices, instructed on use. ___ ___ ___ _____

5. Assessed meal tray for completeness and correct diet, instructed patient about diet, food options, and dysphagia risk. ___ ___ ___ _____

6. Asked patient in which order patient would like to eat meal, helped set up tray if needed. ___ ___ ___ _____

7. Watched patient swallow first bites of food and drink, stayed or returned later as appropriate. ___ ___ ___ _____

8. Helped patient who cannot eat independently:

   a. Assumed comfortable position. ___ ___ ___ _____

   b. Identified food placement as if plate were a clock for visually impaired patient. ___ ___ ___ _____

   c. Asked patient in what order he or she would like to eat, cut food into bite-size pieces. ___ ___ ___ _____

   d. Provided fluids as requested, encouraged patient not to drink all liquid at the beginning of the meal. ___ ___ ___ _____

Copyright © 2018 by Elsevier Inc. All rights reserved.

	S	U	NP	Comments
e. Paced feeding to avoid patient fatigue, interacted with patient during mealtime, encouraged self-feeding attempts.	___	___	___	_____
f. Used the meal as an opportunity to educate patient.	___	___	___	_____
g. Fed patient in a manner that facilitates chewing and swallowing, positioned patient's chin down, placed food on stronger side of the mouth.	___	___	___	_____
9. Used appropriate feeding techniques for patients with special needs.	___	___	___	_____
10. Assisted patient with hand hygiene and mouth care.	___	___	___	_____
11. Helped patient to appropriate position.	___	___	___	_____
12. Returned patient's trays to appropriate place, removed and discarded gloves, performed hand hygiene.	___	___	___	_____

EVALUATION

	S	U	NP	Comments
1. Monitored body weight daily or weekly.	___	___	___	_____
2. Monitored laboratory values as indicated.	___	___	___	_____
3. Monitored I&O and complete intake measurement.	___	___	___	_____
4. Observed patient's ability to self-feed any part of meal.	___	___	___	_____
5. Observed patient choking, coughing, gagging, or food left in mouth during eating.	___	___	___	_____
6. Asked caregiver to describe two ways to help feed patient.	___	___	___	_____
7. Identified unexpected outcomes.	___	___	___	_____

RECORDING AND REPORTING

	S	U	NP	Comments
1. Recorded patient's type of diet, assistance needed, tolerance or diet, amount eaten, and calorie count.	___	___	___	_____
2. Recorded fluid intake on appropriate form.	___	___	___	_____
3. Recorded amount of oral nutritional supplements taken and patient's tolerance.	___	___	___	_____
4. Reported any swallowing difficulties, food dislikes, and refusal to eat.	___	___	___	_____
5. Documented your evaluation of family caregiver learning.	___	___	___	_____

Copyright © 2018 by Elsevier Inc. All rights reserved.

Student _____ Date _____

Instructor _____ Date _____

PERFORMANCE CHECKLIST SKILL 31.3 **ASPIRATION PRECAUTIONS**

	S	U	NP	Comments
ASSESSMENT				
1. Reviewed results of nutritional screening in medical record.	——	——	——	_____
2. Identified patient using at least two identifiers.	——	——	——	_____
3. Asked patient or caregiver if patient has difficulties with chewing or swallowing.	——	——	——	_____
4. Assessed for conditions that cause risk for aspiration, assessed signs of dysphagia.	——	——	——	_____
5. Assessed mental status.	——	——	——	_____
6. Assessed patient's oral health; checked level of dental hygiene, missing teeth, or poorly fitting dentures; applied clean gloves if needed.	——	——	——	_____
7. Observed patient during mealtime for signs of dysphagia, noted if patient was fatigued or had difficulty swallowing.	——	——	——	_____
8. Obtained baseline assessment of oxygen saturation.	——	——	——	_____
9. Indicated in log if dysphagia/aspiration risk is present.	——	——	——	_____
PLANNING				
1. Identified expected outcomes.	——	——	——	_____
2. Provided patient 30 minutes of rest.	——	——	——	_____
3. Explained why patient is being observed while eating.	——	——	——	_____
4. Explained to patient and caregiver what is being done and why.	——	——	——	_____
IMPLEMENTATION				
1. Performed hand hygiene, had patient or caregiver perform hand hygiene.	——	——	——	_____
2. Applied clean gloves, provided oral hygiene.	——	——	——	_____
3. Positioned patient properly.	——	——	——	_____
4. Applied pulse oximeter to patient's finger monitor during feeding.	——	——	——	_____

Copyright © 2018 by Elsevier Inc. All rights reserved.

	S	U	NP	Comments

5. Used penlight and tongue blade to inspect for pockets of food.

6. Added thickener to thin liquids if necessary, encouraged patient to feed self.

7. Had patient assume chin-tuck position, told patient not to tilt head backward while eating or drinking.

8. Placed appropriate amount of food on unaffected side of patient's mouth if patient was unable to feed self, allowed utensils to touch mouth.

9. Provided verbal cueing while feeding, reminded patient to chew and think about swallowing.

10. Avoided mixing food of different textures, alternated liquid and bites of food.

11. Monitored swallowing, observed for respiratory difficulty, observed for throat clearing, coughing, gagging, and drooling, suctioned airway as needed.

12. Minimized distractions, did not rush patient, allowed adequate time for chewing, provided rest as needed.

13. Used sauces to facilitate cohesive food bolus formation.

14. Asked patient to sit upright after meal.

15. Provided oral hygiene after meals.

16. Removed gloves if worn, returned patient's tray to appropriate place, performed hand hygiene.

EVALUATION

1. Monitored patient's ability to swallow foods and fluids without choking.

2. Monitored pulse oximetry readings for high-risk patients when eating.

3. Monitored patient's I&O, calorie count, and food intake.

4. Weighed patient at appropriate intervals.

5. Observed patient's oral cavity after meal.

6. Asked caregiver to describe signs that patient is having trouble swallowing.

7. Identified unexpected outcomes.

Copyright © 2018 by Elsevier Inc. All rights reserved.

	S	U	NP	Comments

RECORDING AND REPORTING

1. Documented all pertinent information in the appropriate log. ____ ____ ____ _____

2. Reported coughing, gagging, choking, or swallowing difficulties to health care provider. ____ ____ ____ _____

3. Communicated about patient dysphagia with other health care staff during hand-off. ____ ____ ____ _____

4. Documented evaluation of caregiver learning. ____ ____ ____ _____

Copyright © 2018 by Elsevier Inc. All rights reserved.

Student _____ Date _____

Instructor _____ Date _____

PERFORMANCE CHECKLIST SKILL 32.1   **INSERTING AND REMOVING A SMALL-BORE NASOGASTRIC OR NASOENTERIC FEEDING TUBE**

	S	U	NP	Comments
ASSESSMENT				
1. Verified order for type of tube and feeding schedule, determined if health care provider wants prokinetic agent given before tube placement.	____	____	____	_____
2. Identified patient using at least two identifiers.	____	____	____	_____
3. Assessed patient's knowledge of procedure.	____	____	____	_____
4. Performed hand hygiene, had patient close each nostril alternately and breathe, examined each naris for patency and skin breakdown.	____	____	____	_____
5. Reviewed patient's medical history for problems that might affect route of nutritional support.	____	____	____	_____
6. Assessed patient's baseline height, weight, hydration, electrolyte balance, caloric needs, and I&O.	____	____	____	_____
7. Assessed patient's mental status, presence of cough and gag reflex, ability to swallow, critical illness, and presence of artificial airway.	____	____	____	_____
8. Performed physical assessment of the abdomen.	____	____	____	_____
PLANNING				
1. Identified expected outcomes.	____	____	____	_____
2. Explained procedure to patient, included sensations he or she would feel.	____	____	____	_____
3. Explained how to communicate during intubation.	____	____	____	_____
IMPLEMENTATION				
1. Performed hand hygiene, prepared supplies at bedside.	____	____	____	_____
2. Stood on same side of bed as naris chosen for insertion, positioned patient appropriately, obtained assistance if necessary.	____	____	____	_____
3. Applied pulse oximeter, measured vital signs, ensured patient stability before inserting tube.	____	____	____	_____
4. Placed bath towel over patient's chest, kept facial tissues within reach.	____	____	____	_____
5. Determined length of tube to be inserted, marked location properly.	____	____	____	_____

Copyright © 2018 by Elsevier Inc. All rights reserved.

		S	U	NP	Comments

6. Prepared NG or nasoenteric tube for intubation:

  a. Obtained order for stylet tube. _____ _____ _____ _____

  b. Injected water from syringe into the tube if tube has guidewire or stylet. _____ _____ _____ _____

  c. Ensured stylet is positioned securely within tube, injected water from syringe into tube. _____ _____ _____ _____

7. Cut hypoallergenic tape or prepared other securing device. _____ _____ _____ _____

8. Applied clean gloves. _____ _____ _____ _____

9. Dipped tube with surface lubricant into room-temperature water or applied lubricant. _____ _____ _____ _____

10. Handed alert patient a cup of water with straw. _____ _____ _____ _____

11. Explained next step, inserted tube through nostril to back of throat, aimed appropriately. _____ _____ _____ _____

12. Had patient flex head toward chest at appropriate time. _____ _____ _____ _____

13. Encouraged patient to swallow with small sips of water, advanced tube as patient swallowed, rotated tube while inserting. _____ _____ _____ _____

14. Reemphasized mouth breathing and swallowing. _____ _____ _____ _____

15. Did not advance tube during inspiration or coughing, monitored oximetry and capnography. _____ _____ _____ _____

16. Advanced tube each time patient swallowed, until desired length had been passed. _____ _____ _____ _____

17. Checked for position of tube in back of throat. _____ _____ _____ _____

18. Anchored tube to nose temporarily. _____ _____ _____ _____

19. Checked placement of tube by aspirating stomach contents. _____ _____ _____ _____

20. Anchored tube to patient's nose, marked exit site on tube, selected appropriate option for anchoring:

  a. Applied membrane dressing or tube fixation device properly. _____ _____ _____ _____

  b. Applied tape properly. _____ _____ _____ _____

21. Fastened end of NG tube properly to patient's gown. _____ _____ _____ _____

22. Assisted patient to a comfortable position. _____ _____ _____ _____

23. Removed gloves, performed hand hygiene. _____ _____ _____ _____

24. Obtained x-ray film of chest/abdomen. _____ _____ _____ _____

Copyright © 2018 by Elsevier Inc. All rights reserved.

	S	U	NP	Comments

25. Performed hand hygiene, applied clean gloves, administered oral hygiene, cleansed tubing at nostril properly. ____ ____ ____ _____

26. Removed gloves, disposed of equipment, performed hand hygiene. ____ ____ ____ _____

27. Removed tube:

    a. Verified order for tube removal. ____ ____ ____ _____

    b. Gathered equipment. ____ ____ ____ _____

    c. Explained procedure to patient. ____ ____ ____ _____

    d. Performed hand hygiene, applied gloves. ____ ____ ____ _____

    e. Positioned patient appropriately. ____ ____ ____ _____

    f. Placed disposable pad over patient's chest. ____ ____ ____ _____

    g. Disconnected tube from feeding administration set. ____ ____ ____ _____

    h. Removed securement device from the patient's nose. ____ ____ ____ _____

    i. Instructed patient to take a deep breath and hold, kinked end of tubing, withdrew tube in one motion, disposed of tube appropriately. ____ ____ ____ _____

    j. Offered tissues to patient. ____ ____ ____ _____

    k. Offered mouth care. ____ ____ ____ _____

    l. Removed gloves, performed hand hygiene. ____ ____ ____ _____

EVALUATION

1. Observed patient's response to tube placement, assessed for signs of placement in the respiratory tract. ____ ____ ____ _____

2. Confirmed x-ray film results with health care provider. ____ ____ ____ _____

3. Removed stylet after verification of placement. ____ ____ ____ _____

4. Routinely checked condition of nares, location of marking on tube, and color and pH of fluid aspirated from tube. ____ ____ ____ _____

5. Assessed patient's LOC after removal. ____ ____ ____ _____

6. Asked patient to explain how he or she will communicate during NG tube insertion. ____ ____ ____ _____

7. Identified unexpected outcomes. ____ ____ ____ _____

RECORDING AND REPORTING

1. Recorded type and size of tube placed, location of distal tip of tube, patient's tolerance of procedure, condition of naris, and confirmation of tube position. ____ ____ ____ _____

Copyright © 2018 by Elsevier Inc. All rights reserved.

	S	U	NP	Comments
2. Recorded removal of tube, condition of naris, and patient's tolerance.	——	——	——	_____
3. Reported any type of unexpected outcome and interventions performed.	——	——	——	_____
4. Documented evaluation of patient learning.	——	——	——	_____

Copyright © 2018 by Elsevier Inc. All rights reserved.

Student _____ Date _____

Instructor _____ Date _____

PERFORMANCE CHECKLIST SKILL 32.2 **VERIFYING FEEDING TUBE PLACEMENT**

	S	U	NP	Comments
ASSESSMENT				
1. Reviewed agency policy and procedure for frequency and method of checking tube placement.	___	___	___	_____
2. Identified patient using at least two identifiers.	___	___	___	_____
3. Observed for signs of respiratory distress during feeding.	___	___	___	_____
4. Identified conditions that increase the risk for spontaneous tube dislocation.	___	___	___	_____
5. Observed external portion of tube for movement of ink mark.	___	___	___	_____
6. Reviewed patient's medication record for orders for continuous feeding or gastric acid inhibitor or a proton pump inhibitor.	___	___	___	_____
7. Reviewed patient's record for history of prior tube displacement.	___	___	___	_____
PLANNING				
1. Identified expected outcomes.	___	___	___	_____
2. Explained procedure to patient.	___	___	___	_____
IMPLEMENTATION				
1. Prepared equipment at patient's bedside, performed hand hygiene, applied clean gloves.	___	___	___	_____
2. Verified tube placement at the appropriate times.	___	___	___	_____
3. Placed feeding on hold, kinked feeding tube, drew up appropriate amount of air into syringe, attached to end of feeding tube, flushed tube with air before attempting to aspirate, repositioned patient if needed.	___	___	___	_____
4. Drew back on syringe slowly, obtained proper amount of gastric aspirate, observed appearance of aspirate.	___	___	___	_____
5. Mixed aspirate in syringe, expelled a few drops into a clean medicine cup, measured pH of aspirated GI contents, compared color of strip with color on the chart.	___	___	___	_____
6. Continued with irrigation as placement is verified or all indicators confirm tube placement.	___	___	___	_____

Copyright © 2018 by Elsevier Inc. All rights reserved.

	S	U	NP	Comments
7. Irrigated tube.	——	——	——	_____
8. Removed and disposed of gloves and supplies, performed hand hygiene.	——	——	——	_____

EVALUATION

	S	U	NP	Comments
1. Observed patient for respiratory distress.	——	——	——	_____
2. Verified that external length of tube, pH, and appearance of aspirate were consistent with initial tube placement.	——	——	——	_____
3. Asked patient to explain importance of gastric pH testing.	——	——	——	_____
4. Identified unexpected outcomes.	——	——	——	_____

RECORDING AND REPORTING

	S	U	NP	Comments
1. Recorded and reported pH and appearance of aspirate.	——	——	——	_____
2. Documented evaluation of patient learning.	——	——	——	_____

Copyright © 2018 by Elsevier Inc. All rights reserved.

Student _____ Date _____

Instructor _____ Date _____

PERFORMANCE CHECKLIST SKILL 32.3   **IRRIGATING A FEEDING TUBE**

	S	U	NP	Comments
ASSESSMENT				
1. Identified patient using at least two identifiers.	___	___	___	_____
2. Performed hand hygiene, inspected volume, color, and character of gastric aspirates.	___	___	___	_____
3. Assessed bowel sounds.	___	___	___	_____
4. Noted ease with which tube feeding infused through tubing.	___	___	___	_____
5. Monitored volume of enteral formula administered during a shift, compared with ordered amount.	___	___	___	_____
6. Referred to agency policies regarding routine irrigation.	___	___	___	_____
PLANNING				
1. Identified expected outcomes.	___	___	___	_____
2. Explained procedure to patient.	___	___	___	_____
3. Positioned patient properly.	___	___	___	_____
IMPLEMENTATION				
1. Performed hand hygiene, prepared equipment at bedside, applied clean gloves.	___	___	___	_____
2. Verified tube placement if fluid could be aspirated for pH testing.	___	___	___	_____
3. Irrigated routinely and before, between, and after final medication; irrigated before intermittent feeding was administered.	___	___	___	_____
4. Drew up water into ENFit syringe, ensured patient had individual bottle of solution.	___	___	___	_____
5. Changed irrigation bottle every 24 hours.	___	___	___	_____
6. Kinked feeding tube while disconnecting from administration tubing or while removing plug at end of tube.	___	___	___	_____
7. Inserted tip of syringe into feeding tube, released kink, slowly instilled irrigation solution.	___	___	___	_____
8. Repositioned patient on left side and tried again if unable to instill fluid.	___	___	___	_____
9. Removed syringe when water is instilled, reinserted tube feeding, or administered medication, flushed medication completely through tube.	___	___	___	_____

Copyright © 2018 by Elsevier Inc. All rights reserved.

	S	U	NP	Comments
10. Removed and discarded gloves, disposed of supplies, performed hand hygiene.	——	——	——	————————

EVALUATION

	S	U	NP	Comments
1. Observed ease with which tube feeding instilled.	——	——	——	————————
2. Monitored patient's caloric intake.	——	——	——	————————
3. Asked patient to explain why it is important to flush tube.	——	——	——	————————
4. Identified unexpected outcomes.	——	——	——	————————

RECORDING AND REPORTING

	S	U	NP	Comments
1. Recorded time of irrigation, amount and type of fluid instilled.	——	——	——	————————
2. Reported if tubing had become clogged.	——	——	——	————————
3. Documented evaluation of patient or caregiver learning.	——	——	——	————————

Copyright © 2018 by Elsevier Inc. All rights reserved.

Student _____ Date _____

Instructor _____ Date _____

PERFORMANCE CHECKLIST SKILL 32.4   **ADMINISTERING ENTERAL NUTRITION: NASOENTERIC, GASTRONOMY, OR JEJUNOSTOMY TUBE**

	S	U	NP	Comments
ASSESSMENT				
1. Identified patient using at least two identifiers.	___	___	___	_____
2. Assessed patient's clinical status to determine potential need for tube feedings, consulted with nutrition support team or health care provider.	___	___	___	_____
3. Assessed patient for food allergies.	___	___	___	_____
4. Performed physical assessment of abdomen.	___	___	___	_____
5. Obtained baseline weight; reviewed serum electrolytes and blood glucose measurement; assessed patient for fluid volume excess or deficit, electrolyte abnormalities, and metabolic abnormalities.	___	___	___	_____
6. Verified health care provider's order for type of formula, rate, route, and frequency.	___	___	___	_____
PLANNING				
1. Identified expected outcomes.	___	___	___	_____
2. Explained procedure to patient.	___	___	___	_____
IMPLEMENTATION				
1. Performed hand hygiene, applied clean gloves.	___	___	___	_____
2. Verified correct formula, checked expiration date, noted integrity of container.	___	___	___	_____
3. Prepared formula for administration:				
a. Had formula at room temperature.	___	___	___	_____
b. Used aseptic technique when manipulating components of feeding system.	___	___	___	_____
c. Shook formula container well, cleaned top of can with alcohol swab.	___	___	___	_____
d. Connected tubing to container for closed system, poured formula from brick pack or can into administration bag.	___	___	___	_____
4. Opened roller clamp, allowed administration tubing to fill, clamped off tubing, hung container on IV pole.	___	___	___	_____
5. Placed patient in appropriate position.	___	___	___	_____

Copyright © 2018 by Elsevier Inc. All rights reserved.

	S	U	NP	Comments

6. Verified tube placement, observed appearance of aspirate, noted pH measure. ___ ___ ___ _____

7. Checked GRV properly before each feeding and appropriately thereafter. ___ ___ ___ _____

8. Used ENFit device when administering enteral feedings. ___ ___ ___ _____

9. Intermittent feeding:

    a. Pinched proximal end of feeding tube, removed cap, connected distal end of tubing to ENFit device, released tubing. ___ ___ ___ _____

    b. Set rate properly, allowed bag to empty gradually, labeled bag properly. ___ ___ ___ _____

    c. Followed feeding with water, covered end of feeding tube with cap, kept bag as clean as possible, changed bag every 24 hours. ___ ___ ___ _____

10. Continuous drip method:

    a. Removed cap, connected distal end of administration set tubing to feeding tube properly. ___ ___ ___ _____

    b. Threaded tubing through feeding pump, set rate and turned pump on. ___ ___ ___ _____

    c. Advanced rate of tube feeding as ordered. ___ ___ ___ _____

11. Flushed tubing with water at appropriate times, had registered dietitian recommend total free water requirement per day, obtained health care provider's order. ___ ___ ___ _____

12. Rinsed bag and tubing with warm water whenever feedings were interrupted, used new administration set every 24 hours. ___ ___ ___ _____

13. Disposed of supplies, performed hand hygiene. ___ ___ ___ _____

EVALUATION

1. Measured GRV per policy, asked if nausea or abdominal cramping was present. ___ ___ ___ _____

2. Monitored I&O at least every 8 hours, calculated daily totals. ___ ___ ___ _____

3. Weighed patient daily or three times per week as appropriate. ___ ___ ___ _____

4. Monitored laboratory values. ___ ___ ___ _____

5. Observed patient's respiratory status. ___ ___ ___ _____

6. Examined and auscultated bowel sounds. ___ ___ ___ _____

7. Inspected site for signs of impaired skin integrity and symptoms of infection, injury, or tightness of tube. ___ ___ ___ _____

Copyright © 2018 by Elsevier Inc. All rights reserved.

	S	U	NP	Comments

8. Observed nasoenteral tube insertion site at least daily, noted skin integrity.   ___ ___ ___ _____

9. Asked patient to describe signs that tube feedings are not being tolerated.   ___ ___ ___ _____

10. Identified unexpected outcomes.   ___ ___ ___ _____

RECORDING AND REPORTING

1. Recorded and reported all pertinent information in the appropriate log.   ___ ___ ___ _____

2. Recorded volume of formula and additional water on I&O form.   ___ ___ ___ _____

3. Reported type of feeding, status of tube, patient's tolerance, and adverse outcomes.   ___ ___ ___ _____

4. Documented evaluation of patient learning.   ___ ___ ___ _____

Copyright © 2018 by Elsevier Inc. All rights reserved.

Student _____ Date _____

Instructor _____ Date _____

PERFORMANCE CHECKLIST PROCEDURAL GUIDELINE 32.1 **CARE OF A GASTROSTOMY OR JEJUNOSTOMY TUBE**

	S	U	NP	Comments
PROCEDURAL STEPS				
1. Determined whether exit site was left to open air or if dressing was indicated, checked order.	——	——	——	_____
2. Identified patient using at least two identifiers.	——	——	——	_____
3. Performed hand hygiene, applied clean gloves.	——	——	——	_____
4. Removed old dressing, folded appropriately, removed gloves inside out over dressing, discarded appropriately.	——	——	——	_____
5. Assessed exit site for evidence of tenderness, leakage, swelling, excoriation, drainage, infection, or bleeding.	——	——	——	_____
6. Cleansed skin around site with water and soap using gauze.	——	——	——	_____
7. Rinsed and dried site completely.	——	——	——	_____
8. Applied thin layer of protective skin barrier to exit site if indicated.	——	——	——	_____
9. Placed drain-gauze over external bar or disc if dressing was ordered.	——	——	——	_____
10. Secured dressing with tape.	——	——	——	_____
11. Placed date, time, and initials on new dressing.	——	——	——	_____
12. Removed gloves, disposed of supplies, performed hand hygiene.	——	——	——	_____
13. Evaluated condition of site routinely.	——	——	——	_____
14. Documented in nurses' notes appearance of exit site, drainage noted, and dressing application.	——	——	——	_____
15. Reported any exit site complications to health care provider.	——	——	——	_____

Copyright © 2018 by Elsevier Inc. All rights reserved.

Student _____ Date _____

Instructor _____ Date _____

PERFORMANCE CHECKLIST SKILL 33.1 **ADMINISTERING CENTRAL PARENTERAL NUTRITION**

	S	U	NP	Comments
ASSESSMENT				
1. Assessed indications of and risks for protein/calorie malnutrition, conferred with nutritional support team.	___	___	___	_____
2. Inspected condition of central vein access site for presence of inflammation, edema, and tenderness; inspected tubing of access device for patency and kinking.	___	___	___	_____
3. Assessed level of serum albumin, total protein, transferrin, prealbumin, and triglycerides; checked blood glucose levels.	___	___	___	_____
4. Assessed patient's medical history for factors influenced by PCN administration and for history of allergies.	___	___	___	_____
5. Assessed vital signs, auscultated lung sounds, measured weight.	___	___	___	_____
6. Consulted with health care provider and dietitian on calculation of calorie, protein, and fluid requirements for patient.	___	___	___	_____
7. Verified order for nutrients, minerals, vitamins, trace elements, added medications, and flow rate; checked for compatibility of added medications.	___	___	___	_____
PLANNING				
1. Identified expected outcomes.	___	___	___	_____
2. Explained purpose of CPN to the patient.	___	___	___	_____
3. Removed solution from refrigeration if needed.	___	___	___	_____
IMPLEMENTATION				
1. Performed hand hygiene.	___	___	___	_____
2. Checked label in CPN bag with order on MAR, checked additives and noted expiration date, removed solution from refrigerator if necessary.	___	___	___	_____
3. Inspected 2:1 CPN solution for particulate matter, inspected 3:1 CPN solution for separation of fat into layer.	___	___	___	_____
4. Checked IV solution using six rights of medication administration, checked label of CPN bag against MAR.	___	___	___	_____

Copyright © 2018 by Elsevier Inc. All rights reserved.

	S	U	NP	Comments

5. Identified patient using at least two identifiers, compared with information on MAR. ___ ___ ___ _____

6. Applied clean gloves, prepared IV tubing for CPN solution. ___ ___ ___ _____

7. Wiped end port of CVAD with alcohol, attached syringe of normal saline to needleless port, aspirated for blood return, flushed saline. ___ ___ ___ _____

8. Removed syringe, connected Luer-Lok end of CPN IV tubing to end port of CVAD, labeled tubing for multilumen lines. ___ ___ ___ _____

9. Placed IV tubing in EID, opened roller clamp, set and regulated flow rate as ordered. ___ ___ ___ _____

10. Infused all IV medications or blood through alternative IV line, did not obtain blood samples or CVP readings through same lumen. ___ ___ ___ _____

11. Hung CPN for appropriate time. ___ ___ ___ _____

12. Changed administration sets every 24 hours and on suspected contamination, discarded used supplies, performed hand hygiene. ___ ___ ___ _____

EVALUATION

1. Monitored and documented flow rate routinely, did not attempt to catch up infusion. ___ ___ ___ _____

2. Monitored I&O every 8 hours. ___ ___ ___ _____

3. Obtained weights daily or as ordered. ___ ___ ___ _____

4. Assessed for fluid retention, palpated skin of extremities, auscultated lung sounds. ___ ___ ___ _____

5. Monitored patient's glucose levels as ordered, monitored other laboratory parameters daily or as ordered. ___ ___ ___ _____

6. Inspected central venous access site for IV patency and signs of infection, infiltration, or phlebitis. ___ ___ ___ _____

7. Monitored for signs of systemic infection. ___ ___ ___ _____

8. Asked patient to describe what signs to report to health care provider. ___ ___ ___ _____

9. Identified unexpected outcomes. ___ ___ ___ _____

RECORDING AND REPORTING

1. Recorded all pertinent information in the appropriate log. ___ ___ ___ _____

2. Notified health care provider if signs of infection, occlusion, fluid retention, or infiltration occurred. ___ ___ ___ _____

3. Documented evaluation of patient or family caregiver learning. ___ ___ ___ _____

Copyright © 2018 by Elsevier Inc. All rights reserved.

Student _____ Date _____

Instructor _____ Date _____

PERFORMANCE CHECKLIST SKILL 33.2 **ADMINISTERING PERIPHERAL PARENTERAL NUTRITION WITH LIPID (FAT) EMULSION**

	S	U	NP	Comments

ASSESSMENT

1. Assessed patient for potential hypertriglyceridemia, obtained a serum triglyceride level before initiation of PPN and weekly thereafter.

2. Selected or initiated appropriate functional IV site, assessed its patency and function.

3. Checked health care provider's order against MAR for volume of fat emulsion, PPN solution, and administration time for fat emulsion.

4. Read label of fat emulsion solution.

5. Assessed blood glucose level.

6. Assessed patient's fluid status.

7. Obtained patient's weight and vital signs before beginning infusion.

PLANNING

1. Identified expected outcomes.

2. Explained purposes of PPN and fat emulsion.

3. Placed patient in comfortable position.

4. Removed solution from refrigerator 1 hour before infusion.

IMPLEMENTATION

1. Performed hand hygiene.

2. Compared label of bag and bottle with MAR and patient's name, checked for correct additives and expiration date.

3. Examined lipid solution for separation of emulsion or presence of froth.

4. Identified patient using two identifiers.

5. Measured patient's vital signs.

6. Applied clean gloves. Prepared IV tubing for PPN solution, ran solution through tubing to remove excess air, turned roller clamp off, added sterile capped needle or placed sterile cap on tubing, followed same procedure with set for lipid infusion.

Copyright © 2018 by Elsevier Inc. All rights reserved.

	S	U	NP	Comments

7. Connected PPN solution to functional peripheral IV, disconnected old tubing from site, inserted adapter of new PPN tubing, opened clamp on new tubing, ensured tubing was patent, regulated IV drip rate. ___ ___ ___ _____

8. Cleaned needleless peripheral line tubing injection port with antimicrobial swab. ___ ___ ___ _____

9. Attached fat emulsion infusion tubing to injection cap of IV line, used Y connector if appropriate, labeled tubing. ___ ___ ___ _____

10. Opened roller clamp completely on fat emulsion infusion, checked flow rate on infusion pump. ___ ___ ___ _____

11. Infused lipids at appropriate rate, increased rate as ordered. ___ ___ ___ _____

12. Began PPN at ordered rate, infused for appropriate length of time. ___ ___ ___ _____

13. Discarded supplies, performed hand hygiene. ___ ___ ___ _____

EVALUATION

1. Monitored flow rate routinely as necessary. ___ ___ ___ _____

2. Measured vital signs and patient comfort every 10 minutes for first 30 minutes. ___ ___ ___ _____

3. Monitored patient's laboratory values daily, performed blood glucose monitoring as ordered, measured serum lipids 4 hours after discontinuing infusion. ___ ___ ___ _____

4. Monitored temperature every 4 hours, inspected venipuncture site for signs of phlebitis or infiltration. ___ ___ ___ _____

5. Assessed patient's weight, I&O, condition of peripheral extremities, and breath sounds. ___ ___ ___ _____

6. Asked patient to explain why nutrition is being received. ___ ___ ___ _____

7. Identified unexpected outcomes. ___ ___ ___ _____

RECORDING AND REPORTING

1. Recorded pertinent information in the appropriate log. ___ ___ ___ _____

2. Recorded adverse reactions in nurses' notes. ___ ___ ___ _____

3. Notified health care provider of signs of fat intolerance, infection, occlusion, fluid retention, or infiltration. ___ ___ ___ _____

4. Documented evaluation of patient or caregiver learning. ___ ___ ___ _____

Copyright © 2018 by Elsevier Inc. All rights reserved.

Student _____ Date _____

Instructor _____ Date _____

PERFORMANCE CHECKLIST PROCEDURAL GUIDELINE 34.1 **ASSISTING WITH USE OF A URINAL**

PROCEDURAL STEPS	S	U	NP	Comments
1. Assessed patient's normal urinary elimination habits.	___	___	___	_____
2. Determined how much assistance was needed to place and remove urinal.	___	___	___	_____
3. Determined if a urine specimen was to be collected.	___	___	___	_____
4. Performed hand hygiene.	___	___	___	_____
5. Explained procedure to patient.	___	___	___	_____
6. Provided privacy.	___	___	___	_____
7. Assessed for distended bladder.	___	___	___	_____
8. Applied clean gloves.	___	___	___	_____
9. Assisted patient into appropriate position.	___	___	___	_____
10. Assisted male patient in holding urinal or positioning penis if necessary.	___	___	___	_____
11. Assisted female patient in positioning urinal if necessary.	___	___	___	_____
12. Covered patient with bed linens, placed call light within reach, provided privacy, removed gloves, performed hand hygiene.	___	___	___	_____
13. Removed urinal and assessed characteristics of urine, assisted patient with washing and drying genitalia.	___	___	___	_____
14. Measured urine, recorded output on I&O if needed.	___	___	___	_____
15. Emptied and cleansed urinal, returned urinal to patient for future use.	___	___	___	_____
16. Assisted patient to perform hand hygiene.	___	___	___	_____
17. Removed and disposed of gloves, performed hand hygiene.	___	___	___	_____

Copyright © 2018 by Elsevier Inc. All rights reserved.

Student _____ Date _____

Instructor _____ Date _____

PERFORMANCE CHECKLIST SKILL 34.1 **INSERTION OF A STRAIGHT OR INDWELLING URINARY CATHETER**

	S	U	NP	Comments
ASSESSMENT				
1. Identified patient using two identifiers.	___	___	___	_____
2. Reviewed patient's medical record, noted previous catheterization.	___	___	___	_____
3. Reviewed medical record for any pathological condition that may impair passage of catheter.	___	___	___	_____
4. Performed hand hygiene, asked patient and checked chart for allergies.	___	___	___	_____
5. Assessed patient's weight, LOC, developmental level, ability to cooperate, and mobility.	___	___	___	_____
6. Assessed patient's gender and age.	___	___	___	_____
7. Assessed patient's knowledge, prior experience with catheterization, and feelings about procedure.	___	___	___	_____
8. Assessed for pain and bladder fullness.	___	___	___	_____
9. Performed hand hygiene, applied gloves, inspected perineal region, removed gloves, performed hand hygiene.	___	___	___	_____
PLANNING				
1. Identified expected outcomes.	___	___	___	_____
2. Explained procedure to patient.	___	___	___	_____
3. Arranged for extra personnel to assist as necessary, organized supplies at bedside.	___	___	___	_____
IMPLEMENTATION				
1. Checked patient's plan of care for size and type of catheter, used smallest size possible.	___	___	___	_____
2. Performed hand hygiene.	___	___	___	_____
3. Provided privacy.	___	___	___	_____
4. Raised bed to appropriate height, raised side rail on opposite side, lowered side rail on working side.	___	___	___	_____
5. Placed waterproof pad under patient.	___	___	___	_____
6. Applied clean gloves; cleaned, rinsed, and dried perineal area, examined patient and identified urinary meatus, removed and discarded gloves, performed hand hygiene.	___	___	___	_____

Copyright © 2018 by Elsevier Inc. All rights reserved.

	S	U	NP	Comments

7. Positioned patient appropriately.   ___ ___ ___ _____

8. Draped patient appropriately.   ___ ___ ___ _____

9. Positioned light to illuminate genitals or had assistant hold light.   ___ ___ ___ _____

10. Opened outer wrapping of catheterization kit, placed inner wrapped kit on appropriate clean surface.   ___ ___ ___ _____

11. Opened inner sterile wrap using sterile technique.   ___ ___ ___ _____

12. Applied sterile gloves.   ___ ___ ___ _____

13. Draped perineum, kept gloves sterile:

    a. Draped female patient:

        (1) Unfolded square drape without touching unsterile surfaces, allowed top edge to form cuff over both hands, placed drape shiny side down between patient's thighs, asked patient to lift hips, slipped cuffed edge just under buttocks, applied new gloves if old gloves are contaminated.   ___ ___ ___ _____

        (2) Unfolded fenestrated sterile drape without touching unsterile surfaces, allowed top edge to form cuff over both hands, draped over perineum, exposed labia.   ___ ___ ___ _____

    b. Draped male patient:

        (1) Unfolded square drape without touching unsterile surfaces, placed over thighs just below penis, placed fenestrated drape with opening centered over penis.   ___ ___ ___ _____

14. Arranged supplies on sterile field, maintained sterility of gloves, placed loaded sterile tray on sterile drape:

    a. Poured antiseptic solution over cotton balls if necessary.   ___ ___ ___ _____

    b. Opened sterile specimen container if specimen was to be obtained.   ___ ___ ___ _____

    c. Opened inner sterile wrapper of catheter, attached drainage bag if part of a closed system, ensured clamp on drainage port of bag was closed, attached catheter to drainage tubing if part of sterile tray.   ___ ___ ___ _____

    d. Opened lubricant, squeezed onto sterile field, lubricated catheter in gel appropriately.   ___ ___ ___ _____

Copyright © 2018 by Elsevier Inc. All rights reserved.

		S	U	NP	Comments

15. Cleansed urethral meatus:

   a. For female patient:

      (1) Separated labia with fingers of nondominant hand. ___ ___ ___ _____

      (2) Maintained position of nondominant hand throughout procedure. ___ ___ ___ _____

      (3) Cleansed labia with one cotton ball using forceps, cleaned labia and urinary meatus appropriately. ___ ___ ___ _____

   b. For male patient:

      (1) Retracted foreskin if present with nondominant hand, held penis appropriately. ___ ___ ___ _____

      (2) Used uncontaminated hand to appropriately cleanse meatus. ___ ___ ___ _____

      (3) Repeated cleaning 3 times using clean cotton ball each time. ___ ___ ___ _____

16. Held catheter properly away from catheter tip with catheter coiled in hand, positioned urine tray appropriately if necessary. ___ ___ ___ _____

17. Inserted catheter, explained to patient that feeling for burning or pressure is normal and will go away:

   a. For female patient:

      (1) Asked patient to bear down, inserted catheter slowly through urethral meatus. ___ ___ ___ _____

      (2) Advanced catheter appropriately or until urine flows out end. ___ ___ ___ _____

      (3) Released labia, held catheter securely with nondominant hand. ___ S U NP _____

   b. For male patient:

      (1) Applied upward traction to penis as it was held at 90-degree angle from body. ___ ___ ___ _____

      (2) Asked patient to bear down, slowly inserted catheter through urethral meatus. ___ ___ ___ _____

      (3) Advanced catheter appropriately or until urine flows out end. ___ ___ ___ _____

      (4) When urine appears in indwelling catheter, advances to bifurcation. ___ ___ ___ _____

      (5) Lowered penis, held catheter securely. ___ ___ ___ _____

Copyright © 2018 by Elsevier Inc. All rights reserved.

	S	U	NP	Comments

18. Allowed bladder to empty fully unless volume was restricted. ___ ___ ___ _____

19. Collected urine specimen as needed, labeled and bagged specimen in front of patient according to agency policy, sent to laboratory as soon as possible. ___ ___ ___ _____

20. If straight catheterization, withdrew catheter slowly until removed. ___ ___ ___ _____

21. Inflated catheter balloon with designated amount of fluid:

   a. Continued to hold catheter with nondominant hand. ___ ___ ___ _____

   b. Connected prefilled syringe to injection port with free dominant hand. ___ ___ ___ _____

   c. Injected total amount of solution. ___ ___ ___ _____

   d. Released catheter after inflating balloon, pulled catheter gently until resistance was felt, advanced catheter slightly. ___ ___ ___ _____

   e. Connected drainage tubing to catheter if not preconnected. ___ ___ ___ _____

22. Secured indwelling catheter with securement device, left enough slack to allow leg movement, attached device just at the catheter bifurcation:

   a. For female patient, secured tubing to inner thigh, allowed enough slack. ___ ___ ___ _____

   b. For male patient, secured catheter tubing to upper thigh or lower abdomen, allowed enough slack, replaced foreskin if retracted. ___ ___ ___ _____

23. Clipped drainage tubing to edge of mattress, positioned bag lower than bladder, did not attach side rails of bed. ___ ___ ___ _____

24. Ensured there was no obstruction to urine flow, coiled excess tubing on bed, fastened to bottom sheet with securement device. ___ ___ ___ _____

25. Provided hygiene as needed, assisted patient to comfortable position. ___ ___ ___ _____

26. Disposed of supplies in appropriate receptacles. ___ ___ ___ _____

27. Measured urine and recorded the amount. ___ ___ ___ _____

28. Removed gloves, performed hand hygiene. ___ ___ ___ _____

Copyright © 2018 by Elsevier Inc. All rights reserved.

	S	U	NP	Comments

EVALUATION

1. Palpated bladder for distention or used bladder scan.

2. Asked patient to describe level of comfort.

3. Observed character and amount of urine in drainage system for indwelling catheter.

4. Ensured there was no urine leaking from catheter or tubing connections for indwelling catheter.

5. Asked patient to describe how to keep urine flowing out of catheter.

6. Identified unexpected outcomes.

RECORDING AND REPORTING

1. Recorded and reported all pertinent information in the appropriate log.

2. Recorded amount of urine on I&O flow sheet record.

3. Reported persistent catheter-related pain, inadequate urine output, and discomfort to health care provider.

Copyright © 2018 by Elsevier Inc. All rights reserved.

Student _____ Date _____

Instructor _____ Date _____

PERFORMANCE CHECKLIST SKILL 34.2   **CARE AND REMOVAL OF AN INDWELLING CATHETER**

	S	U	NP	Comments
ASSESSMENT				
1. Identified patient using two identifiers.	___	___	___	_____
2. Performed hand hygiene.	___	___	___	_____
3. Assessed need for catheter care:				
a. Observed urinary output and urine characteristics.	___	___	___	_____
b. Assessed for history or presence of bowel incontinence.	___	___	___	_____
c. Observed for any discharge, redness, bleeding, or presence of tissue trauma around urethral meatus.	___	___	___	_____
d. Assessed patient's knowledge of catheter care.	___	___	___	_____
4. Assessed need for catheter removal:				
a. Reviewed patient's medical record, noted length of time catheter was in place.	___	___	___	_____
b. Assessed patient's knowledge and prior experience with catheter removal.	___	___	___	_____
c. Assessed urine color, clarity, odor, and amount; noted any urethral discharge, irritation, or trauma.	___	___	___	_____
d. Determined size of catheter inflation balloon by looking at valve.	___	___	___	_____
PLANNING				
1. Identified expected outcomes following catheter care.	___	___	___	_____
2. Identified expected outcomes following catheter removal.	___	___	___	_____
3. Explained procedure to patient, discussed signs and symptoms of UTI, taught patient how to perform catheter hygiene.	___	___	___	_____
IMPLEMENTATION				
1. Provided privacy.	___	___	___	_____
2. Performed hand hygiene.	___	___	___	_____
3. Raised bed to appropriate working height, lowered side rails on working side.	___	___	___	_____
4. Organized equipment for perineal care and/or removal of catheter.	___	___	___	_____

Copyright © 2018 by Elsevier Inc. All rights reserved.

	S	U	NP	Comments

5. Positioned patient with waterproof pad under buttocks, covered with bath blanket, exposed genital area and catheter only. ____ ____ ____ _____

6. Applied gloves. ____ ____ ____ _____

7. Removed catheter securement device while maintaining connection with drainage tubing. ____ ____ ____ _____

8. Performed catheter care:

   a. Separated labia or retracted foreskin to expose meatus, maintained position throughout procedure. ____ ____ ____ _____

   b. Grasped catheter with two fingers to stabilize it. ____ ____ ____ _____

   c. Assessed urethral meatus and surrounding tissues for inflammation, swelling, discharge, or tissue trauma; asked patient if burning or discomfort was present. ____ ____ ____ _____

   d. Provided perineal hygiene with soap and water. ____ ____ ____ _____

   e. Cleaned catheter properly with clean washcloth. ____ ____ ____ _____

   f. Reapplied catheter securement device, allowed slack in catheter. ____ ____ ____ _____

9. Checked drainage tubing and bag routinely for proper securement and positioning. ____ ____ ____ _____

10. Performed catheter removal:

    a. Loosened syringe, withdrew plunger, inserted hub of syringe into inflation valve, allowed balloon fluid to drain into syringe, ensured entire amount of fluid was removed. ____ ____ ____ _____

    b. Pulled catheter appropriately, ensured catheter was whole, did not use force. ____ ____ ____ _____

    c. Wrapped contaminated catheter in waterproof pad, unhooked bag and drainage tubing from bed. ____ ____ ____ _____

    d. Emptied, measured, and recorded urine present in drainage bag. ____ ____ ____ _____

    e. Encouraged patient to maintain or increase fluid intake. ____ ____ ____ _____

    f. Initiated voiding record or bladder diary, instructed patient to tell you when need to empty bladder occurred and that all urine was measured, ensured patient knew how to use collection container. ____ ____ ____ _____

Copyright © 2018 by Elsevier Inc. All rights reserved.

	S	U	NP	Comments

g. Explained that many patients experience mild burning, discomfort, or small-volume voiding, which will subside. ⎯ ⎯ ⎯ ⎯⎯⎯⎯⎯⎯⎯⎯⎯

h. Informed patient to report signs of UTI. ⎯ ⎯ ⎯ ⎯⎯⎯⎯⎯⎯⎯⎯⎯

i. Ensured easy access to toilet or bedpan, placed urine "hat" on toilet seat, placed call bell within easy reach. ⎯ ⎯ ⎯ ⎯⎯⎯⎯⎯⎯⎯⎯⎯

11. Repositioned patient, provided hygiene, lowered bed and positioned side rails. ⎯ ⎯ ⎯ ⎯⎯⎯⎯⎯⎯⎯⎯⎯

12. Disposed of all contaminated supplies in appropriate receptacle, performed hand hygiene. ⎯ ⎯ ⎯ ⎯⎯⎯⎯⎯⎯⎯⎯⎯

EVALUATION

1. Inspected catheter and genital area for soiling, irritation, and skin breakdown; asked patient about discomfort. ⎯ ⎯ ⎯ ⎯⎯⎯⎯⎯⎯⎯⎯⎯

2. Observed time and measured amount of first voiding after catheter removal. ⎯ ⎯ ⎯ ⎯⎯⎯⎯⎯⎯⎯⎯⎯

3. Evaluated patient for signs and symptoms of UTI. ⎯ ⎯ ⎯ ⎯⎯⎯⎯⎯⎯⎯⎯⎯

4. Asked patient to describe preventive measures against UTIs. ⎯ ⎯ ⎯ ⎯⎯⎯⎯⎯⎯⎯⎯⎯

5. Identified unexpected outcomes. ⎯ ⎯ ⎯ ⎯⎯⎯⎯⎯⎯⎯⎯⎯

RECORDING AND REPORTING

1. Recorded time for catheter care and appearance of urine, described condition of meatus and catheter. ⎯ ⎯ ⎯ ⎯⎯⎯⎯⎯⎯⎯⎯⎯

2. Recorded and reported time of catheter removal; amount of water removed from balloon; condition of urethral meatus and catheter; and time, amount, and characteristics of first voided urine. ⎯ ⎯ ⎯ ⎯⎯⎯⎯⎯⎯⎯⎯⎯

3. Recorded teaching related to catheter care, catheter removal, and fluid intake. ⎯ ⎯ ⎯ ⎯⎯⎯⎯⎯⎯⎯⎯⎯

4. Reported hematuria, dysuria, inability or difficulty voiding, or any new incontinence after catheter removal. ⎯ ⎯ ⎯ ⎯⎯⎯⎯⎯⎯⎯⎯⎯

5. Reported signs of UTI to health care provider. ⎯ ⎯ ⎯ ⎯⎯⎯⎯⎯⎯⎯⎯⎯

Copyright © 2018 by Elsevier Inc. All rights reserved.

Student _____ Date _____

Instructor _____ Date _____

PERFORMANCE CHECKLIST PROCEDURAL GUIDELINE 34.2 **BLADDER SCAN AND CATHETERIZATION TO DETERMINE RESIDUAL URINE**

	S	U	NP	Comments
PROCEDURAL STEPS				
1. Identified patient using two identifiers.	___	___	___	_____
2. Assessed I&O record to determine urine output trends, verified correct timing of the bladder scan measurement.	___	___	___	_____
3. Performed hand hygiene, applied clean gloves.	___	___	___	_____
4. Provided privacy.	___	___	___	_____
5. Discussed procedure with patient, asked patient to void, measured voided urine value if measurement was for PVR.	___	___	___	_____
6. Measured PVR with bladder scan:				
a. Assisted patient to appropriate position, raised bed to working height, lowered side rail on working side.	___	___	___	_____
b. Exposed patient's lower abdomen.	___	___	___	_____
c. Turned on scanner per manufacturer's guidelines.	___	___	___	_____
d. Set gender designation per manufacturer's guidelines.	___	___	___	_____
e. Wiped scanner head with cleanser, allowed to air dry.	___	___	___	_____
f. Palpated patient's symphysis pubis, applied ultrasound gel to midline abdomen.	___	___	___	_____
g. Placed scanner head on gel, ensured scanner head was oriented properly.	___	___	___	_____
h. Applied light pressure, kept head steady, pointed scanner head toward bladder, pressed and released scan button.	___	___	___	_____
i. Verified accurate aim, completed scan, printed image.	___	___	___	_____
7. Removed ultrasound gel from patient's abdomen.	___	___	___	_____
8. Removed ultrasound gel from scanner head, wiped with cleanser, let air dry.	___	___	___	_____

Copyright © 2018 by Elsevier Inc. All rights reserved.

	S	U	NP	Comments
9. Assisted patient to comfortable position, lowered bed, replaced side rails accordingly.	___	___	___	_____
10. Removed gloves, performed hand hygiene.	___	___	___	_____
11. Measured PVR using straight/intermittent catheterization.	___	___	___	_____
12. Reviewed prescriber's order to determine how often to assess residual urine.	___	___	___	_____
13. Reviewed I&O record to determine urine output trends.	___	___	___	_____

Copyright © 2018 by Elsevier Inc. All rights reserved.

Student _____ Date _____

Instructor _____ Date _____

PERFORMANCE CHECKLIST SKILL 34.3 **PERFORMING CLOSED URINARY CATHETER IRRIGATION**

	S	U	NP	Comments
ASSESSMENT				
1. Identified patient using two identifiers.	___	___	___	_____
2. Verified order for irrigation method, type, and amount of irrigant, as well as type of catheter in place.	___	___	___	_____
3. Performed hand hygiene, palpated bladder for distention and tenderness.	___	___	___	_____
4. Assessed patient for abdominal pain or spasms, sensation of bladder fullness, or catheter bypassing.	___	___	___	_____
5. Observed urine for color, amount, clarity, and presence of mucus, clots, or sediment.	___	___	___	_____
6. Monitored I&O.	___	___	___	_____
7. Assessed patient's knowledge regarding purpose of performing catheter irrigation.	___	___	___	_____
PLANNING				
1. Identified expected outcomes.	___	___	___	_____
2. Explained procedure to patient.	___	___	___	_____
IMPLEMENTATION				
1. Performed hand hygiene.	___	___	___	_____
2. Provided privacy.	___	___	___	_____
3. Raised bed to working height, lowered side rail on working side.	___	___	___	_____
4. Positioned patient properly, exposed catheter junctions.	___	___	___	_____
5. Removed catheter securement device.	___	___	___	_____
6. Organized supplies according to type of irrigation prescribed, applied gloves.	S	U	NP	_____
7. Closed continuous irrigation:				
a. Closed clamp on irrigation tubing, hung bag of irrigation solution on IV pole, inserted tip of sterile irrigation tubing into port of solution bag.	___	___	___	_____
b. Filled drip chamber half full, allowed solution to flow through tubing, closed clamp and recapped end of tubing once fluid had completely filled tubing.	___	___	___	_____

Copyright © 2018 by Elsevier Inc. All rights reserved.

	S	U	NP	Comments

c. Connected tubing securely to drainage port into double-/triple-lumen catheter using aseptic technique.

d. Adjusted clamp on tubing to begin flow of solution into bladder, calculated drip rate and adjusted at roller clamp, increased irrigation rate if necessary.

e. Observed for outflow of fluid into drainage bag, emptied catheter drainage bag as needed.

8. Closed intermittent irrigation:

   a. Poured prescribed irrigation solution into sterile container.

   b. Drew prescribed volume of irrigant into syringe using aseptic technique, placed sterile cap on tip of needleless syringe.

   c. Clamped catheter tubing appropriately with screw clamp.

   d. Cleaned catheter port with antiseptic swab.

   e. Inserted tip of needleless syringe properly into port.

   f. Injected solution properly.

   g. Removed syringe, removed clamp to allow solution to drain into bag.

9. Anchored catheter with catheter securement device.

10. Assisted patient to safe and comfortable position, lowered bed, placed side rail appropriately.

11. Disposed of all contaminated supplies appropriately, removed gloves, performed hand hygiene.

EVALUATION

1. Measured actual urine output properly.

2. Reviewed I&O flow sheet to verify appropriate hourly output.

3. Inspected urine for blood clots and sediment, ensured tubing was not kinked or occluded.

4. Assessed patient comfort.

5. Assessed for signs of infection.

6. Asked patient to explain reason for irrigation.

7. Identified unexpected outcomes.

Copyright © 2018 by Elsevier Inc. All rights reserved.

	S	U	NP	Comments

RECORDING AND REPORTING

1. Recorded all pertinent information in the appropriate log. ___ ___ ___ _____

2. Reported catheter occlusion, sudden bleeding, infection, or increased pain to health care provider. ___ ___ ___ _____

3. Recorded I&O on appropriate flow sheet. ___ ___ ___ _____

4. Documented evaluation of patient learning. ___ ___ ___ _____

Copyright © 2018 by Elsevier Inc. All rights reserved.

Student _____ Date _____

Instructor _____ Date _____

PERFORMANCE CHECKLIST SKILL 34.4 **APPLYING A CONDOM-TYPE EXTERNAL CATHETER**

	S	U	NP	Comments
ASSESSMENT				
1. Identified patient using two identifiers.	___	___	___	_____
2. Reviewed medical record, assessed urinary pattern, ability to empty bladder, and degree of urinary incontinence.	___	___	___	_____
3. Reviewed medical record for allergy to rubber or latex, checked patient's allergy wristband.	___	___	___	_____
4. Performed hand hygiene, applied clean gloves, assessed skin of penis for rashes, erythema, and/or open areas, removed gloves, performed hand hygiene.	___	___	___	_____
5. Assessed patient's mental status, knowledge of purpose for use of condom-type catheter, and ability to apply the device; included family members if appropriate.	___	___	___	_____
6. Verified patient's size and type of catheter properly.	___	___	___	_____
PLANNING				
1. Identified expected outcomes.	___	___	___	_____
2. Explained procedure to patient.	___	___	___	_____
IMPLEMENTATION				
1. Identified patient using two identifiers.	___	___	___	_____
2. Performed hand hygiene.	___	___	___	_____
3. Provided privacy.	___	___	___	_____
4. Raised bed to working height, lowered side rail on working side.	___	___	___	_____
5. Prepared drainage collection bag and tubing, clamped off drainage bag port, placed nearby ready to attach.	___	___	___	_____
6. Assisted patient to appropriate position, placed bath blanket over upper torso, folded sheets so only penis was exposed.	___	___	___	_____
7. Applied gloves, provided perineal care, dried thoroughly, ensured foreskin was in normal position, did not apply barrier cream.	___	___	___	_____

416

Copyright © 2018 by Elsevier Inc. All rights reserved.

	S	U	NP	Comments
8. Clipped hair at base of penis as necessary, applied hair guard or paper towel if appropriate.	___	___	___	_____
9. Applied condom catheter properly.	___	___	___	_____
10. Applied appropriate securement device as indicated in manufacturer's guidelines.	___	___	___	_____
11. Removed hair guard, connected drainage tubing to end of condom catheter, ensured condom was not twisted, placed excess tubing on bed and secured.	___	___	___	_____
12. Assisted patient to appropriate position, lowered bed, placed side rail accordingly.	___	___	___	_____
13. Disposed of contaminated supplies, removed gloves, performed hand hygiene.	___	___	___	_____
14. Removed and reapplied daily unless extended-wear device was used, removed condom properly when appropriate.	___	___	___	_____

EVALUATION

	S	U	NP	Comments
1. Observed urinary drainage.	___	___	___	_____
2. Inspected penis with condom catheter in place after application, assessed for swelling and discoloration, asked patient if there was any discomfort.	___	___	___	_____
3. Inspected skin on shaft for signs of breakdown or irritation appropriately.	___	___	___	_____
4. Asked patient to explain how to keep catheter from slipping off.	___	___	___	_____
5. Identified unexpected outcomes.	___	___	___	_____

RECORDING AND REPORTING

	S	U	NP	Comments
1. Recorded condom application; condition of penis, skin, and scrotum; urinary output; and voiding pattern in the appropriate log.	___	___	___	_____
2. Reported penile erythema, rashes, and/or skin breakdown.	___	___	___	_____
3. Documented evaluation of patient/caregiver learning.	___	___	___	_____

Copyright © 2018 by Elsevier Inc. All rights reserved.

Student _____ Date _____

Instructor _____ Date _____

PERFORMANCE CHECKLIST SKILL 34.5 **SUPRAPUBIC CATHETER CARE**

	S	U	NP	Comments
ASSESSMENT				
1. Identified patient using two identifiers.	___	___	___	_____
2. Assessed urine in drainage bag for amount, clarity, color, odor, and sediment.	___	___	___	_____
3. Performed hand hygiene, applied, clean gloves, observed dressing for drainage and intactness.	___	___	___	_____
4. Assessed catheter insertion site for signs of inflammation, asked patient if there was any pain at site, removed gloves, performed hand hygiene.	___	___	___	_____
5. Assessed for elevated temperature and chills.	___	___	___	_____
6. Assessed patient's knowledge of purpose of catheter and its care.	___	___	___	_____
7. Checked for allergies.	___	___	___	_____
PLANNING				
1. Identified expected outcomes.	___	___	___	_____
2. Explained procedure to patient and caregiver.	___	___	___	_____
IMPLEMENTATION				
1. Performed hand hygiene.	___	___	___	_____
2. Provided privacy.	___	___	___	_____
3. Raised bed to working height, lowered side rail on working side.	___	___	___	_____
4. Prepared supplies properly.	___	___	___	_____
5. Applied gloves, removed existing dressing, noted type and presence of drainage, removed gloves, performed hand hygiene.	___	___	___	_____
6. Cleansed using sterile technique for newly established catheter:				
a. Applied sterile gloves.	___	___	___	_____
b. Held catheter with nondominant hand, used gauze and saline to cleanse skin appropriately.	___	___	___	_____

Copyright © 2018 by Elsevier Inc. All rights reserved.

	S	U	NP	Comments
c. Cleansed base of catheter properly with fresh, moistened gauze.	___	___	___	_____
d. Applied drain dressing with sterile gloved hand around catheter, taped in place.	___	___	___	_____
7. Cleansed using aseptic technique for new or established catheter:				
a. Applied clean gloves.	___	___	___	_____
b. Held catheter with nondominant hand, cleansed properly with soap and water.	___	___	___	_____
c. Cleansed base of catheter properly with fresh washcloth or gauze.	___	___	___	_____
d. Applied drain dressing around catheter if necessary, taped in place.	___	___	___	_____
8. Secured catheter to lateral abdomen with tape or Velcro.	___	___	___	_____
9. Coiled excess tubing on bed, kept drainage bag below level of bladder.	___	___	___	_____
10. Disposed of all contaminated supplies properly, removed gloves, performed hand hygiene.	___	___	___	_____

EVALUATION

	S	U	NP	Comments
1. Asked patient to rate pain or discomfort.	___	___	___	_____
2. Monitored for signs of infection.	___	___	___	_____
3. Observed catheter insertion site for erythema, edema, discharge, and tenderness; checked dressing at least every 8 hours.	___	___	___	_____
4. Asked patient to describe care of suprapubic catheter.	___	___	___	_____
5. Identified unexpected outcomes.	___	___	___	_____

RECORDING AND REPORTING

	S	U	NP	Comments
1. Recorded and reported character of urine, type of dressing, and patient's comfort level.	___	___	___	_____
2. Recorded urine output on I&O flow sheet properly.	___	___	___	_____
3. Documented evaluation of patient learning.	___	___	___	_____
4. Reported signs of UTI or infection to health care provider.	___	___	___	_____

Copyright © 2018 by Elsevier Inc. All rights reserved.

Student _____ Date _____

Instructor _____ Date _____

PERFORMANCE CHECKLIST SKILL 35.1   **PROVIDING A BEDPAN**

	S	U	NP	Comments
ASSESSMENT				
1. Assessed patient's normal bowel elimination habits.	___	___	___	_____
2. Performed hand hygiene, auscultated abdomen for bowel sounds, palpated lower abdomen for distention.	___	___	___	_____
3. Assessed patient's level of mobility.	___	___	___	_____
4. Assessed patient's level of comfort; noted rectal or abdominal pain, presence of hemorrhoids, or irritation of skin surrounding anus.	___	___	___	_____
5. Applied clean gloves, inspected condition of perianal and perineal skin, remove gloves, performed hand hygiene.	___	___	___	_____
6. Determined need for stool specimen.	___	___	___	_____
PLANNING				
1. Identified expected outcomes.	___	___	___	_____
2. Explained procedure to patient, including self-help tips.	___	___	___	_____
3. Obtained assistance from additional nursing personnel as warranted.	___	___	___	_____
IMPLEMENTATION				
1. Performed hand hygiene.	___	___	___	_____
2. Provided privacy.	___	___	___	_____
3. Raised bed on opposite side.	___	___	___	_____
4. Raised bed horizontally according to nurses' height.	___	___	___	_____
5. Had patient assume supine position.	___	___	___	_____
6. Placed patient who can assist on bedpan:				
a. Applied clean gloves, raised head of patient's bed appropriately.	___	___	___	_____
b. Removed upper bed linens, did not expose patient.	___	___	___	_____
c. Instructed patient in how to flex knees and lift hips upward.	___	___	___	_____

Copyright © 2018 by Elsevier Inc. All rights reserved.

	S	U	NP	Comments

d. Placed hand under patient's sacrum to assist lifting, asked patient to bend knees and raise hips, slipped bedpan under patient with other hand, ensured open rim faced foot of bed, did not force. ____ ____ ____ _____

7. Placed patient with mobility restrictions on bedpan:

   a. Applied clean gloves, lowered head of bed appropriately. ____ ____ ____ _____

   b. Removed top linens as necessary. ____ ____ ____ _____

   c. Assisted patient with rolling onto side, placed bedpan on buttocks and down into mattress, ensured open rim faced foot of bed. ____ ____ ____ _____

   d. Kept one hand against bedpan and other around patient's far hip, asked patient to roll onto bedpan, did not force the pan under the patient. ____ ____ ____ _____

   e. Raised patient's head properly. ____ ____ ____ _____

   f. Had patient bend knees unless contra-indicated. ____ ____ ____ _____

8. Maintained patient's comfort and safety, covered patient for warmth, placed pillow or towel under lumbar curve of back, stayed close by. ____ ____ ____ _____

9. Had call bell and toilet tissue within reach of patient. ____ ____ ____ _____

10. Ensured that bed was in lowest position, raised upper side rails. ____ ____ ____ _____

11. Removed and discarded gloves, performed hand hygiene. ____ ____ ____ _____

12. Allowed patient to be alone, monitored status and responded promptly. ____ ____ ____ _____

13. Performed hand hygiene, applied clean gloves. ____ ____ ____ _____

14. Removed bedpan:

   a. Placed patient's bedside chair close to working side of bed. ____ ____ ____ _____

   b. Maintained privacy, determined if patient is able to wipe own perineal area, used toilet tissue or washcloths if nurse is needed to cleanse perineal area, cleansed patient properly. ____ ____ ____ _____

Copyright © 2018 by Elsevier Inc. All rights reserved.

	S	U	NP	Comments

c. Deposited contaminated tissue in bed-pan if appropriate, removed gloves and performed hand hygiene. ____ ____ ____ _____

d. For mobile patient, asked patient to flex knees and lift buttocks up, placed hand properly for support, had patient lift and remove bedpan, placed bedpan on draped chair, covered bedpan. ____ ____ ____ _____

e. For immobile patient, lowered head of bed, assisted patient with rolling off bedpan, held bedpan flat while patient rolled, placed bedpan on bedside chair, covered bedpan. ____ ____ ____ _____

15. Allowed patient to perform hand hygiene, changed soiled linens, removed gloves, and returned patient to comfortable position. ____ ____ ____ _____

16. Placed bed in its lowest position; ensured call bell, phone, water, and personal items are within reach. ____ ____ ____ _____

17. Obtained stool specimen as ordered, wore gloves when emptying bedpan, used spray faucet to rinse bedpan, used disinfectant if required, removed gloves. ____ ____ ____ _____

18. Performed hand hygiene. ____ ____ ____ _____

EVALUATION

1. Assessed characteristics of stool and urine. ____ ____ ____ _____

2. Evaluated patient's ability to use bedpan. ____ ____ ____ _____

3. Inspected patient's perineal area and surrounding skin while removing bedpan. ____ ____ ____ _____

4. Asked patient to demonstrate use of trapeze. ____ ____ ____ _____

5. Identified unexpected outcomes. ____ ____ ____ _____

RECORDING AND REPORTING

1. Recorded type of assistance needed, patient's tolerance, character and amount of stool, and urine output in appropriate log. ____ ____ ____ _____

2. Completed laboratory requisition, sent specimen to lab, recorded type of specimen sent. ____ ____ ____ _____

Copyright © 2018 by Elsevier Inc. All rights reserved.

Student _____ Date _____

Instructor _____ Date _____

PERFORMANCE CHECKLIST SKILL 35.2 **REMOVING FECAL IMPACTION DIGITALLY**

	S	U	NP	Comments
ASSESSMENT				
1. Identified patient using at least two identifiers.	___	___	___	_____
2. Asked patient about normal and current bowel elimination pattern.	___	___	___	_____
3. Inspected patient's abdomen for distention.	___	___	___	_____
4. Auscultated all four quadrants for presence of bowel sounds.	___	___	___	_____
5. Palpated patient's abdomen for distention, discomfort, and masses.	___	___	___	_____
6. Measured patient's current vital signs and comfort level.	___	___	___	_____
7. Did not interrupt routine of patient with spinal cord injury.	___	___	___	_____
8. Performed hand hygiene, applied clean gloves, observed consistency of stool, observed anal area for signs of irritation or hemorrhoids, removed gloves, performed hand hygiene.	___	___	___	_____
9. Determined if patient is receiving anticoagulant therapy or has a past history of rectal surgery.	___	___	___	_____
10. Checked patient's record for order for digital removal of impaction and use of anesthetic lubricant.	___	___	___	_____
PLANNING				
1. Identified expected outcomes.	___	___	___	_____
2. Explained procedure to patient.	___	___	___	_____
3. Performed hand hygiene, arranged supplies at bedside.	___	___	___	_____
IMPLEMENTATION				
1. Obtained assistance to help change patient's position if necessary, raised bed to working height.	___	___	___	_____
2. Provided privacy.	___	___	___	_____
3. Lowered side rail on patient's right side, assisted patient to appropriate position.	___	___	___	_____

Copyright © 2018 by Elsevier Inc. All rights reserved.

	S	U	NP	Comments
4. Draped patient's trunk and lower extremities with bath blanket, placed waterproof pad under patient's buttocks.	___	___	___	_____
5. Performed hygiene, applied clean gloves, placed bedpan next to patient.	___	___	___	_____
6. Lubricated gloved fingers of dominant hand.	___	___	___	_____
7. Instructed patient to take slow deep breaths, inserted index finger properly, inserted middle finger when appropriate.	___	___	___	_____
8. Advanced fingers slowly along rectal wall toward umbilicus.	___	___	___	_____
9. Loosened fecal mass appropriately, worked fingers into hardened mass.	___	___	___	_____
10. Worked stool downward, removed small sections of feces, discarded in bedpan.	___	___	___	_____
11. Observed patient's response, assessed heart rate, looked for signs of fatigue.	___	___	___	_____
12. Continued to clear rectum, allowed patient to rest at intervals.	___	___	___	_____
13. Performed perineal hygiene after removal of impaction.	___	___	___	_____
14. Removed bedpan, inspected feces for color and consistency, disposed of feces in toilet.	___	___	___	_____
15. Assisted patient to toilet if needed, cleaned and stored bedpan.	___	___	___	_____
16. Removed gloves and disposed of properly, performed hand hygiene.	___	___	___	_____

EVALUATION

	S	U	NP	Comments
1. Applied clean gloves. Performed rectal examination, observed anal and perianal area for irritation or breakdown, removed and disposed of gloves, performed hand hygiene.	___	___	___	_____
2. Reassessed vital signs, compared to baseline values, monitored patient for bradycardia for 1 hour.	___	___	___	_____
3. Auscultated bowel sounds.	___	___	___	_____
4. Palpated abdomen to determine if it is soft and nontender.	___	___	___	_____
5. Asked patient to describe what kinds of food to add to diet.	___	___	___	_____
6. Identified unexpected outcomes.	___	___	___	_____

Copyright © 2018 by Elsevier Inc. All rights reserved.

	S	U	NP	Comments

RECORDING AND REPORTING

1. Recorded patient's tolerance to procedure, amount and consistency of stool, vital signs, and adverse effects in appropriate log. ___ ___ ___ _____

2. Recorded understanding of necessary dietary changes. ___ ___ ___ _____

3. Reported any change in vital signs and adverse effects to health care provider. ___ ___ ___ _____

Copyright © 2018 by Elsevier Inc. All rights reserved.

Student _____ Date _____

Instructor _____ Date _____

PERFORMANCE CHECKLIST SKILL 35.3 **ADMINISTERING AN ENEMA**

	S	U	NP	Comments
ASSESSMENT				
1. Identified patient using at least two identifiers.	___	___	___	_____
2. Reviewed health care provider's order for enema, clarified reason for administration.	___	___	___	_____
3. Assessed last bowel movement, normal versus most recent bowel pattern, presence of hemorrhoids, and presence of abdominal pain or cramping.	___	___	___	_____
4. Assessed patient's mobility and ability to turn and position on side.	___	___	___	_____
5. Inspected abdomen for presence of distention, auscultated for bowel sounds.	___	___	___	_____
6. Assessed patient for allergy to active ingredients of Fleet enema.	___	___	___	_____
7. Determined patient's level of understanding of purpose of enema.	___	___	___	_____
PLANNING				
1. Identified expected outcomes.	___	___	___	_____
2. Performed hand hygiene, arranged supplies at bedside.	___	___	___	_____
IMPLEMENTATION				
1. Checked accuracy and completeness of each MAR with written order, compared MAR with label of solution.	___	___	___	_____
2. Provided privacy.	___	___	___	_____
3. Placed bedpan or bedside commode in accessible position, ensured toilet, nonskid slippers, and bathrobe are accessible.	___	___	___	_____
4. Performed hand hygiene.	___	___	___	_____
5. Assisted patient to appropriate position, encouraged patient to remain in position until procedure is complete.	___	___	___	_____
6. Applied clean gloves, placed waterproof pad under hips and buttocks, covered patient with bath blanket, exposed only rectal area.	___	___	___	_____

Copyright © 2018 by Elsevier Inc. All rights reserved.

	S	U	NP	Comments

7. Separated buttocks, examined perianal region for abnormalities. — — — _____

8. Administered enema:

  a. Administered prepackaged disposable enema.

    (1) Removed cap from container, applied more water-soluble lubricant as needed. — — — _____

    (2) Gently separated buttocks, instructed patient to relax by breathing out through the mouth. — — — _____

    (3) Expelled any air from enema container. — — — _____

    (4) Inserted lubricated tip of container properly into anal canal. — — — _____

    (5) Rolled bottle until all of solution entered rectum, instructed patient to retain solution until urge to defecate occurs. — — — _____

  b. Administered enema in standard enema bag.

    (1) Added warmed solution to enema bag properly, checked temperature of solution on inner wrist. — — — _____

    (2) Added castile soap if SSE is ordered. — — — _____

    (3) Raised container, released clamp, allowed solution to flow until tubing was filled. — — — _____

    (4) Reclamped tubing. — — — _____

    (5) Lubricated tip of rectal tube. — — — _____

    (6) Separated buttocks, instructed patient to relax by breathing out through the mouth, touched patient's skin next to anus with tip of tube. — — — _____

    (7) Inserted tip of rectal tube appropriately. — — — _____

    (8) Held tubing constantly until end of fluid instillation. — — — _____

    (9) Opened regulating clamp, allowed solution to enter properly. — — — _____

    (10) Raised height of enema container to appropriate level above anus. — — — _____

    (11) Instilled all solution, clamped tubing, told patient that procedure is complete and you will be removing tubing. — — — _____

Copyright © 2018 by Elsevier Inc. All rights reserved.

	S	U	NP	Comments

9. Placed layers of toilet tissue around anus, withdrew rectal tube and tip.

10. Explained to patient that distention and abdominal cramping is normal, asked patient to retain solution as long as possible, stayed at beside, had patient lie quietly in bed if possible.

11. Discarded enema container and tubing in proper receptacle, removed gloves, performed hand hygiene.

12. Assisted patient to bathroom or with bedpan if possible.

13. Observed character of stool and solution, cautioned patient against flushing toilet before inspection.

14. Assisted patient as needed with washing anal area with soap and water.

15. Removed and discarded gloves, performed hand hygiene.

EVALUATION

1. Inspected color, consistency, and amount of stool, odor, and fluid passed.

2. Assessed for abdominal distention.

3. Asked patient to describe how to position self for Fleet enema.

4. Identified unexpected outcomes.

RECORDING AND REPORTING

1. Recorded all pertinent information in the appropriate log.

2. Recorded patient's understanding of self-administration of a Fleet enema.

3. Reported failure of patient to defecate and any adverse effects to health care provider.

Copyright © 2018 by Elsevier Inc. All rights reserved.

Student _____ Date _____

Instructor _____ Date _____

PERFORMANCE CHECKLIST PROCEDURAL GUIDELINE 35.1 **APPLYING A FECAL MANAGEMENT SYSTEM**

	S	U	NP	Comments
ASSESSMENT				
1. Identified patient using at least two identifiers.	____	____	____	_____
2. Reviewed medical record for contraindications for use of an FMS.	____	____	____	_____
3. Assessed for diarrhea over the last 24 to 48 hours.	____	____	____	_____
4. Assessed patient for allergy to silicone.	____	____	____	_____
5. Performed hand hygiene, applied clean gloves, performed perineal hygiene, observed patient's anal region for conditions that contraindicate use of device.	____	____	____	_____
6. Changed gloves, performed rectal examination, ensured there is no rectal impaction, removed and discarded gloves.	____	____	____	_____
7. Applied new gloves.	____	____	____	_____
8. Applied the FMS:				
a. Connected collection bag to catheter tube assembly.	____	____	____	_____
b. Deflated cuff with syringe in kit.	____	____	____	_____
c. Filled syringe with tap water, attached syringe to inflation port, did not inflate.	____	____	____	_____
d. Positioned patient appropriately.	____	____	____	_____
e. Placed protective bed pad under patient's hip.	____	____	____	_____
f. Folded and lubricated cuff properly.	____	____	____	_____
g. Lubricated anal sphincter.	____	____	____	_____
h. Separated patient's buttocks, exposed perineal area for entire procedure, ensured area is clean and dry.	____	____	____	_____
i. Inserted cuff, depressed syringe plunger to inflate cuff, removed syringe, ensured cuff seats against rectal floor.	____	____	____	_____
j. Noted position of indicator line, repositioned cuff if needed, removed gloves, performed hand hygiene.	____	____	____	_____
9. Irrigated and repositioned cuff as needed.	____	____	____	_____

Copyright © 2018 by Elsevier Inc. All rights reserved.

	S	U	NP	Comments

10. If stool sample is needed, applied clean gloves, collected sample from sample port, closed port when finished. ____ ____ ____ _____

11. Replaced collection bag as needed, performed hand hygiene, applied clean gloves:

   a. Disconnected tubing from collection bag. ____ ____ ____ _____

   b. Attached bag plug into collection bag hub if necessary. ____ ____ ____ _____

   c. Connected new bag to tubing. ____ ____ ____ _____

   d. Disposed of fecal contents appropriately, removed gloves and performed hand hygiene. ____ ____ ____ _____

12. Removed FMS, performed hand hygiene, applied clean gloves:

   a. Attached depressed syringe to cuff infusion port, withdrew all water. ____ ____ ____ _____

   b. Grasped catheter and slowly slid out of anus. ____ ____ ____ _____

   c. Disposed of FMS, removed gloves, performed hand hygiene. ____ ____ ____ _____

13. Positioned patient comfortably, performed any hygiene as needed. ____ ____ ____ _____

14. Monitored patient for diarrhea, recorded amounts on I&O record. ____ ____ ____ _____

15. Recorded application of device and appearance of skin in the appropriate log. ____ ____ ____ _____

Copyright © 2018 by Elsevier Inc. All rights reserved.

Student _____ Date _____

Instructor _____ Date _____

PERFORMANCE CHECKLIST SKILL 35.4 **INSERTION, MAINTENANCE, AND REMOVAL OF A NASOGASTRIC TUBE FOR GASTRIC DECOMPRESSION**

	S	U	NP	Comments
ASSESSMENT				
1. Identified patient using at least two identifiers.	——	——	——	_____
2. Performed hand hygiene, inspected condition of patient's nasal and oral cavity.	——	——	——	_____
3. Asked if patient has history of nasal surgery or congestion and allergies, noted if deviated nasal septum is present.	——	——	——	_____
4. Auscultated for bowel sounds; palpated patient's abdomen for distention, pain, and rigidity, removed and discarded gloves.	——	——	——	_____
5. Assessed patient's LOC and ability to follow instructions.	——	——	——	_____
6. Determined if patient had previous NG tube and which naris was used.	——	——	——	_____
7. Verified order for type of NG tube and whether tube is to be attached to suction or drainage bag.	——	——	——	_____
PLANNING				
1. Identified expected outcomes.	——	——	——	_____
2. Informed patient that procedure may make him or her gag and there will be a burning sensation in the nasopharynx, developed hand signal with patient.	——	——	——	_____
3. Performed hand hygiene, arranged supplies at bedside.	——	——	——	_____
IMPLEMENTATION				
1. Positioned patient appropriately.	——	——	——	_____
2. Placed bath towel over patient's chest, gave facial tissue to patient, allowed patient to blow nose if necessary, placed emesis basin within reach.	——	——	——	_____
3. Provided privacy.	——	——	——	_____
4. Washed bridge of nose with soap and water or alcohol, dried thoroughly.	——	——	——	_____
5. Stood on appropriate side of patient.	——	——	——	_____

Copyright © 2018 by Elsevier Inc. All rights reserved.

	S	U	NP	Comments

6. Instructed patient to relax and breathe normally while occluding one naris then the other, selected naris with greater airflow. ___ ___ ___ _____

7. Measured distance to insert tubing using NEX method. ___ ___ ___ _____

8. Marked length to be inserted with tape. ___ ___ ___ _____

9. Prepared tube fixation materials. ___ ___ ___ _____

10. Performed hand hygiene, applied clean gloves. ___ ___ ___ _____

11. Applied pulse oximetry/capnography device, measured vital signs, monitored during insertion. ___ ___ ___ _____

12. Lubricated end of tube with water-soluble lubricant if necessary. ___ ___ ___ _____

13. Handed patient cup of water, explained that tube is about to be inserted. ___ ___ ___ _____

14. Inserted tube properly into naris to back of throat. ___ ___ ___ _____

15. Had patient relax and flex head toward chest after tube passes nasopharynx. ___ ___ ___ _____

16. Encouraged patient to swallow with the water, advanced tube as patient swallows, rotated tube while inserting. ___ ___ ___ _____

17. Emphasized need to mouth breathe. ___ ___ ___ _____

18. Did not advance tube during inspiration or coughing, continued to monitor oximetry/capnography. ___ ___ ___ _____

19. Advanced tube each time patient swallows until desired length is reached. ___ ___ ___ _____

20. Used penlight and tongue blade, ensured tube is not positioned in back of throat. ___ ___ ___ _____

21. Anchored tube to nose with tape. ___ ___ ___ _____

22. Verified tube placement:

   a. Followed order for bedside x-ray film, notified radiology for examination of chest and abdomen. ___ ___ ___ _____

   b. Aspirated gastric contents using Asepto or catheter-tipped syringe, observed amount, color, and quality of return. ___ ___ ___ _____

   c. Used gastric pH paper to measure aspirate for pH. ___ ___ ___ _____

Copyright © 2018 by Elsevier Inc. All rights reserved.

	S	U	NP	Comments

23. Anchored tube:

   a. Applied tape.

     (1) Applied tincture of benzoin to bridge of nose, allowed to become tacky. ___ ___ ___ _____

     (2) Printed date and time on top of tape. ___ ___ ___ _____

     (4) Wrapped bottom end of tape around tube as it exits nose. ___ ___ ___ _____

   b. Applied tube fixation device using shaped adhesive patch.

     (1) Applied wide end of patch to bridge of nose. ___ ___ ___ _____

     (2) Slipped connector around tube as it exits nose. ___ ___ ___ _____

24. Fastened end of NG tube to patient's gown properly, did not use safety pins. ___ ___ ___ _____

25. Elevated head of bed unless contraindicated. ___ ___ ___ _____

26. Assisted radiology as needed in obtaining x-ray film. ___ ___ ___ _____

27. Removed gloves, performed hand hygiene, helped patient to comfortable position. ___ ___ ___ _____

28. Placed a mark where tube exits nose or measured length of tube from nares to connector and documented length of tube in patient's record. ___ ___ ___ _____

29. Attached NG tube to suction as ordered. ___ ___ ___ _____

30. Performed NG tube irrigation:

   a. Performed hand hygiene, applied clean gloves. ___ ___ ___ _____

   b. Checked for tube placement in stomach, clamped tube or reconnected connecting tube, removed syringe. ___ ___ _____

   c. Emptied syringe of aspirate, used to draw up normal saline. ___ ___ _____

   d. Disconnected NG from connecting tube, laid end of connection tubing on towel. ___ ___ ___ _____

   e. Inserted tip of irrigating syringe into end of NG tube, removed clamp, held syringe properly, injected saline slowly, did not force solution. ___ ___ ___ _____

   f. Checked for kinks in tubing if resistance occurred, turned patient onto left side, reported repeated resistance. ___ ___ ___ _____

Copyright © 2018 by Elsevier Inc. All rights reserved.

	S	U	NP	Comments

g. Aspirated fluid after instilling saline, recorded any difference in output or intake.

h. Placed air into blue pigtail with Asepto syringe.

i. Repeated irrigation if solution did not return. Reconnected NG tube to drain or suction.

31. Removed NG tube:

   a. Verified order to remove NG tube.

   b. Auscultated abdomen for presence of bowel sounds.

   c. Explained procedure to patient, reassured that removal is less distressing than insertion.

   d. Performed hand hygiene, applied clean gloves.

   e. Turned off suction, disconnected NG tube from drainage bag or suction, inserted air into lumen of NG tube with irrigating syringe, removed tape or fixation device, unpinned tube from gown.

   f. Handed patient facial tissue, placed towel across chest, instructed patient to take and hold breath.

   g. Clamped or kinked tubing, pulled tube out into towel.

   h. Inspected intactness of tube.

   i. Measured amount of drainage, noted character of content, disposed of tube and drainage equipment appropriately.

   j. Cleaned nares, provided mouth care.

   k. Positioned patient comfortably, explained procedure for drinking fluids, instructed patient to notify you if nausea occurs.

32. Cleaned equipment, returned to proper place, placed soiled linen in proper receptacle.

33. Removed and discarded gloves, performed hand hygiene.

434

Copyright © 2018 by Elsevier Inc. All rights reserved.

	S	U	NP	Comments

EVALUATION

1. Observed amount and character of contents draining from NG tube, asked if patient feels nauseated.

2. Auscultated for presence of bowel sounds, turned off suction while auscultated.

3. Palpated patient's abdomen periodically; noted distention, pain, and rigidity.

4. Inspected nares and nose.

5. Observed position of tubing.

6. Explained it is normal if patient feels sore throat or irritation in pharynx.

7. Asked if patient understands why it is important to report nausea.

8. Identified unexpected outcomes.

RECORDING AND REPORTING

1. Recorded all pertinent information in the appropriate log.

2. Recorded patient understanding of what to report to nurse and purpose of NG tube in appropriate log.

3. Recorded difference between saline instilled and gastric aspirate on I&O sheet, recorded amount and character of contents draining from NG tube every shift.

4. Recorded removal of tube intact, patient's tolerance, and final amount and character of drainage.

Copyright © 2018 by Elsevier Inc. All rights reserved.

Student _____ Date _____

Instructor _____ Date _____

PERFORMANCE CHECKLIST SKILL 36.1 **POUCHING A COLOSTOMY OR AN ILEOSTOMY**

	S	U	NP	Comments

ASSESSMENT

1. Identified patient using at least two identifiers. ___ ___ ___ _____

2. Performed hand hygiene, applied gloves. ___ ___ ___ _____

3. Observed existing skin barrier and pouch for leakage, changed pouch at appropriate intervals, removed to fully observe stoma in case of opaque pouch, disposed of pouch properly. ___ ___ ___ _____

4. Observed amount of effluent in the pouch, emptied pouch properly if necessary, noted consistency of effluent, recorded I&O. ___ ___ ___ _____

5. Observed stoma for type, location, color, swelling, sutures, trauma, healing, or irritation. ___ ___ ___ _____

6. Observed placement of stoma in relation to abdominal contours and presence of scars, removed gloves, performed hand hygiene. ___ ___ ___ _____

7. Explored patient's attitude, perceptions, knowledge, and acceptance of stoma, discussed interest in self-care, identified others who would be assisting patient after leaving the hospital. ___ ___ ___ _____

PLANNING

1. Identified expected outcomes. ___ ___ ___ _____

2. Explained procedure to patient, encouraged patient's interactions and questions. ___ ___ ___ _____

3. Assembled equipment, provided privacy. ___ ___ ___ _____

IMPLEMENTATION

1. Positioned patient properly, provided patient with mirror. ___ ___ ___ _____

2. Performed hand hygiene, applied clean gloves. ___ ___ ___ _____

3. Placed towel or waterproof barrier under patient and across patient's lower abdomen. ___ ___ ___ _____

4. Removed used pouch and skin barrier if necessary, used adhesive remover if necessary, emptied pouch and disposed of it in appropriate receptacle, measured output if needed. ___ ___ ___ _____

Copyright © 2018 by Elsevier Inc. All rights reserved.

	S	U	NP	Comments
5. Cleansed peristomal skin with warm water and washcloth, did not scrub, patted skin dry.	—	—	—	——————
6. Measured stoma.	—	—	—	——————
7. Traced pattern on pouch backing or skin barrier.	—	—	—	——————
8. Cut opening on backing or skin barrier, ensured opening was slightly larger than stoma.	—	—	—	——————
9. Removed protective backing from adhesive.	—	—	—	——————
10. Applied pouch over stoma, pressed into place around stoma and outside edges.	—	—	—	——————
11. Closed end of pouch, removed drape from patient, assisted patient to comfortable position.	—	—	—	——————
12. Removed gloves, performed hand hygiene.	—	—	—	——————

EVALUATION

	S	U	NP	Comments
1. Observed condition of skin barrier and adherence to abdominal surface.	—	—	—	——————
2. Observed appearance of stoma, peristomal skin, abdominal contours, and suture line during pouch change.	—	—	—	——————
3. Noted presence of flatus during pouch change.	—	—	—	——————
4. Observed patient's and caregiver's willingness to view stoma and ask questions.	—	—	—	——————
5. Asked patient how to prevent skin from being irritated and frequency with which pouch should be emptied.	—	—	—	——————
6. Identified unexpected outcomes.	—	—	—	——————

RECORDING AND REPORTING

	S	U	NP	Comments
1. Recorded all pertinent information in the appropriate log.	—	—	—	——————
2. Recorded patient/family level of participation, teaching that was done, and response to teaching.	—	—	—	——————
3. Reported abnormal appearance of stoma, suture line, peristomal skin, or character of output to nurse in charge or health care provider.	—	—	—	——————

Copyright © 2018 by Elsevier Inc. All rights reserved.

Student _____ Date _____

Instructor _____ Date _____

PERFORMANCE CHECKLIST SKILL 36.2 **POUCHING A UROSTOMY**

	S	U	NP	Comments

ASSESSMENT

1. Identified patient using at least two identifiers. ___ ___ ___ _____

2. Performed hand hygiene, applied clean gloves. ___ ___ ___ _____

3. Observed existing barrier and pouch for leakage and length of time in place, changed at appropriate intervals or if necessary. ___ ___ ___ _____

4. Observed characteristics or urine in pouch or drainage bag, emptied pouch if necessary. ___ ___ ___ _____

5. Observed stoma for color, swelling, sutures, trauma, and healing of peristomal skin; assessed type of stoma; removed and disposed of gloves. ___ ___ ___ _____

6. Explored patient's perceptions, acceptance, and knowledge of stoma and attitude toward learning self-care, identified others who would be assisting patient after leaving the hospital. ___ ___ ___ _____

PLANNING

1. Identified expected outcomes. ___ ___ ___ _____

2. Explained procedure to patient, encouraged patient's interaction and questions. ___ ___ ___ _____

3. Assembled equipment, provided privacy. ___ ___ ___ _____

IMPLEMENTATION

1. Positioned patient appropriately, provided patient with a mirror. ___ ___ ___ _____

2. Performed hand hygiene, applied clean gloves. ___ ___ ___ _____

3. Placed towel or waterproof barrier under patient and across patient's lower abdomen. ___ ___ ___ _____

4. Removed used pouch and barrier, pulled pouch around stents and laid towel underneath when stents were present, emptied pouch and measured output, disposed of pouch in appropriate receptacle. ___ ___ ___ _____

5. Placed rolled gauze at stoma opening, maintained gauze at the stoma opening continuously during pouch measurement and change. ___ ___ ___ _____

6. Cleansed peristomal skin with warm water and washcloth, did not scrub, patted skin dry. ___ ___ ___ _____

438

Copyright © 2018 by Elsevier Inc. All rights reserved.

	S	U	NP	Comments
7. Measured stoma, ensured opening was slightly larger than stoma.	___	___	___	_____
8. Traced pattern on pouch backing or barrier.	___	___	___	_____
9. Cut opening in pouch, customized pouch to fit stoma.	___	___	___	_____
10. Removed protective backing from adhesive surface.	___	___	___	_____
11. Applied pouch, pressed into place around stoma and outside edges, had patient hold hand over pouch.	___	___	___	_____
12. Used adapter to connect pouch to urinary bag.	___	___	___	_____
13. Removed drape from patient, removed gloves and performed hand hygiene.	___	___	___	_____

EVALUATION

	S	U	NP	Comments
1. Observed appearance of stoma, peristomal skin, and suture line.	___	___	___	_____
2. Evaluated character and volume of urinary drainage.	___	___	___	_____
3. Observed patient's and caregiver's willingness to view stoma and ask questions.	___	___	___	_____
4. Asked patient to describe how and when to empty pouch.	___	___	___	_____
5. Identified unexpected outcomes.	___	___	___	_____

RECORDING AND REPORTING

	S	U	NP	Comments
1. Recorded all pertinent information in the appropriate log.	___	___	___	_____
2. Recorded urinary output on I&O form.	___	___	___	_____
3. Recorded patient's and caregiver's reaction to stoma and level of participation.	___	___	___	_____
4. Documented evaluation of patient learning.	___	___	___	_____
5. Reported abnormalities in stoma or peristomal skin and absence of urinary output to nurse in charge or health care provider.	___	___	___	_____

Copyright © 2018 by Elsevier Inc. All rights reserved.

Student _____ Date _____

Instructor _____ Date _____

PERFORMANCE CHECKLIST SKILL 36.3 **CATHETERIZING A URINARY DIVERSION**

	S	U	NP	Comments

ASSESSMENT

1. Identified patient using at least two identifiers.

2. Observed for signs and symptoms of UTI.

3. Obtained order for catheterization.

4. Assessed patient's understanding of need for procedure and how procedure was done.

PLANNING

1. Identified expected outcomes.

2. Assembled equipment, provided privacy.

3. Explained procedure to patient, obtained specimen when patient was due to change pouch if using one-piece system.

IMPLEMENTATION

1. Positioned patient appropriately, draped towel across lower abdomen.

2. Performed hand hygiene, put on clean gloves.

3. Removed pouch, left barrier attached if patient uses two-piece system.

4. Removed gloves, performed hand hygiene.

5. Opened catheterization set or opened needed equipment and arranged on sterile barrier or placed gauze pad with lubricant on sterile field if did not use catheterization kit; applied sterile gloves.

6. Had patient hold absorbent gauze wick on stoma if necessary.

7. Cleansed surface of stoma with antiseptic, wiped off excess antiseptic with dry gauze.

8. Removed lid from sterile specimen container.

9. Lubricated tip of catheter, kept catheter sterile.

440

Copyright © 2018 by Elsevier Inc. All rights reserved.

	S	U	NP	Comments
10. Inserted catheter tip into stoma with dominant hand, did not force, placed distal end of catheter into specimen container, used gentle but firm pressure, had patient cough or turn slightly.	____	____	____	_____
11. Held container below level of stoma, waited long enough to get adequate amount of urine.	____	____	____	_____
12. Withdrew catheter properly, placed absorbent pad over stoma.	____	____	____	_____
13. Put lid on specimen container.	____	____	____	_____
14. Reapplied new pouch or reattached pouch if patient uses a two-piece system.	____	____	____	_____
15. Disposed of used pouch and equipment properly.	____	____	____	_____
16. Removed gloves, performed hand hygiene, labeled specimen in presence of patient, placed in biohazard bag, sent to laboratory at once.	____	____	____	_____

EVALUATION

	S	U	NP	Comments
1. Compared results of culture and sensitivity with expected findings.	____	____	____	_____
2. Asked patient to describe signs of UTI.	____	____	____	_____
3. Identified unexpected outcomes.	____	____	____	_____

RECORDING AND REPORTING

	S	U	NP	Comments
1. Recorded time specimen collected; patient's tolerance; and appearance of urine, skin, and stoma.	____	____	____	_____
2. Documented evaluation of patient learning.	____	____	____	_____
3. Reported results of laboratory test to nurse in charge or health care provider.	____	____	____	_____

Copyright © 2018 by Elsevier Inc. All rights reserved.

Student _____ Date _____

Instructor _____ Date _____

PERFORMANCE CHECKLIST SKILL 37.1 **PREOPERATIVE ASSESSMENT**

	S	U	NP	Comments
ASSESSMENT				
1. Identified patient using at least two identifiers.	___	___	___	_____
2. Performed hand hygiene, prepared equipment and room for assessment.	___	___	___	_____
3. Determined any communication impairments and mental competency, obtained professional interpreter if needed.	___	___	___	_____
4. Assessed patient's understanding of intended surgery and anesthesia.	___	___	___	_____
5. Asked if patient has advance directive.	___	___	___	_____
6. Collected nursing history, identified surgical risk factors:				
a. Condition requiring surgery.	___	___	___	_____
b. Chronic illnesses and associated risks.	___	___	___	_____
c. Obstructive sleep apnea.	___	___	___	_____
d. Date of last menstrual period.	___	___	___	_____
e. Previous hospitalizations.	___	___	___	_____
f. Full medication history.	___	___	___	_____
g. Previous experience with and outcomes from surgery and anesthesia.	___	___	___	_____
h. Family history of complications from surgery or anesthesia.	___	___	___	_____
i. Allergies to medications, food, or tape.	___	___	___	_____
j. Physical impairment.	___	___	___	_____
k. Prostheses and implants.	___	___	___	_____
l. Smoking, alcohol, and drug use.	___	___	___	_____
m. Occupation.	___	___	___	_____
7. Obtained patient's weight, height, and vital signs.	___	___	___	_____
8. Assessed patient's respiratory status.	___	___	___	_____

Copyright © 2018 by Elsevier Inc. All rights reserved.

	S	U	NP	Comments
9. Auscultated heart sounds, evaluated patient's circulatory status.	___	___	___	_____
10. Assessed patient's risk for postoperative thrombus formation.	___	___	___	_____
11. Completed gastrointestinal assessment, identified time of patient's last food or drink.	___	___	___	_____
12. Completed neurologic assessment.	___	___	___	_____
13. Assessed patient's musculoskeletal system.	___	___	___	_____
14. Examined patient's skin, identified breaks in integrity, determined level of hydration.	___	___	___	_____
15. Assessed patient's emotional status.	___	___	___	_____
16. Reviewed results of laboratory tests.	___	___	___	_____

PLANNING
1. Identified expected outcomes. ___ ___ ___ _____

IMPLEMENTATION
1. Communicated risk factors to preoperative team. ___ ___ ___ _____
2. Presented preoperative instruction to patient and caregiver as appropriate. ___ ___ ___ _____

EVALUATION
1. Determined if patient information is complete, verified unclear information with caregiver. ___ ___ ___ _____
2. Evaluated patient's ability to cooperate. ___ ___ ___ _____
3. Asked patient to describe when surgery is scheduled and the reason for the surgery. ___ ___ ___ _____
4. Identified unexpected outcomes. ___ ___ ___ _____

RECORDING AND REPORTING
1. Documented preoperative notes in appropriate log. ___ ___ ___ _____
2. Reported abnormal laboratory values or concerns to surgeon or anesthesiologist. ___ ___ ___ _____
3. Documented evaluation of patient learning. ___ ___ ___ _____

Copyright © 2018 by Elsevier Inc. All rights reserved.

Student _____ Date _____

Instructor _____ Date _____

PERFORMANCE CHECKLIST SKILL 37.2 **PREOPERATIVE TEACHING**

	S	U	NP	Comments
ASSESSMENT				
1. Identified patient using at least two identifiers.	___	___	___	_____
2. Asked about patient's previous experiences with surgery and anesthesia.	___	___	___	_____
3. Determined if patient and caregiver understand surgery.	___	___	___	_____
4. Identified patient's cognitive level, language, and culture; obtained interpreter's assistance if needed.	___	___	___	_____
5. Assessed patient's risk of postoperative respiratory complications.	___	___	___	_____
6. Assessed patient's anxiety related to surgery.	___	___	___	_____
7. Assessed caregiver's willingness to learn and support patient following surgery.	___	___	___	_____
8. Assessed patient's medical orders.	___	___	___	_____
PLANNING				
1. Identified expected outcomes.	___	___	___	_____
IMPLEMENTATION				
1. Performed hand hygiene; informed patient and caregiver of date, time, location, and length of surgery, postanesthesia recovery time, and waiting area.	___	___	___	_____
2. Answered questions patient and caregiver ask.	___	___	___	_____
3. Instructed patient about preoperative bowel or skin preparations, checked medical orders regarding preoperative showers, instructed patient to rinse and dry following showers, ensured patient donned clean clothing.	___	___	___	_____
4. Instructed patient on extent and purpose of food and fluid restrictions.	___	___	___	_____
5. Described preoperative routines.	___	___	___	_____
6. Described planned effect of preoperative medications.	___	___	___	_____
7. Reviewed which routine medications patient needs to discontinue before surgery.	___	___	___	_____

Copyright © 2018 by Elsevier Inc. All rights reserved.

	S	U	NP	Comments
8. Described perioperative sensations.	___	___	___	_____
9. Described pain control methods to be used after surgery.	___	___	___	_____
10. Described what patient will experience after surgery.	___	___	___	_____
11. Instructed patient on turning and sitting up:				
a. Instructed patient on how to properly turn onto right side and reverse process for left side.	___	___	___	_____
b. Instructed patient to turn every 2 hours while awake, ensured patient has assistance when needed.	___	___	___	_____
c. Instructed patient in sitting up on the side of bed with nurse's help.	___	___	___	_____
12. Taught patient coughing and deep breathing:				
a. Positioned patient appropriately.	___	___	___	_____
b. Instructed patient to place palms along lower border of rib cage.	___	___	___	_____
c. Explained and demonstrated breathing and feeling of diaphragm.	___	___	___	_____
d. Had patient avoid using chest and shoulder muscles while inhaling.	___	___	___	_____
e. Had patient deep breathe slowly and exhale through mouth.	___	___	___	_____
f. Had patient repeat exercise 3 to 5 times.	___	___	___	_____
g. Had patient take two slow deep breaths through nose, exhaling through pursed lips.	___	___	___	_____
h. Had patient inhale deeply, hold breath, and then cough fully.	___	___	___	_____
i. Cautioned patient against clearing throat.	___	___	___	_____
j. Had patient practice coughing; instructed patient to perform turning, coughing, and deep breathing every 2 hours; had caregiver coach patient to exercise.	___	___	___	_____
13. Taught patient use of incentive spirometer:				
a. Positioned patient appropriately.	___	___	___	_____
b. Indicated volume level to be reached with each breath.	___	___	___	_____
c. Explained how to position mouthpiece, had patient demonstrate until position is correct.	___	___	___	_____

Copyright © 2018 by Elsevier Inc. All rights reserved.

	S	U	NP	Comments

d. Instructed patient to exhale completely, position mouthpiece properly, and maintain flow until reaching goal volume. ____ ____ ____ _____

e. Had patient hold breath once maximum inspiration is reached, had patient hold breath for 2 to 3 seconds and exhale slowly. ____ ____ ____ _____

f. Instructed patient to breathe normally between 10 breaths on incentive spirometer, repeated every hour while awake. ____ ____ ____ _____

14. Taught patient PEP therapy and "huff" coughing:

a. Set PEP device correctly. ____ ____ ____ _____

b. Positioned patient correctly, applied nose clip to patient's nose. ____ ____ ____ _____

c. Had patient place lips around mouthpiece, instructed patient to hake full breath and exhale 2 or 3 times longer than inhalation, repeated pattern for 10 to 20 breaths. ____ ____ ____ _____

d. Removed device from mouth, had patient take slow deep breath and hold for 3 seconds. ____ ____ ____ _____

e. Instructed patient to exhale in quick forced "huffs" and to repeat exercise every 2 hours while awake. ____ ____ ____ _____

15. Taught patient controlled coughing:

a. Explained importance of maintaining position. ____ ____ ____ _____

b. Demonstrated coughing, had patient inhale through nose and exhale through mouth twice. ____ ____ ____ _____

c. Instructed patient to inhale deeply a third time, hold to count of three, and cough fully. ____ ____ ____ _____

d. Cautioned patient against clearing throat instead of coughing. ____ ____ ____ _____

e. Taught patient to press hands over incisional area during exercises. ____ ____ ____ _____

f. Instructed patient to cough 2 to 3 times every 2 hours while awake. ____ ____ ____ _____

g. Instructed patient to examine sputum for changes that indicate pulmonary complications and notify nurse if changes are noted. ____ ____ ____ _____

Copyright © 2018 by Elsevier Inc. All rights reserved.

	S	U	NP	Comments

16. Taught patient leg exercises:

   a. Instructed and encouraged patient in leg exercises.

   b. Positioned patient appropriately.

   c. Instructed patient to rotate each ankle in a complete circle and draw circles with big toe 5 times.

   d. Alternated dorsiflexion and plantar flexion 5 times.

   e. Performed quadriceps setting 5 times.

   f. Instructed patient to alternate raising legs straight up from bed surface, repeated 5 times.

17. Had patient continue to practice exercises before surgery every 2 hours while awake, taught patient to coordinate turning and exercises with breathing and use of incentive spirometer.

18. Ensured patient's expectations of surgery are realistic.

19. Reinforced therapeutic coping strategies or encouraged alternatives if strategies are unsuccessful.

EVALUATION

1. Observed patient demonstrating all learned skills.

2. Asked family to identify location of waiting room and validated.

3. Asked caregiver if he or she is able to help prepare patient for surgery.

4. Observed level of emotional support caregiver provides patient.

5. Ensured patient understands what medications should be discontinued before surgery.

6. Identified unexpected outcomes.

RECORDING AND REPORTING

1. Documented all preoperative teaching and response in the appropriate log.

Copyright © 2018 by Elsevier Inc. All rights reserved.

Student _____ Date _____

Instructor _____ Date _____

PERFORMANCE CHECKLIST SKILL 37.3 **PHYSICAL PREPARATION FOR SURGERY**

	S	U	NP	Comments
ASSESSMENT				
1. Identified patient using at least two identifiers.	___	___	___	_____
2. Completed preoperative assessment.	___	___	___	_____
3. Assessed and recorded patient's heart rate, BP, respiratory rate, oxygen saturation, and temperature.	___	___	___	_____
4. Validated that admissions preparations were completed as ordered.	___	___	___	_____
5. Asked if patient had advance directive, placed it in medical record if so.	___	___	___	_____
PLANNING				
1. Identified expected outcomes.	___	___	___	_____
IMPLEMENTATION				
1. Performed hand hygiene, helped patient to put on hospital gown and remove personal items, explained sensations patient will feel.	___	___	___	_____
2. Instructed patient to remove makeup, nail polish, hairpins, and jewelry.	___	___	___	_____
3. Ensured money and valuables have been locked up or given to caregiver.	___	___	___	_____
4. Ensured patient has followed appropriate fluid and food restrictions.	___	___	___	_____
5. Verified presence of allergies, ensured safety armbands are present.	___	___	___	_____
6. Verified that patient had followed instructions about medications.	___	___	___	_____
7. Verified that bowel preparation has been completed.	___	___	___	_____
8. Ensured medical history and physical examination results are in patient's record.	___	___	___	_____
9. Verified that all consents are complete and all necessary signatures are present.	___	___	___	_____
10. Ensured necessary lab work, ECG, and chest x-ray studies are completed and results are on chart.	___	___	___	_____

Copyright © 2018 by Elsevier Inc. All rights reserved.

	S	U	NP	Comments

11. Verified that blood type and cross-match are completed if ordered and that blood transfusions are available. ____ ____ ____ _____

12. Instructed patient to void. ____ ____ ____ _____

13. Started IV line properly. ____ ____ ____ _____

14. Administered preoperative medications as ordered. ____ ____ ____ _____

15. Applied compression stockings. ____ ____ ____ _____

16. Applied ICD if ordered. ____ ____ ____ _____

17. Performed hand hygiene, applied clean gloves, cleaned and prepared surgical site. ____ ____ ____ _____

18. Performed hand hygiene, inserted urinary catheter if ordered. ____ ____ ____ _____

19. Allowed patient to wear glasses or hearing aids as long as possible, noted all items removed before proceeding. ____ ____ ____ _____

20. Placed cap over patient's head and hair. ____ ____ ____ _____

21. Placed patient on bed with call light within reach, allowed family to remain at bedside until patient is transferred to surgical area, maintained quiet and relaxing environment. ____ ____ ____ _____

22. Helped patient onto stretcher for transport to OR. ____ ____ ____ _____

EVALUATION

1. Had patient describe surgical procedure and its risks and benefits. ____ ____ ____ _____

2. Had patient repeat preoperative instructions. ____ ____ ____ _____

3. Monitored patient for signs and symptoms of anxiety, asked how patient and family are feeling. ____ ____ ____ _____

4. Asked patient to describe what he or she expects to happen in the recovery room. ____ ____ ____ _____

5. Identified unexpected outcomes. ____ ____ ____ _____

RECORDING AND REPORTING

1. Documented preoperative physical preparation on preoperative checklist. ____ ____ ____ _____

2. Recorded disposition of patient valuables and belongings in appropriate log. ____ ____ ____ _____

3. Reported lack of signed consent form or failure of patient to maintain NPO status. ____ ____ ____ _____

Copyright © 2018 by Elsevier Inc. All rights reserved.

Student _____ Date _____

Instructor _____ Date _____

PERFORMANCE CHECKLIST SKILL 37.4 **PROVIDING IMMEDIATE ANESTHESIA RECOVERY IN THE POSTANESTHESIA CARE UNIT**

	S	U	NP	Comments
ASSESSMENT				
1. Identified patient using at least two identifiers.	___	___	___	_____
2. Received hand-off report from circulating nurse and anesthesia provider.	___	___	___	_____
3. Reviewed surgeon's orders on patient's arrival in PACU.	___	___	___	_____
4. Considered type of surgical procedure, restrictions to movement, and type of anesthesia used.	___	___	___	_____
5. Performed hand hygiene; performed thorough patient assessment; assessed patient's surgical site and drains, skin integrity, safety, and anxiety.	___	___	___	_____
6. Took vital signs, monitored pulse oximetry during initial stabilization.	___	___	___	_____
7. Assessed all criteria for discharged from phase I level of care properly.	___	___	___	_____
PLANNING				
1. Identified expected outcomes.	___	___	___	_____
2. Performed hand hygiene, prepared equipment for continued monitoring and care activities.	___	___	___	_____
IMPLEMENTATION				
1. Attached oxygen tubing to regulator, hung IV fluids, and checked IV flow when patient enters PACU; connected tubing to gravity drainage or suction as needed; attached cardiac monitor; ensured indwelling catheter and bag are in drainage position and patent.	___	___	___	_____
2. Continued ongoing assessment as needed, compared findings with patient's baseline, provided blankets as needed.	___	___	___	_____
3. Maintained patent airway after general anesthesia:				
a. Positioned patient appropriately.	___	___	___	_____

Copyright © 2018 by Elsevier Inc. All rights reserved.

	S	U	NP	Comments

b. Placed towel or pillow under patient's head, positioned patient appropriately, had emesis basin available if patient becomes nauseated. ____ ____ ____ _____

c. Encouraged patient to cough and deep breathe on awakening and at appropriate intervals. ____ ____ ____ _____

d. Suctioned artificial airway and oral cavity. ____ ____ ____ _____

e. Had patient spit out oral airway once gag reflex returns. ____ ____ ____ _____

f. Avoided position changes if necessary, ensured appropriate position, maintained IV infusion, encouraged fluid intake. ____ ____ ____ _____

4. Called patient by name in normal tone of voice, gently touched patient if needed, explained that surgery is over and patient is in recovery area. ____ ____ ____ _____

5. Assessed circulatory perfusion, palpated for skin temperature, tested for capillary refill. ____ ____ ____ _____

6. Inspected color of nail beds and skin, palpated for skin temperature. ____ ____ ____ _____

7. Assessed signs of complications from general anesthesia, monitored laboratory findings. ____ ____ ____ _____

8. Introduced self and oriented patient to surroundings as patient wakes from general anesthesia. ____ ____ ____ _____

9. Monitored responses after spinal or epidural anesthesia:

a. Monitored hypotension, bradycardia, and nausea/vomiting. ____ ____ ____ _____

b. Maintained adequate IV infusion. ____ ____ ____ _____

c. Kept patient in appropriate position. ____ ____ ____ _____

d. Observed patient in PACU until patient regained movement in extremities. ____ ____ ____ _____

e. Assessed respiratory status, level of spinal sensation, and mobility in lower extremities; tested sensation along sensory dermatomes; had patient identify warm or cold; reminded patient lost sensation will return in several hours. ____ ____ ____ _____

Copyright © 2018 by Elsevier Inc. All rights reserved.

	S	U	NP	Comments

10. Monitored source of intake and output:

   a. Observed dressing and drains for evidence of bright red blood, inspected surgical incision for swelling or discoloration, noted condition of surgical dressing, marked dressing with circle around drainage, noted changes and vital signs over time. ____ ____ ____ _____

   b. Reinforced pressure dressing or changed simple dressing if ordered; continued monitoring incision, tissue, and drainage. ____ ____ ____ _____

   c. Informed surgeon of unexpected bloody drainage, reinforced dressing as indicated, applied direct pressure, monitored for decreased BP and increased pulse. ____ ____ ____ _____

   d. Inspected condition and contents of drainage tubes and collecting devices, noted character and volume of drainage. ____ ____ ____ _____

   e. Observed amount, color, and appearance of urine. ____ ____ ____ _____

   f. Assessed drainage of NG tube if present, checked placement and irrigated if necessary. ____ ____ ____ _____

   g. Monitored and maintained IV fluid rates, observed IV site for signs of infiltration. ____ ____ ____ _____

11. Promoted comfort:

   a. Provided mouth care. ____ ____ ____ _____

   b. Provided blankets or therapy to promote warmth and minimize shivering. ____ ____ ____ _____

   c. Helped with position changes, provided supportive pillows. ____ ____ ____ _____

12. Continued monitoring pain until transfer to surgical unit or discharge, provided pain medication as ordered. ____ ____ ____ _____

13. Explained patient's condition to patient, informed patient of transfer plans. ____ ____ ____ _____

14. Contacted anesthesiologist to approve transfer or release when patient's condition stabilizes. ____ ____ ____ _____

15. Provided written and verbal instructions before discharge. ____ ____ ____ _____

Copyright © 2018 by Elsevier Inc. All rights reserved.

	S	U	NP	Comments

EVALUATION

1. Compared all vital signs with patient's baseline and expected normal levels.   ____ ____ ____ _____

2. Inspected surgical wound and dressings for drainage, assessed for wound drainage under patient.   ____ ____ ____ _____

3. Measured I&O.   ____ ____ ____ _____

4. Auscultated bowel sounds, asked if patient has passed flatus.   ____ ____ ____ _____

5. Measured patient's perception of pain after implementing pain relief measures.   ____ ____ ____ _____

6. Completed system-specific physical assessments as appropriate.   ____ ____ ____ _____

7. Asked patient to explain signs and symptoms of infection.   ____ ____ ____ _____

8. Identified unexpected outcomes.   ____ ____ ____ _____

RECORDING AND REPORTING

1. Documented patient's arrival, vital signs, LOC, pain severity, condition of dressings and tubes, character of drainage, and nursing measures in appropriate log.   ____ ____ ____ _____

2. Recorded vital signs and I&O on appropriate flow sheets.   ____ ____ ____ _____

3. Reported abnormal assessment findings and signs of complications to surgeon.   ____ ____ ____ _____

Copyright © 2018 by Elsevier Inc. All rights reserved.

Student _____ Date _____

Instructor _____ Date _____

PERFORMANCE CHECKLIST SKILL 37.5 **PROVIDING EARLY POSTOPERATIVE AND CONVALESCENT PHASE RECOVERY**

	S	U	NP	Comments
ASSESSMENT				
1. Obtained phone report from PACU nurse summarizing patient's current status.	___	___	___	_____
2. Identified patient using at least two identifiers.	___	___	___	_____
3. Collected more detailed hand-off report from nurse on patient's arrival.	___	___	___	_____
4. Reviewed patient chart for all relevant information.	___	___	___	_____
5. Reviewed postoperative medical orders.	___	___	___	_____
6. Assessed patient's and family's knowledge and expectations of surgical recovery.	___	___	___	_____
PLANNING				
1. Identified expected outcomes.	___	___	___	_____
2. Performed hand hygiene, arranged equipment at bedside.	___	___	___	_____
3. Prepared patient properly for transfer.	___	___	___	_____
IMPLEMENTATION				
1. Early recovery and initial postoperative care:				
a. Assisted in moving patient to bed, identified patient using at least two identifiers.	___	___	___	_____
b. Attached existing oxygen tubing, positioned IV fluids, verified flow-rate settings, checked drainage tubes.	___	___	___	_____
c. Maintained airway, kept lethargic patient positioned properly.	___	___	___	_____
d. Conducted initial assessment of LOC and vital signs, compared with recovery area vital signs and patient's baseline values, continued monitoring.	___	___	___	_____
e. Encouraged coughing, deep breathing, use of incentive spirometer, and PEP device.	___	___	___	_____
f. Assessed GI system for return of bowel sounds.	___	___	___	_____

Copyright © 2018 by Elsevier Inc. All rights reserved.

	S	U	NP	Comments
g. Checked placement and irrigated NG tube, connected to proper drainage device, connected and secured all other tubing.	___	___	___	_____
h. Assessed patient's surgical dressing for appearance, presence, and character of drainage; outlined drainage and reassessed after 1 hour or inspected condition of wound.	___	___	___	_____
i. Palpated abdomen for bladder distention, used bladder ultrasound when available, checked placement and function of any catheter.	___	___	___	_____
j. Explained that voiding within 8 hours of surgery is expected if no drainage system is present.	___	___	___	_____
k. Measured all sources of fluid I&O.	___	___	___	_____
l. Described purpose of equipment and observations to patient and significant others.	___	___	___	_____
m. Positioned patient for comfort and alignment, avoided tension on wound site.	___	___	___	_____
n. Placed call light in reach and raised side rails, instructed patient to call for help to get out of bed.	___	___	___	_____
o. Assessed patient's level of pain, assessed time of last analgesic, medicated patient as ordered, explained pain control plan to patient.	___	___	___	_____
2. Continued postoperative care:				
a. Assessed vital signs as ordered.	___	___	___	_____
b. Monitored progress of wound healing, changed dressings as ordered.	___	___	___	_____
c. Monitored drainage, maintained drainage devices, emptied and recharged as needed.	___	___	___	_____
d. Provided oral care at least every 2 hours, offered ice chips if permitted.	___	___	___	_____
e. Encouraged patient to turn, cough, deep breathe, and use incentive spirometer and PEP device.	___	___	___	_____
f. Monitored function of sequential compression devices, applied elastic stockings if ordered, explained that compression device will inflate and deflate.	___	___	___	_____

Copyright © 2018 by Elsevier Inc. All rights reserved.

	S	U	NP	Comments

g. Promoted ambulation and activity as ordered, assessed tolerance.

h. Progressed to regular diet as tolerated.

i. Included patient and caregiver in decision making, answered questions.

j. Provided opportunity for patient to verbalize feelings about changes in appearance or function.

3. Convalescent phase:

a. Assessed patient's home environment for safety, cleanliness, and availability for resources.

b. Provided instruction on care activities to be performed at home.

c. Kept patient and caregiver informed of progress toward recovery, explained time expected for discharge from hospital, provided answers to questions.

EVALUATION

1. Auscultated breath sounds bilaterally.

2. Monitored vital signs trending.

3. Evaluated I&O records, assessed time of patient's first postoperative urination.

4. Auscultated bowel sounds.

5. Asked patient to describe pain after moderate activity.

6. Inspected incision.

7. Had patient or caregiver describe incision care, dietary or activity modifications, medication schedule, and follow-up plans.

8. Asked patient to describe how to increase activity level during first week at home.

9. Identified unexpected outcomes.

RECORDING AND REPORTING

1. Documented patient's arrival at nursing unit, vital signs, assessment findings, and nursing measures in appropriate log.

2. Continued to document factors at appropriate intervals.

3. Recorded vital signs and I&O in appropriate log.

4. Reported abnormal assessment findings and signs of complications to surgeon.

Copyright © 2018 by Elsevier Inc. All rights reserved.

Student _____ Date _____

Instructor _____ Date _____

PERFORMANCE CHECKLIST SKILL 38.1   **SURGICAL HAND ANTISEPSIS**

	S	U	NP	Comments
ASSESSMENT				
1. Determined type and length of time for hand hygiene.	___	___	___	_____
2. Removed bracelets, rings, and watches.	___	___	___	_____
3. Inspected fingernails, removed nail polish and artificial or extended nails.	___	___	___	_____
4. Inspected condition of cuticles, hands, and forearms for presence of abrasions, cuts, or open lesions.	___	___	___	_____
PLANNING				
1. Identified expected outcomes.	___	___	___	_____
IMPLEMENTATION				
1. Donned surgical shoe covers, cap or hood, face mask, and protective eyewear.	___	___	___	_____
2. Performed a prescrub wash at beginning of work shift:				
a. Turned water on using foot or knee, adjusted temperature.	___	___	___	_____
b. Wet hands thoroughly with water, applied soap.	___	___	___	_____
c. Rubbed hands, covered all surfaces, washed for at least 15 seconds.	___	___	___	_____
d. Rinsed well, dried hands thoroughly with disposable towel, discarded towel.	___	___	___	_____
3. Performed surgical hand scrub:				
a. Turned on water using foot or knee, cleaned properly under nails, rinsed hands and forearms under water.	___	___	___	_____
b. Dispensed antimicrobial scrub agent, applied to hands and forearms using sponge.	___	___	___	_____
c. Timed a 3- to 5-minute scrub; washed all surfaces; kept hand elevated and elbow down; repeated for other hand, fingers, and arm.	___	___	___	_____
d. Avoided splashing surgical attire, discarded sponges appropriately.	___	___	___	_____
e. Rinsed hands and arms in running water, kept hands higher than elbows.	___	___	___	_____

Copyright © 2018 by Elsevier Inc. All rights reserved.

	S	U	NP	Comments

f. Turned off water using foot or knee, backed into OR, held hands above elbows and away from surgical attire. ⎯⎯ ⎯⎯ ⎯⎯ ⎯⎯⎯⎯⎯⎯⎯⎯⎯⎯⎯⎯

g. Approached sterile setup, grasped sterile towel, did not drip water on the sterile field. ⎯⎯ ⎯⎯ ⎯⎯ ⎯⎯⎯⎯⎯⎯⎯⎯⎯⎯⎯⎯

h. Kept hands and arms above waist, dried one hand and elbow with one end of towel. ⎯⎯ ⎯⎯ ⎯⎯ ⎯⎯⎯⎯⎯⎯⎯⎯⎯⎯⎯⎯

i. Used opposite end of towel to dry other hand. ⎯⎯ ⎯⎯ ⎯⎯ ⎯⎯⎯⎯⎯⎯⎯⎯⎯⎯⎯⎯

j. Dropped towel into linen hamper or circulating nurse's hand. ⎯⎯ ⎯⎯ ⎯⎯ ⎯⎯⎯⎯⎯⎯⎯⎯⎯⎯⎯⎯

4. Performed spongeless surgical hand scrub with alcohol-based hand-rub product:

a. Turned on water using foot or knee, cleaned properly under nails, rinsed hands and forearms under water, dried hands thoroughly with paper towel, turned off water. ⎯⎯ ⎯⎯ ⎯⎯ ⎯⎯⎯⎯⎯⎯⎯⎯⎯⎯⎯⎯

b. Dispensed hand preparation, applied properly to hands and forearms. ⎯⎯ ⎯⎯ ⎯⎯ ⎯⎯⎯⎯⎯⎯⎯⎯⎯⎯⎯⎯

c. Repeated application if indicated. ⎯⎯ ⎯⎯ ⎯⎯ ⎯⎯⎯⎯⎯⎯⎯⎯⎯⎯⎯⎯

d. Rubbed thoroughly until dry, proceeded to OR to don gloves. ⎯⎯ ⎯⎯ ⎯⎯ ⎯⎯⎯⎯⎯⎯⎯⎯⎯⎯⎯⎯

EVALUATION

1. Monitored patient postoperatively for signs of surgical site infection. ⎯⎯ ⎯⎯ ⎯⎯ ⎯⎯⎯⎯⎯⎯⎯⎯⎯⎯⎯⎯

2. Identified unexpected outcomes. ⎯⎯ ⎯⎯ ⎯⎯ ⎯⎯⎯⎯⎯⎯⎯⎯⎯⎯⎯⎯

Copyright © 2018 by Elsevier Inc. All rights reserved.

Student _____ Date _____

Instructor _____ Date _____

PERFORMANCE CHECKLIST SKILL 38.2 **DONNING A STERILE GOWN AND CLOSED GLOVING**

	S	U	NP	Comments
ASSESSMENT				
1. Selected proper size and type of sterile gloves.	___	___	___	_____
2. Asked about patient's previous experiences with surgery and anesthesia.	___	___	___	_____
PLANNING				
1. Identified expected outcomes.	___	___	___	_____
IMPLEMENTATION				
1. Donned sterile gown:				
a. Opened sterile gown and glove package on clean, dry, flat surface.	___	___	___	_____
b. Performed surgical hand antisepsis, dried hand thoroughly.	___	___	___	_____
c. Picked up gown grasping inside surface of gown at collar.	___	___	___	_____
d. Lifted folded gown upwards, stepped away from table.	___	___	___	_____
e. Located neckband, grasped inside front of gown just below neckband.	___	___	___	_____
f. Allowed gown to unfold with inside of gown toward body, did not touch outside of gown or allow gown to touch the floor.	___	___	___	_____
g. Slipped both arms into armholes with hands at shoulder level, did not allow hands to move through cuff opening, had circulating nurse pull gown over shoulders.	___	___	___	_____
h. Had circulating nurse tie neck and waist.	___	___	___	_____
2. Applied gloves using closed-glove method:				
a. Kept hands covered by gown cuffs and sleeves, opened sterile glove package.	___	___	___	_____
b. Grasped folded cuff of gloves for dominant hand with nondominant hand.	___	___	___	_____
c. Extended dominant forearm forward palm up, placed palm of glove against palm of hand.	___	___	___	_____
d. Grasped back of glove cuff with nondominant hand, turned glove cuff over end of dominant hand and gown cuff.	___	___	___	_____

Copyright © 2018 by Elsevier Inc. All rights reserved.

	S	U	NP	Comments

e. Grasped top of glove and sleeve with nondominant hand, extended fingers into glove, ensured glove cuff covered gown cuff. ___ ___ ___ _____

f. Gloved nondominant hand in same manner, ensured fingers were fully extended into both gloves. ___ ___ ___ _____

3. Donned a wraparound gown:

   a. Grasped sterile front flap or tab with gloved hands, untied. ___ ___ ___ _____

   b. Passed sterile tab to a member of the team, kept gown tie in hand, turned as circulating nurse stood still. ___ ___ ___ _____

   c. Turned to left covering back with extended gown flap, retrieved sterile tie from team member, secured both ties. ___ ___ ___ _____

EVALUATION

1. Monitored patient postoperatively for signs of surgical site infection. ___ ___ ___ _____

2. Identified unexpected outcomes. ___ ___ ___ _____

Copyright © 2018 by Elsevier Inc. All rights reserved.

Student _____ Date _____

Instructor _____ Date _____

PERFORMANCE CHECKLIST SKILL 39.1 **RISK ASSESSMENT, SKIN ASSESSMENT, AND PREVENTION STRATEGIES**

	S	U	NP	Comments
ASSESSMENT				
1. Identified patient using at least two identifiers.	___	___	___	_____
2. Identified patient characteristics that might be risk factors for pressure injury formation.	___	___	___	_____
3. Selected risk assessment tool, performed risk assessment when patient entered health care setting, repeated on a regular basis or with significant change in patient's condition.	___	___	___	_____
4. Obtained risk score, evaluated meaning based on patient's unique characteristics.	___	___	___	_____
5. Assessed condition of patient's skin over regions of pressure, applied gloves if necessary.	___	___	___	_____
6. Assessed patient for additional areas of potential pressure injury.	___	___	___	_____
7. Observed patient for preferred positions when in bed or chair.	___	___	___	_____
8. Observed ability of patient to initiate and assist with position changes.	___	___	___	_____
9. Assessed patient's and caregiver's understanding of risks for development of pressure injuries.	___	___	___	_____
PLANNING				
1. Identified expected outcomes.	___	___	___	_____
2. Explained procedure and purpose to patient and caregiver.	___	___	___	_____
IMPLEMENTATION				
1. Implemented prevention guidelines adapted from WOCN Society's *Guideline for Prevention and Management of Pressure Ulcers.*	___	___	___	_____
2. Provided privacy, performed hand hygiene.	___	___	___	_____
3. Applied clean gloves if necessary.	___	___	___	_____
4. Inspected skin at least once a day:				
a. Observed patient's skin, paying particular attention to bony prominences, gently pressed any reddened area to check for blanching, rechecked in 1 hour any area that does not blanch.	___	___	___	_____

Copyright © 2018 by Elsevier Inc. All rights reserved.

	S	U	NP	Comments

b. Looked for color changes that differ from the patient's normal skin color in patient with darkly pigmented skin.   ___ ___ ___ _____

5. Checked all treatment and assistive devices for potential pressure points, removed gloves.   ___ ___ ___ _____

6. Reviewed patient's pressure injury risk score.   ___ ___ ___ _____

7. Considered appropriate intervention if patient's immobility, inactivity, or poor sensory perception was a risk factor.   ___ ___ ___ _____

8. Considered appropriate intervention if friction and shear were identified as risk factors.   ___ ___ ___ _____

9. Considered appropriate intervention if patient received a low score on a moisture subscale.   ___ ___ ___ _____

10. Educated patient and family caregiver regarding pressure injury risk and prevention.   ___ ___ ___ _____

11. Removed gloves, discarded appropriately, performed hand hygiene.   ___ ___ ___ _____

EVALUATION

1. Observed patient's skin for areas at risk for tissue damage; noted change in color, appearance, or texture.   ___ ___ ___ _____

2. Observed tolerance of patient for position change.   ___ ___ ___ _____

3. Compared subsequent risk assessment scores and skin assessments.   ___ ___ ___ _____

4. Asked patient to explain why skin is being checked on a regular basis.   ___ ___ ___ _____

5. Identified unexpected outcomes.   ___ ___ ___ _____

RECORDING AND REPORTING

1. Recorded skin changes, risk score, and skin assessment; described pertinent information and patient's response to interventions in appropriate log.   ___ ___ ___ _____

2. Recorded patient's understanding of need for frequent assessments.   ___ ___ ___ _____

3. Reported need for additional consultations to health care provider.   ___ ___ ___ _____

Copyright © 2018 by Elsevier Inc. All rights reserved.

Student _____ Date _____

Instructor _____ Date _____

PERFORMANCE CHECKLIST SKILL 39.2   **TREATMENT OF PRESSURE INJURIES**

	S	U	NP	Comments
ASSESSMENT				
1. Identified patient using at least two identifiers.	___	___	___	_____
2. Assessed patient's level of comfort and need for pain medication.	___	___	___	_____
3. Determined if patient had allergies to topical agents.	___	___	___	_____
4. Reviewed the order for topical agent(s) or dressings.	___	___	___	_____
5. Provided privacy.	___	___	___	_____
6. Positioned patient to allow dressing removal, positioned plastic bag for dressing removal.	___	___	___	_____
7. Performed hand hygiene, applied clean gloves, removed and discarded old dressing.	___	___	___	_____
8. Removed wound dressing; assessed patient's wounds using wound parameters: location, stage, size, presence of undermining, presence of sinus tracts, presence of tunnels, condition of wound bed, volume of exudate, condition of periwound skin, and wound edges.	___	___	___	_____
9. Assessed periwound skin, checked for maceration, redness, and denuded tissue.	___	___	___	_____
10. Removed gloves, discarded appropriately, performed hand hygiene.	___	___	___	_____
11. Assessed for factors affecting wound healing (i.e., poor perfusion, immunosuppression, preexisting infection).	___	___	___	_____
12. Assessed patient's nutritional status.	___	___	___	_____
13. Assessed patient's and caregiver's understanding of prevention, treatment, and factors contributing to recurrence of pressure injuries.	___	___	___	_____
PLANNING				
1. Identified expected outcomes.	___	___	___	_____
2. Explained procedure to patient and caregiver, individualized teaching.	___	___	___	_____
3. Prepared all necessary equipment and supplies.	___	___	___	_____

Copyright © 2018 by Elsevier Inc. All rights reserved.

	S	U	NP	Comments

IMPLEMENTATION

1. Assembled supplies at bedside, provided privacy. ____ ____ ____ _____

2. Performed hand hygiene, applied gloves, opened sterile packages and topical containers, kept dressings sterile, wore PPE if necessary. ____ ____ ____ _____

3. Removed bed linens, arranged patient's gown to expose injury and surrounding skin only. ____ ____ ____ _____

4. Cleansed wound thoroughly with saline or prescribed agent from least contaminated to most contaminated area, removed gloves and discarded. ____ ____ ____ _____

5. Performed hand hygiene, changed gloves. ____ ____ ____ _____

6. Applied topical agents if prescribed:

  a. Applied enzymes.

   (1) Applied small amount of enzyme debridement ointment directly to necrotic areas, *did not apply enzyme to surrounding skin.* ____ ____ ____ _____

   (2) Placed moist gauze directly over injury, taped in place, followed manufacturer's recommendation for type of dressing material. ____ ____ ____ _____

  b. Applied antibacterials. ____ ____ ____ _____

7. Applied prescribed wound dressing:

  a. Applied hydrogel.

   (1) Covered surface of injury with hydrogel or cut a sheet to fit wound base. ____ ____ ____ _____

   (2) Applied secondary dressing such as dry gauze, taped in place. ____ ____ ____ _____

   (3) Packed impregnated gauze loosely into wound if used, covered with secondary gauze dressing and tape. ____ ____ ____ _____

  b. Applied calcium alginate.

   (1) Packed wound with alginate properly. ____ ____ ____ _____

   (2) Applied secondary dressing and tape in place. ____ ____ ____ _____

  c. Applied transparent film dressing, hydrocolloid, and foam dressings. ____ ____ ____ _____

8. Repositioned patient comfortably off pressure injury. ____ ____ ____ _____

9. Removed gloves, disposed of soiled supplies, performed hand hygiene. ____ ____ ____ _____

Copyright © 2018 by Elsevier Inc. All rights reserved.

	S	U	NP	Comments

EVALUATION

1. Observed skin surrounding ulcer for inflammation, edema, and tenderness.

2. Inspected dressings and exposed ulcers; observed for drainage, foul odor, and tissue necrosis; monitored patient for signs of infection.

3. Compared subsequent injury measurements.

4. Asked patient why wound will be measured and examined at each dressing change.

5. Identified unexpected outcomes.

RECORDING AND REPORTING

1. Recorded type of wound tissue, measurements, periwound skin condition, presence of drainage, topical agent used, dressing applied, and patient response in appropriate log.

2. Recorded patient's understanding of reasons for frequent observation and measuring of wound.

3. Reported any deterioration in injury appearance to nurse in charge or health care provider.

Copyright © 2018 by Elsevier Inc. All rights reserved.

Student _____ Date _____

Instructor _____ Date _____

PERFORMANCE CHECKLIST PROCEDURAL GUIDELINE 40.1 **PERFORMING A WOUND ASSESSMENT**

	S	U	NP	Comments
ASSESSMENT				
1. Identified patient using two identifiers.	___	___	___	_____
2. Examined medical record for last wound assessment, reviewed record to determine etiology of the wound.	___	___	___	_____
3. Determined agency wound assessment tool, reviewed frequency of assessment, examined last wound assessment for comparison.	___	___	___	_____
4. Assessed comfort level or pain, identified symptoms of anxiety, offered pain medication if indicated.	___	___	___	_____
5. Provided privacy, positioned patient, exposed only wound.	___	___	___	_____
6. Explained procedure of wound assessment to patient.	___	___	___	_____
7. Performed hand hygiene, formed cuff on waterproof biohazard bag, placed near bed.	___	___	___	_____
8. Applied clean gloves, removed soiled dressings.	___	___	___	_____
9. Examined dressings for quality of drainage, presence or absence of odor, quantity of drainage; discarded dressings in waterproof biohazard bag, discarded gloves.	___	___	___	_____
10. Performed hand hygiene, applied clean gloves.	___	___	___	_____
11. Inspected wound, determined type of wound healing.	___	___	___	_____
12. Used agency-approved assessment tool, assessed the following:				
a. Wound healing by primary intention.				
(1) Assessed anatomical location of wound on body.	___	___	___	_____
(2) Noted if wound margins were approximated or closed together.	___	___	___	_____
(3) Observed for presence of drainage.	___	___	___	_____
(4) Looked for evidence of infection.	___	___	___	_____
(5) Palpated along incision to feel a healing ridge.	___	___	___	_____

Copyright © 2018 by Elsevier Inc. All rights reserved.

	S	U	NP	Comments

b. Wound healing by secondary intention.

   (1) Assessed anatomical location of wound.   —— —— —— ————————————

   (2) Assessed wound dimensions properly, discarded measuring guide and applicator in trash bag.   —— —— —— ————————————

   (3) Assessed for undermining, documented number of centimeters that area extends from wound edge.   —— —— —— ————————————

   (4) Assessed extent of tissue loss.   —— —— —— ————————————

   (5) Observed tissue type, including percentage of granulation, slough, and necrotic tissue.   —— —— —— ————————————

   (6) Noted presence of exudates, indicated amount.   —— —— —— ————————————

   (7) Noted if wound edges were rounded toward the wound bed, described presence of epithelialization at wound edges.   —— —— —— ————————————

13. Inspected periwound skin, described skin integrity.   —— —— —— ————————————

14. Reapplied dressings as per order; placed time, date, and initials on new dressing.   —— —— —— ————————————

15. Reassessed patient's pain and level of comfort at wound site after dressing was applied.   —— —— —— ————————————

16. Discarded biohazard bag, soiled supplies, and gloves properly; performed hand hygiene.   —— —— —— ————————————

17. Recorded wound assessment findings, compared assessment with previous wound assessments.   —— —— —— ————————————

Copyright © 2018 by Elsevier Inc. All rights reserved.

Student _____ Date _____

Instructor _____ Date _____

PERFORMANCE CHECKLIST SKILL 40.1 **PERFORMING A WOUND IRRIGATION**

	S	U	NP	Comments
ASSESSMENT				
1. Identified patient using at least two identifiers.	__	__	__	_____
2. Reviewed order for irrigation and type of solution to be used.	__	__	__	_____
3. Assessed patient's level of comfort, offered analgesic at least 30 minutes before removal.	__	__	__	_____
4. Reviewed medical record for symptoms related to patient's open wound.	__	__	__	_____
5. Assessed patient for history of allergies to antiseptics, medication, tapes, or dressing material.	__	__	__	_____
PLANNING				
1. Identified expected outcomes.	__	__	__	_____
2. Administered analgesic 30 to 45 minutes before procedure if needed.	__	__	__	_____
3. Educated patient and family about procedure.	__	__	__	_____
4. Gathered appropriate supplies.	__	__	__	_____
5. Provided privacy, performed hand hygiene, positioned patient.	__	__	__	_____
IMPLEMENTATION				
1. Performed hand hygiene.	__	__	__	_____
2. Formed cuff on waterproof biohazard bag and placed near bed.	__	__	__	_____
3. Applied PPE, used sterile precautions if needed, discarded old dressing and gloves, performed hand hygiene.	__	__	__	_____
4. Performed hand hygiene, applied clean gloves, performed wound assessment, and examined recent charted assessment of patient's room.	__	__	__	_____
5. Exposed area near wound only.	__	__	__	_____
6. Irrigated wound with wide opening:				
a. Filled syringe with irrigation solution.	__	__	__	_____
b. Attached 19-gauge angiocatheter.	__	__	__	_____
c. Held syringe tip above upper end of wound and over area being cleansed.	__	__	__	_____
d. Flushed wound using continuous pressure until solution draining was clear.	__	__	__	_____

468

Copyright © 2018 by Elsevier Inc. All rights reserved.

	S	U	NP	Comments

7. Irrigated deep wound with small opening:

   a. Attached soft catheter to filled syringe. _____ _____ _____ _____

   b. Inserted tip of catheter into opening. _____ _____ _____ _____

   c. Flushed wound using slow, continuous pressure. _____ _____ _____ _____

   d. Pinched off catheter below syringe while in place. _____ _____ _____ _____

   e. Removed and refilled syringe, reconnected to catheter, repeated until solution draining was clear. _____ _____ _____ _____

8. Applied clean gloves, cleansed wound with hand-held shower:

   a. Performed hand hygiene, applied clean gloves, adjusted spray with patient seated, ensured water was warm. _____ _____ _____ _____

   b. Showered for 5 to 10 minutes. _____ _____ _____ _____

9. Obtained cultures after cleansing with nonbacteriostatic saline when indicated. _____ _____ _____ _____

10. Dried wound edges with gauze, dried patient. _____ _____ _____ _____

11. Applied appropriate dressing, labeled with time, date, and nurse's initials. _____ _____ _____ _____

12. Removed mask, goggles, and gown. _____ _____ _____ _____

13. Disposed of equipment and soiled supplies, removed gloves, performed hand hygiene. _____ _____ _____ _____

14. Helped patient to comfortable position. _____ _____ _____ _____

EVALUATION

1. Had patient rate level of comfort. _____ _____ _____ _____

2. Monitored type of tissue in wound bed. _____ _____ _____ _____

3. Inspected dressing periodically. _____ _____ _____ _____

4. Evaluated periwound skin integrity. _____ _____ _____ _____

5. Observed for presence of retained irrigant. _____ _____ _____ _____

6. Asked patient to explain importance of wound irrigation. _____ _____ _____ _____

7. Identified unexpected outcomes. _____ _____ _____ _____

RECORDING AND REPORTING

1. Recorded all findings in appropriate log. _____ _____ _____ _____

2. Recorded patient's understanding for reasons for wound irrigations. _____ _____ _____ _____

3. Reported to health care provider any evidence of fresh bleeding, sharp increase in pain, retention of irrigant, or signs of shock immediately. _____ _____ _____ _____

Copyright © 2018 by Elsevier Inc. All rights reserved.

Student _____ Date _____

Instructor _____ Date _____

PERFORMANCE CHECKLIST SKILL 40.2   **REMOVING SUTURES AND STAPLES**

	S	U	NP	Comments

ASSESSMENT

1. Identified patient using at least two identifiers. ___ ___ ___ _____

2. Reviewed patient's medical record for the following:

   a. Health care provider's order. ___ ___ ___ _____

   b. Specific directions related to removal. ___ ___ ___ _____

   c. History of conditions that may pose risk for impaired wound healing. ___ ___ ___ _____

3. Assessed patient for history of allergies. ___ ___ ___ _____

4. Assessed patient's comfort level or pain. ___ ___ ___ _____

5. Inspected incision for healing ridge and skin integrity of suture line for uniform closure, normal color, and absence of drainage and inflammation. ___ ___ ___ _____

PLANNING

1. Identified expected outcomes. ___ ___ ___ _____

2. Explained to patient that suture removal is not usually painful but patient may feel tugging. ___ ___ ___ _____

IMPLEMENTATION

1. Provided privacy. ___ ___ ___ _____

2. Positioned patient comfortably, exposed suture line, ensured direct lighting was on suture line. ___ ___ ___ _____

3. Performed hand hygiene. ___ ___ ___ _____

4. Placed cuffed waterproof disposal bag within easy reach. ___ ___ ___ _____

5. Prepared materials needed:

   a. Opened sterile kit. ___ ___ ___ _____

   b. Opened antiseptic swabs, placed on inside surface of kit. ___ ___ ___ _____

   c. Obtained gloves, sterile if necessary. ___ ___ ___ _____

6. Performed hand hygiene, applied clean gloves, removed dressing, discarded dressing and gloves in disposal bag. ___ ___ ___ _____

7. Inspected incision and suture line. ___ ___ ___ _____

8. Performed hand hygiene, applied clean or sterile gloves as appropriate. ___ ___ ___ _____

470

Copyright © 2018 by Elsevier Inc. All rights reserved.

	S	U	NP	Comments
9. Cleansed sutures or staples and healed incisions with antiseptic, used clean swab for each swipe.	——	——	——	_____
10. Removed staples:				
a. Placed lower tip of extractor under first staple, closed handles to extract ends.	——	——	——	_____
b. Controlled staple extractor carefully.	——	——	——	_____
c. Moved staple away from surface when both ends were visible.	——	——	——	_____
d. Dropped staple into refuse bag.	——	——	——	_____
e. Repeated steps a–d until all staples were removed.	——	——	——	_____
11. Removed interrupted sutures:				
a. Placed gauze a few inches from suture line, held scissors and forceps appropriately.	——	——	——	_____
b. Grasped knot with forceps, pulled while slipping tip of scissors under suture.	——	——	——	_____
c. Snipped suture as close to skin as possible.	——	——	——	_____
d. Grasped knotted end, pulled suture through from other side, placed removed sutures on gauze.	——	——	——	_____
e. Repeated steps a–d until every other (alternating) suture was removed.	——	——	——	_____
f. Observed healing level, determined whether remaining sutures were to be removed, if so removed all.	——	——	——	_____
g. Stopped and notified health care provider if in doubt.	——	——	——	_____
12. Removed continuous and blanket stitch sutures:				
a. Placed gauze a few inches from suture line, held scissors and forceps appropriately.	——	——	——	_____
b. Snipped first suture close to skin surface distal to knot.	——	——	——	_____
c. Snipped second suture on same side.	——	——	——	_____
d. Grasped knotted end, removed suture, placed suture on gauze compress.	——	——	——	_____
e. Repeated steps a–d until entire line was removed.	——	——	——	_____
13. Inspected incision, ensured all sutures were removed, identified trouble areas, wiped suture line with antiseptic swab.	——	——	——	_____

Copyright © 2018 by Elsevier Inc. All rights reserved.

	S	U	NP	Comments

14. Applied Steri-Strips if any separation greater than two stitches or two staples wide:

    a. Cut strips to appropriate length.   ____   ____   ____   _____

    b. Removed backing, applied across incision.   ____   ____   ____   _____

    c. Instructed patient to take showers rather than soak in bathtub.   ____   ____   ____   _____

15. Applied light dressing, exposed to air if clothing would not come into contact, instructed patient about applying own dressing.   ____   ____   ____   _____

16. Discarded contaminated materials, removed and disposed of gloves.   ____   ____   ____   _____

17. Disposed of sharps properly, performed hand hygiene.   ____   ____   ____   _____

EVALUATION

1. Assessed site where sutures or staples were removed, inspected condition of soft tissues, looked for pieces of removed suture left behind.   ____   ____   ____   _____

2. Determined if patient had pain along incision.   S   U   NP   _____

3. Asked patient to describe signs of infection to be reported to health care provider.   ____   ____   ____   _____

4. Identified unexpected outcomes.   ____   ____   ____   _____

RECORDING AND REPORTING

1. Recorded all pertinent information in the appropriate log.   ____   ____   ____   _____

2. Recorded patient's understanding of why sutures were removed.   ____   ____   ____   _____

3. Reported signs of suture line separation, dehiscence, evisceration, bleeding, or purulent drainage.   ____   ____   ____   _____

Copyright © 2018 by Elsevier Inc. All rights reserved.

Student _____ Date _____

Instructor _____ Date _____

PERFORMANCE CHECKLIST SKILL 40.3 **MANAGING WOUND DRAINAGE EVACUATION**

	S	U	NP	Comments
ASSESSMENT				
1. Identified patient using at least two identifiers.	___	___	___	_____
2. Identified presence, location, and purpose of closed wound drain and drainage system, assessed drainage on patient's dressing.	___	___	___	_____
3. Identified number of wound drain tubes and what each was draining, labeled each drain tube.	___	___	___	_____
4. Determined if drain tube needed self-suction, wall suction, or no suction by checking orders.	___	___	___	_____
5. Inspected system to determine presence of straight or Y-tube arrangement.	___	___	___	_____
6. Inspected system to ensure proper functioning.	___	___	___	_____
7. Identified type of drainage container patient has.	___	___	___	_____
PLANNING				
1. Identified expected outcomes.	___	___	___	_____
2. Explained procedure to patient.	___	___	___	_____
IMPLEMENTATION				
1. Provided privacy.	___	___	___	_____
2. Performed hand hygiene, applied clean gloves.	___	___	___	_____
3. Placed open specimen container or measuring graduate on bed between you and patient.	___	___	___	_____
4. Emptied Hemovac or ConstaVac:				
a. Maintained asepsis while opening proper plug on port, tilted suction container in direction of plug, squeezed flat surfaces together, tilted toward measuring container.	___	___	___	_____
b. Drained contents into measuring container.	___	___	___	_____
c. Placed suction device properly on flat surface, pressed down until bottom and top were in contact.	___	___	___	_____
d. Held surfaces with one hand, cleaned opening and plug, replaced plug, secured suction device on patient's bed.	___	___	___	_____
e. Checked device for reestablishment of vacuum, patency of drainage tubing, and absence of stress on tubing.	___	___	___	_____

Copyright © 2018 by Elsevier Inc. All rights reserved.

	S	U	NP	Comments

5. Emptied Hemovac with wall suction:

   a. Turned off suction. ___ ___ ___ _____

   b. Disconnected suction tubing from Hemovac port. ___ ___ ___ _____

   c. Emptied Hemovac as described in step 4. ___ ___ ___ _____

   d. Cleansed port opening and end of suction tubing. ___ ___ ___ _____

   e. Set suction level appropriately or as prescribed. ___ ___ ___ _____

6. Emptied JP suction drain:

   a. Opened port on top of bulb-shaped reservoir. ___ ___ ___ _____

   b. Tilted bulb in direction of port, drained away from opening, emptied drainage into measuring container, cleansed end of port and plugged with alcohol. ___ ___ ___ _____

   c. Compressed bulb over drainage container, replaced plug immediately. ___ ___ ___ _____

7. Placed secure drainage system below site with safety pin on gown, ensured there was slack in tubing. ___ ___ ___ _____

8. Noted characteristics of drainage. ___ ___ ___ _____

9. Discarded soiled supplies, removed gloves, performed hand hygiene. ___ ___ ___ _____

10. Applied clean gloves, proceeded with dressing change and inspection of skin if indicated or ordered. ___ ___ ___ _____

11. Discarded contaminated materials, performed hand hygiene. ___ ___ ___ _____

EVALUATION

1. Observed for drainage in suction device. ___ ___ ___ _____

2. Inspected wound for drainage or collection of fluid under skin. ___ ___ ___ _____

3. Measured drainage, emptied drainage system, recorded on I&O form. ___ ___ ___ _____

4. Assessed patient's level of comfort. ___ ___ ___ _____

5. Asked patient to explain when reservoir should be emptied. ___ ___ ___ _____

6. Identified unexpected outcomes. ___ ___ ___ _____

RECORDING AND REPORTING

1. Recorded all pertinent information in the appropriate log. ___ ___ ___ _____

2. Recorded amount of drainage on I&O record. ___ ___ ___ _____

3. Documented evaluation of patient learning. ___ ___ ___ _____

4. Reported sudden change in amount of drainage, pungent odor of drainage or new signs of purulence, severe pain, or dislodgment of tube to health care provider immediately. ___ ___ ___ _____

Copyright © 2018 by Elsevier Inc. All rights reserved.

Student _____ Date _____

Instructor _____ Date _____

PERFORMANCE CHECKLIST SKILL 40.4 **NEGATIVE-PRESSURE WOUND THERAPY**

	S	U	NP	Comments
ASSESSMENT				
1. Identified patient using at least two identifiers.	——	——	——	_____
2. Reviewed health care provider's orders for frequency of dressing change, amount of negative pressure, type of foam or gauze, and pressure cycle.	——	——	——	_____
3. Reviewed medical record for signs related to condition of patient's wound.	——	——	——	_____
4. Assessed patient's level of comfort on pain scale, administered prescribed analgesic 30 minutes before dressing change.	——	——	——	_____
5. Assessed location, appearance, and size of wound.	——	——	——	_____
6. Assessed patient's and caregiver's knowledge of purpose of dressing and whether they will participate in dressing wound.	——	——	——	_____
PLANNING				
1. Identified expected outcomes.	——	——	——	_____
2. Explained procedure to patient.	——	——	——	_____
IMPLEMENTATION				
1. Provided privacy.	——	——	——	_____
2. Positioned patient comfortably, draped to expose only wound site, instructed patient not to touch wound or sterile supplies.	——	——	——	_____
3. Cuffed top of disposable waterproof bag, placed within reach of work area.	——	——	——	_____
4. Performed hand hygiene, applied clean gloves and appropriate PPE.	——	——	——	_____
5. Followed manufacturer's directions for removal and replacement of NPWT, turned off NPWT unit:				
a. Kept tube connectors attached to unit, raised tubing connectors, disconnected tubes and drained fluids into drainage collector.	——	——	——	_____
b. Tightened clamp on canister tube, disconnected canister and dressing tubing at connection points.	——	——	——	_____

Copyright © 2018 by Elsevier Inc. All rights reserved.

	S	U	NP	Comments

6. Removed transparent film properly. ___ ___ ___ _____

7. Removed old dressing one layer at a time and discarded, observed drainage on dressing, avoided tension on drains. ___ ___ ___ _____

8. Performed wound assessment, observed surface area and tissue character within wound, measured length, width, and depth of wound as ordered. ___ ___ ___ _____

9. Removed and discarded gloves in waterproof bag, avoided letting patient see old dressing, performed hand hygiene. ___ ___ ___ _____

10. Cleaned wound:

    a. Applied clean or sterile gloves as appropriate. ___ ___ ___ _____

    b. Irrigated wound with appropriate solution if ordered, blotted periwound with gauze to dry thoroughly. ___ ___ ___ _____

11. Applied appropriate seal to periwound skin. ___ ___ ___ _____

12. Filled uneven skin surfaces with skin barrier product. ___ ___ ___ _____

13. Removed and discarded gloves, performed hand hygiene. ___ ___ ___ _____

14. Applied sterile or new clean gloves depending on wound. ___ ___ ___ _____

15. Applied NPWT:

    a. Prepared filler dressing, consulted with wound-care expert for appropriate type. ___ ___ ___ _____

    b. Placed filler dressing in wound properly, ensured filler is in contact with entire wound base, margins, tunneled, and undermined areas, documented number of dressings. ___ ___ ___ _____

    c. Placed suction device properly. ___ ___ ___ _____

    d. Trimmed and applied NPWT transparent dressings over foam wound dressing, secured tubing to transparent film, did not apply tension. ___ ___ ___ _____

16. Connected tubing from dressing to tubing from canister and NPWT unit after wound is covered, set at ordered suction level. ___ ___ ___ _____

17. Inspected NPWT system:

    a. Verified that system is on. ___ ___ ___ _____

    b. Verified that all clamps are open and all tubing is patent. ___ ___ ___ _____

    c. Ensured seal is intact and therapy is working. ___ ___ ___ _____

Copyright © 2018 by Elsevier Inc. All rights reserved.

	S	U	NP	Comments

d. Used transparent film to patch areas around edges of wound if a leak is present. ___ ___ ___ _____

18. Recorded initials, date, and time on new dressing. ___ ___ ___ _____

19. Helped patient to comfortable position. ___ ___ ___ _____

20. Discarded gloves, disposed of dressing material, performed hand hygiene. ___ ___ ___ _____

EVALUATION

1. Inspected condition of wound on ongoing basis, noted drainage and odor. ___ ___ ___ _____

2. Asked patient to rate pain on pain scale. ___ ___ ___ _____

3. Verified airtight dressing seal and corrected negative-pressure setting. ___ ___ ___ _____

4. Measured wound drainage output in canister on regular basis. ___ ___ ___ _____

5. Asked patient to demonstrate how to replace filler dressings into wound. ___ ___ ___ _____

6. Identified unexpected outcomes. ___ ___ ___ _____

RECORDING AND REPORTING

1. Recorded appearance of wound, character of drainage, placement of NPWT, and patient response in appropriate log. ___ ___ ___ _____

2. Documented evaluation of patient learning. ___ ___ ___ _____

3. Reported brisk bright-red bleeding, evidence of poor wound healing, evisceration or dehiscence, or possible wound infection to health care provider. ___ ___ ___ _____

Copyright © 2018 by Elsevier Inc. All rights reserved.

Student _____ Date _____

Instructor _____ Date _____

PERFORMANCE CHECKLIST SKILL 41.1 **APPLYING A DRESSING (DRY AND DAMP-TO-DRY)**

	S	U	NP	Comments
ASSESSMENT				
1. Identified patient using at least two identifiers.	___	___	___	_____
2. Assessed patient for allergies, acquired orders for dressing change.	___	___	___	_____
3. Asked patient to rate pain level and assess character of pain, administered analgesic if necessary.	___	___	___	_____
4. Assessed size, location, and condition of the wound; reviewed previous notes.	___	___	___	_____
5. Assessed patient's and caregiver's knowledge of purpose of dressing change.	___	___	___	_____
6. Assessed need, readiness, and willingness for patient or caregiver to participate in dressing wound.	___	___	___	_____
7. Reviewed medical orders for dressing change procedure.	___	___	___	_____
8. Identified patient with risk factors for wound healing problems.	___	___	___	_____
PLANNING				
1. Identified expected outcomes.	___	___	___	_____
2. Explained procedure to patient.	___	___	___	_____
IMPLEMENTATION				
1. Provided privacy.	___	___	___	_____
2. Positioned patient comfortably, draped to expose only wound site, instructed patient not to touch wound or supplies.	___	___	___	_____
3. Placed disposable biohazard bag within reach, folded top to make cuff, performed hand hygiene and put on clean gloves, applied necessary PPE.	___	___	___	_____
4. Removed tape, bandages, or ties properly; got permission to clip or shave hair if necessary; removed adhesive from skin.	___	___	___	_____
5. Removed dressing properly one layer at a time, observed appearance and drainage of dressing, avoided tension on drainage devices, kept soiled undersurface from patient's sight, freed dressing sticking to wound appropriately.	___	___	___	_____

478

Copyright © 2018 by Elsevier Inc. All rights reserved.

	S	U	NP	Comments

6. Assessed condition of wound and periwound, used measuring guide or ruler to measure size of wound, palpated wound edges for bogginess or patient report of increased pain. ___ ___ ___ _____

7. Folded dressings with drainage inside, removed gloves inside out, folded gloves over dressing if appropriate, disposed of gloves and dressing appropriately, covered wound with sterile gauze, performed hand hygiene. ___ ___ ___ _____

8. Described appearance of wound and indications of healing to patient. ___ ___ ___ _____

9. Created sterile field on over-bed tray, poured prescribed solution into sterile basin. ___ ___ ___ _____

10. Cleaned wound:

 a. Performed hand hygiene, applied clean gloves, used gauze or cotton ball with saline or antiseptic or sprayed wound with wound cleaner. ___ ___ ___ _____

 b. Cleaned from least to most contaminated area. ___ ___ ___ _____

 c. Cleaned appropriately around any drain. ___ ___ ___ _____

11. Used dry gauze to blot the wound dry. ___ ___ ___ _____

12. Applied antiseptic ointment properly if ordered, disposed of gloves, performed hand hygiene. ___ ___ ___ _____

13. Applied dressing:

 a. Dry sterile dressing.

 (1) Applied clean gloves. ___ ___ ___ _____

 (2) Applied loose woven gauze as a contact layer. ___ ___ ___ _____

 (3) Applied split gauze around drain if present. ___ ___ ___ _____

 (4) Applied additional layers of gauze as needed. ___ ___ ___ _____

 (5) Applied thicker woven pad. ___ ___ ___ _____

 b. Moist-to-dry dressing.

 (1) Applied sterile gloves. ___ ___ ___ _____

 (2) Placed mesh or gauze in container of prescribed solution, wrung out excess solution. ___ ___ ___ _____

 (3) Applied damp fine-mesh or gauze as a single layer onto wound surface, packed gauze into wound properly if necessary, ensured gauze did not touch periwound skin. ___ ___ ___ _____

Copyright © 2018 by Elsevier Inc. All rights reserved.

	S	U	NP	Comments
(4) Applied dry sterile gauze over moist gauze.	___	___	___	_____
(5) Covered with ABD pad, Surgipad, or gauze.	___	___	___	_____
14. Secured dressing properly with tape, Montgomery ties, or protective window.	___	___	___	_____
15. Disposed of all dressing supplies, removed PPE and disposed properly.	___	___	___	_____
16. Labeled tape over dressing with initials, changed dressing date.	___	___	___	_____
17. Helped patient to comfortable position.	___	___	___	_____
18. Performed hand hygiene.	___	___	___	_____

EVALUATION

	S	U	NP	Comments
1. Observed appearance of wound for healing.	___	___	___	_____
2. Asked patient to rate pain.	___	___	___	_____
3. Inspected condition of dressing at least every shift.	___	___	___	_____
4. Asked patient to explain importance of changing dressing and how often it should be done.	___	___	___	_____
5. Identified unexpected outcomes.	___	___	___	_____

RECORDING AND REPORTING

	S	U	NP	Comments
1. Recorded all pertinent information in the appropriate log.	___	___	___	_____
2. Recorded patient's understanding through teach-back for effective dressing change.	___	___	___	_____
3. Reported unexpected appearance of wound drainage, accidental removal of drain, bright red bleeding, or evidence of wound dehiscence or evisceration.	___	___	___	_____

Copyright © 2018 by Elsevier Inc. All rights reserved.

Student _____ Date _____

Instructor _____ Date _____

PERFORMANCE CHECKLIST SKILL 41.2 **APPLYING A PRESSURE BANDAGE**

	S	U	NP	Comments
ASSESSMENT				
1. Identified patient using at least two identifiers.	——	——	——	————————
2. Anticipated patients at risk for unexpected bleeding.	——	——	——	————————
3. Assessed location where hemorrhage occurred.	——	——	——	————————
4. Assessed patient for allergies to antiseptics, tape, or latex; used other supplies if necessary.	——	——	——	————————
5. Assessed patient's anxiety level.	——	——	——	————————
6. Assessed patient's baseline vital signs before onset of hemorrhage.	——	——	——	————————
PLANNING				
1. Identified expected outcomes.	——	——	——	————————
IMPLEMENTATION				
1. Identified external bleeding site, looked underneath patient with large abdominal dressings.	——	——	——	————————
2. Immediately applied manual pressure to site of bleeding.	——	——	——	————————
3. Sought assistance.	——	——	——	————————
4. Identified source of bleeding quickly.	——	——	——	————————
5. Elevated affected body part if possible.	——	——	——	————————
6. Continued to apply pressure as first nurse, while second nurse unwrapped roller bandage and cut tape appropriately.	——	——	——	————————
7. In coordinated actions:				
a. Covered bleeding area with multiple gauze compresses, first nurse slips fingers out, second nurse exerts pressure.	——	——	——	————————
b. Placed two adhesive strips appropriately over dressing with even pressure, secured tapes properly.	——	——	——	————————
c. Removed fingers, covered center area with third piece of tape.	——	——	——	————————

Copyright © 2018 by Elsevier Inc. All rights reserved.

	S	U	NP	Comments
d. Continued reinforcing area with tape and applying pressure as needed.	___	___	___	_____
e. Applied roller gauze properly over pressure bandage, compressed over bleeding site, removed finger pressure and applied roller gauze over center, continued with figure-eight turns, secured end with two circular turns and adhesive.	___	___	___	_____

EVALUATION

	S	U	NP	Comments
1. Observed dressing for control of bleeding.	___	___	___	_____
2. Evaluated adequacy of circulation.	___	___	___	_____
3. Estimated volume of blood loss.	___	___	___	_____
4. Measured vital signs.	___	___	___	_____
5. Identified unexpected outcomes.	___	___	___	_____

RECORDING AND REPORTING

	S	U	NP	Comments
1. Reported details of incident immediately to health care provider.	___	___	___	_____
2. Recorded assessment, application of pressure dressing, and patient response in appropriately log.	___	___	___	_____

Copyright © 2018 by Elsevier Inc. All rights reserved.

Student _____ Date _____

Instructor _____ Date _____

PERFORMANCE CHECKLIST SKILL 41.3 **APPLYING A TRANSPARENT DRESSING**

	S	U	NP	Comments
ASSESSMENT				
1. Identified patient using at least two identifiers.	___	___	___	_____
2. Assessed location, appearance, and size of wound; reviewed previous nurses' notes.	___	___	___	_____
3. Reviewed health care provider's orders for frequency and type of dressing change.	___	___	___	_____
4. Assessed patient for allergies to antiseptics, tape, or latex.	___	___	___	_____
5. Asked patient to rate pain level and assessed character of pain, administered prescribed analgesic at the appropriate time.	___	___	___	_____
6. Assessed patient's knowledge of purpose of dressing.	___	___	___	_____
7. Assessed patient's risk for impaired wound healing.	___	___	___	_____
PLANNING				
1. Identified expected outcomes.	___	___	___	_____
2. Explained procedure to patient.	___	___	___	_____
3. Positioned patient comfortably, allowed access to dressing site.	___	___	___	_____
IMPLEMENTATION				
1. Provided privacy, kept body parts that did not require exposure draped.	___	___	___	_____
2. Exposed wound site, minimized exposure, instructed patient not to touch wound or supplies.	___	___	___	_____
3. Placed biohazard bag within reach of work area.	___	___	___	_____
4. Performed hand hygiene, applied clean gloves and PPE.	___	___	___	_____
5. Removed old dressing appropriately.	___	___	___	_____
6. Disposed of soiled dressing in waterproof bag, removed gloves inside out and disposed of in bag, performed hand hygiene.	___	___	___	_____
7. Applied sterile gloves if skin is broken or clean gloves.	___	___	___	_____
8. Prepared dressing supplies, used sterile supplies for new wounds.	___	___	___	_____

Copyright © 2018 by Elsevier Inc. All rights reserved.

	S	U	NP	Comments

9. Poured prescribed solution over sterile gauze pads. ___ ___ ___ _____

10. Cleaned wound and periwound area with gauze and saline or sprayed with wound cleaner. ___ ___ ___ _____

11. Patted skin around wound thoroughly dry with gauze. ___ ___ ___ _____

12. Inspected wound for tissue type, color, odor, and drainage; measured if indicated. ___ ___ ___ _____

13. Removed gloves, performed hand hygiene. ___ ___ ___ _____

14. Applied transparent dressing properly; applied clean gloves; labeled dressing with date, initials, and time of dressing change. ___ ___ ___ _____

15. Discarded soiled dressing materials properly, removed gloves inside out, discarded appropriately, performed hand hygiene. ___ ___ ___ _____

16. Helped patient to comfortable position. ___ ___ ___ _____

EVALUATION

1. Inspected appearance of wound, amount of drainage, and size. ___ ___ ___ _____

2. Inspected periwound areas. ___ ___ ___ _____

3. Asked patient to rate pain. ___ ___ ___ _____

4. Asked patient to demonstrate how to apply dressing. ___ ___ ___ _____

5. Identified unexpected outcomes. ___ ___ ___ _____

RECORDING AND REPORTING

1. Recorded appearance of wound, presence and characteristics of drainage or odor in appropriate log. ___ ___ ___ _____

2. Recorded patient's understanding of application of dressing. ___ ___ ___ _____

3. Reported any signs of infection to health care provider. ___ ___ ___ _____

Copyright © 2018 by Elsevier Inc. All rights reserved.

Student _____ Date _____

Instructor _____ Date _____

PERFORMANCE CHECKLIST SKILL 41.4 **APPLYING A HYDROCOLLOID, HYDROGEL, FOAM, OR ALGINATE DRESSING**

	S	U	NP	Comments

ASSESSMENT

1. Identified patient using at least two identifiers. ⎯⎯ ⎯⎯ ⎯⎯ _____

2. Assessed for presence of allergies to antiseptics, tape, or latex. ⎯⎯ ⎯⎯ ⎯⎯ _____

3. Inspected location, size, and condition of wound. ⎯⎯ ⎯⎯ ⎯⎯ _____

4. Asked patient to rate pain and assess character of pain, administered prescribed analgesic at the appropriate time. ⎯⎯ ⎯⎯ ⎯⎯ _____

5. Reviewed health care provider's orders for frequency and type of dressing change. ⎯⎯ ⎯⎯ ⎯⎯ _____

6. Considered using customized shape or size of dressing. ⎯⎯ ⎯⎯ ⎯⎯ _____

7. Assessed patient's knowledge of purpose of dressing, determined need to include caregiver in dressing wound. ⎯⎯ ⎯⎯ ⎯⎯ _____

PLANNING

1. Identified expected outcomes. ⎯⎯ ⎯⎯ ⎯⎯ _____

2. Explained procedure to patient. ⎯⎯ ⎯⎯ ⎯⎯ _____

3. Positioned patient comfortably to allow access to dressing site. ⎯⎯ ⎯⎯ ⎯⎯ _____

IMPLEMENTATION

1. Provided privacy. ⎯⎯ ⎯⎯ ⎯⎯ _____

2. Exposed wound site, draped patient, instructed patient not to touch wound or supplies. ⎯⎯ ⎯⎯ ⎯⎯ _____

3. Cuffed top of biohazard bag, placed within reach. ⎯⎯ ⎯⎯ ⎯⎯ _____

4. Performed hand hygiene, put on clean gloves, applied appropriate PPE. ⎯⎯ ⎯⎯ ⎯⎯ _____

5. Removed tape, bandages, or ties of existing dressing appropriately; removed all adhesive from the skin. ⎯⎯ ⎯⎯ ⎯⎯ _____

6. Removed old dressing one layer at a time, noted amount and character of drainage, used caution to avoid tension on any drains. ⎯⎯ ⎯⎯ ⎯⎯ _____

Copyright © 2018 by Elsevier Inc. All rights reserved.

	S	U	NP	Comments

7. Disposed of soiled dressings in bag, removed clean gloves inside out, disposed of them in bag, covered wound with gauze, performed hand hygiene. ___ ___ ___ _____

8. Prepared sterile field on over-bed table, poured solution into sterile bowl. ___ ___ ___ _____

9. Removed gauze cover over wound. ___ ___ ___ _____

10. Cleaned wound:

   a. Performed hand hygiene, applied clean gloves, used antiseptic swab or wound cleaner to clean wound. ___ ___ ___ _____

   b. Cleaned from least contaminated area to most contaminated. ___ ___ ___ _____

   c. Cleaned around drain, moved outward from insertion site. ___ ___ ___ _____

11. Used gauze to blot dry the wound bed and skin around wound. ___ ___ ___ _____

12. Inspected appearance and condition of wound, measured wound size and depth. ___ ___ ___ _____

13. Removed gloves and performed hand hygiene. ___ ___ ___ _____

14. Applied dressing properly:

   a. Hydrocolloid dressings.

   (1) Selected proper size wafer. ___ ___ ___ _____

   (2) Applied hydrocolloid granules, impregnated gauze, or paste if necessary. ___ ___ ___ _____

   (3) Removed paper backing, placed over wound, avoided wrinkles, held in place after application. ___ ___ ___ _____

   (4) Taped edges if necessary. ___ ___ ___ _____

   b. Hydrogel dressings.

   (1) Applied skin barrier wipe to skin that would come in contact with adhesive or gel. ___ ___ ___ _____

   (2) Applied gel into wound properly, covered with appropriate dressing. ___ ___ ___ _____

   (3) Cut hydrogel sheet containing glycerin so it extended over wound to intact skin, cut secondary dressing as needed. ___ ___ ___ _____

   (4) Secured dressing as necessary. ___ ___ ___ _____

Copyright © 2018 by Elsevier Inc. All rights reserved.

	S	U	NP	Comments
c. Foam dressings.				
(1) Knew removal and application characteristics of dressing.	——	——	——	_____
(2) Applied skin barrier to skin that would come in contact with adhesive.	——	——	——	_____
(3) Cut foam to proper size, verified orientation.	——	——	——	_____
(4) Cut foam to fit around drain or tube.	——	——	——	_____
(5) Covered foam dressing with secondary dressing if needed.	——	——	——	_____
d. Alginate dressing.				
(1) Cut sheet or rope to fit wound or packed into wound space.	——	——	——	_____
(2) Applied secondary dressing properly.	——	——	——	_____
15. Labeled dressing with your initials and date dressing changed.	——	——	——	_____
16. Discarded soiled dressing materials properly, removed gloves inside out, discarded in bags, performed hand hygiene.	——	——	——	_____
17. Assisted patient to comfortable position.	——	——	——	_____

EVALUATION

	S	U	NP	Comments
1. Inspected condition of wound and character of drainage, palpated around wound for tenderness.	——	——	——	_____
2. Evaluated patient's level of comfort.	——	——	——	_____
3. Inspected condition of dressing at least every shift.	——	——	——	_____
4. Asked patient to explain why dressing in use is the best option for the wound.	——	——	——	_____
5. Identified unexpected outcomes.	——	——	——	_____

RECORDING AND REPORTING

	S	U	NP	Comments
1. Recorded all pertinent information in appropriate log.	——	——	——	_____
2. Graphed wound area or volume if wound was chronic.	——	——	——	_____
3. Recorded patient understanding of proper wound dressing.	——	——	——	_____
4. Reported signs of infection, necrosis, or deteriorating wound status to health care provider immediately.	——	——	——	_____

Copyright © 2018 by Elsevier Inc. All rights reserved.

Student _____ Date _____

Instructor _____ Date _____

PERFORMANCE CHECKLIST PROCEDURE GUIDELINE 41.1 **APPLYING GAUZE AND ELASTIC BANDAGES**

	S	U	NP	Comments

PROCEDURAL STEPS

1. Identified patient using at least two identifiers. ____ ____ ____ _____

2. Reviewed patient's medical record for specific orders related to application of gauze or elastic bandage. ____ ____ ____ _____

3. Assessed patient's level of comfort, administered prescribed analgesic as needed before dressing change. ____ ____ ____ _____

4. Observed adequacy of circulation, skin color, and movement of body part to be wrapped. ____ ____ ____ _____

5. Applied clean gloves, inspected area of skin to be bandaged for alterations in integrity, paid attention to bony prominences. ____ ____ ____ _____

6. Inspected condition of any wound for appearance, size, and presence and character of drainage; reapplied dressing if necessary; removed clean gloves and performed hand hygiene. ____ ____ ____ _____

7. Assessed for size of bandage. ____ ____ ____ _____

8. Identified patient's and caregiver's knowledge level and ability to manipulate bandage. ____ ____ ____ _____

9. Provided privacy, positioned patient appropriately. ____ ____ ____ _____

10. Performed hand hygiene, applied clean gloves if drainage is present. ____ ____ ____ _____

11. Applied gauze or elastic bandage to secure dressings:

    a. Elevated dependent extremity before applying elastic bandage. ____ ____ ____ _____

    b. Ensured primary dressing over wound is securely in place. ____ ____ ____ _____

    c. Wrapped bandage from distal body part, held bandage properly. ____ ____ ____ _____

    d. Applied even tension during application, maintained even tension while wrapping. ____ ____ ____ _____

    e. Used appropriate turns to cover body parts, overlapped bandage properly. ____ ____ ____ _____

Copyright © 2018 by Elsevier Inc. All rights reserved.

	S	U	NP	Comments
f. Double-checked tension, ensured bandage is snug and positioned correctly.	___	___	___	_____
g. Stretched bandage while unrolling, explained benefits of smooth bandage to patient.	___	___	___	_____
h. Ended bandage with two circular turns, secured end of bandage appropriately	___	___	___	_____
12. Applied elastic bandage over stump:				
a. Elevated stump.	___	___	___	_____
b. Secured bandage appropriately around patient's stump or waist.	___	___	___	_____
c. Made half turn with bandage perpendicular to its edge.	___	___	___	_____
d. Brought body of bandage over distal end of stump.	___	___	___	_____
e. Folded bandage from distal to proximal points.	___	___	___	_____
f. Secured with clips, Velcro, or tape.	___	___	___	_____
13. Removed gloves, performed hand hygiene.	___	___	___	_____
14. Assessed degree of tightness of bandage, wrinkles, looseness, and presence of drainage.	___	___	___	_____
15. Evaluated distal circulation at appropriate intervals:				
a. Observed skin color for pallor or cyanosis.	___	___	___	_____
b. Palpated skin for warmth.	___	___	___	_____
c. Palpated distal pulses, compared bilaterally.	___	___	___	_____
d. Asked patient to rate pain on scale and describe any numbness or discomfort.	___	___	___	_____
16. Observed mobility of extremity.	___	___	___	_____
17. Asked patient to demonstrate how to apply elastic roll.	___	___	___	_____
18. Recorded patient's LOC, circulation status, bandage applied, presence of swelling, and ROM at baseline and after bandage application in the appropriate log.	___	___	___	_____
19. Reported change in neurologic or circulatory status to health care provider.	___	___	___	_____

Copyright © 2018 by Elsevier Inc. All rights reserved.

Student _____ Date _____

Instructor _____ Date _____

PERFORMANCE CHECKLIST PROCEDURAL GUIDELINE 41.2 **APPLYING AN ABDOMINAL BINDER**

	S	U	NP	Comments

PROCEDURAL STEPS

1. Identified patient using at least two identifiers. ⎯⎯ ⎯⎯ ⎯⎯ _____

2. Reviewed medical record for order for binder. ⎯⎯ ⎯⎯ ⎯⎯ _____

3. Observed patient's ability to breathe deeply, cough effectively, and turn or move independently. ⎯⎯ ⎯⎯ ⎯⎯ _____

4. Inspected skin for alterations in integrity; observed for irritation, abrasion, and skin surfaces that rub against one another. ⎯⎯ ⎯⎯ ⎯⎯ _____

5. Inspected any surgical dressing for intactness, drainage, and coverage of incision; changed any soiled dressing before applying binder. ⎯⎯ ⎯⎯ ⎯⎯ _____

6. Determined patient's level of comfort, administered prescribed analgesic before dressing change. ⎯⎯ ⎯⎯ ⎯⎯ _____

7. Gathered necessary data to ensure proper fit of binder. ⎯⎯ ⎯⎯ ⎯⎯ _____

8. Determined patient's knowledge of purpose of binder. ⎯⎯ ⎯⎯ ⎯⎯ _____

9. Provided privacy. ⎯⎯ ⎯⎯ ⎯⎯ _____

10. Performed hand hygiene and applied clean gloves. ⎯⎯ ⎯⎯ ⎯⎯ _____

11. Applied abdominal binder:

   a. Positioned patient appropriately. ⎯⎯ ⎯⎯ ⎯⎯ _____

   b. Helped patient roll on side while supporting incision and dressing with hands, fanfolded far side of binder toward midline. ⎯⎯ ⎯⎯ ⎯⎯ _____

   c. Placed binder flat on bed, fanfolded far side of binder toward midline of binder. ⎯⎯ ⎯⎯ ⎯⎯ _____

   d. Placed fanfolded ends of binder under patient. ⎯⎯ ⎯⎯ ⎯⎯ _____

   e. Helped patient roll overfolded binder, obtained help if needed. ⎯⎯ ⎯⎯ ⎯⎯ _____

   f. Unfolded and stretched ends out on far side, then near side. ⎯⎯ ⎯⎯ ⎯⎯ _____

   g. Instructed patient to roll back into supine position. ⎯⎯ ⎯⎯ ⎯⎯ _____

Copyright © 2018 by Elsevier Inc. All rights reserved.

	S	U	NP	Comments
h. Adjusted binder so supine patient is centered.	——	——	——	————————————
i. Padded iliac prominences with gauze if necessary.	——	——	——	————————————
j. Closed binder properly and secured, provided continuous wound support and comfort.	——	——	——	————————————
12. Assessed patient's comfort level, adjusted binder as necessary.	——	——	——	————————————
13. Removed gloves, performed hand hygiene.	——	——	——	————————————
14. Asked patient to rate pain on a scale of 0 to 10.	——	——	——	————————————
15. Removed binder and dressing, assessed skin and wound characteristics at appropriate intervals.	——	——	——	————————————
16. Evaluated patient's ability to ventilate properly at appropriate intervals.	——	——	——	————————————
17. Recorded baseline and post binder condition of skin, circulation, integrity of underlying dressing, and patient's comfort level.	——	——	——	————————————
18. Reported complications to nurse in charge.	——	——	——	————————————
19. Reported reduced ventilation to health care provider immediately.	——	——	——	————————————

Copyright © 2018 by Elsevier Inc. All rights reserved.

Student _____ Date _____

Instructor _____ Date _____

PERFORMANCE CHECKLIST SKILL 42.1 **APPLICATION OF MOIST HEAT (COMPRESS AND SITZ BATH)**

	S	U	NP	Comments
ASSESSMENT				
1. Identified patient using at least two identifiers.	___	___	___	_____
2. Referred to health care provider's order for type of moist heat application, location and duration of application, desired temperature, and agency policies regarding temperature.	___	___	___	_____
3. Performed hand hygiene and assessed skin around area to be treated, performed neurovascular assessments for sensitivity to temperature and pain.	___	___	___	_____
4. Referred to patient's medical record to identify contraindications to moist heat application.	___	___	___	_____
5. Inspected wound for size, color, drainage, tenderness, and odor.	___	___	___	_____
6. Assessed patient's blood pressure and pulse.	___	___	___	_____
7. Assessed patient's mobility.	___	___	___	_____
8. Assessed patient's level of comfort.	___	___	___	_____
9. Assessed patient's and family member's understanding of application and related safety factors.	___	___	___	_____
PLANNING				
1. Identified expected outcomes.	___	___	___	_____
2. Assembled and prepared equipment and supplies.	___	___	___	_____
3. Explained steps of procedure and purpose to patient, described sensations patient would feel and precautions to prevent burning.	___	___	___	_____
IMPLEMENTATION				
1. Provided privacy.	___	___	___	_____
2. Positioned patient in bed, kept affected body part in proper alignment, exposed body part to be covered, draped patient as needed.	___	___	___	_____
3. Performed hand hygiene, applied clean gloves.	___	___	___	_____
4. Placed waterproof pad under patient if appropriate.	___	___	___	_____

Copyright © 2018 by Elsevier Inc. All rights reserved.

	S	U	NP	Comments

5. Applied moist sterile compress:

a. Heated solution to desired temperature properly. ___ ___ ___ _____

b. Prepared aquathermia pad if needed, set temperature if needed. ___ ___ ___ _____

c. Removed any dressing present, inspected condition of wound and surrounding skin, disposed of gloves and dressings in biohazard bag. ___ ___ ___ _____

d. Performed hand hygiene. ___ ___ ___ _____

e. Prepared compress.

(1) Poured warm solution into container, used sterile technique if needed. ___ ___ ___ _____

(2) Opened gauze, used sterile technique if needed. ___ ___ ___ _____

(3) Added gauze to container of solution to immerse gauze, used proper aseptic technique. ___ ___ ___ _____

(4) Followed instructions for warming using commercially prepared compress. ___ ___ ___ _____

f. Applied sterile or clean gloves as appropriate. ___ ___ ___ _____

g. Picked up one layer of gauze, wrung out excess solution, applied to wound, avoided surrounding skin. ___ ___ ___ _____

h. Lifted edge of gauze to assess for redness. ___ ___ ___ _____

i. Packed gauze snugly if patient tolerated compress, covered all wound surfaces with compress. ___ ___ ___ _____

j. Covered moist compress with dry sterile dressing and bath towel, pinned or tied in place, removed and disposed of gloves, performed hand hygiene. ___ ___ ___ _____

k. Applied aquathermia, heat pack, or waterproof heating pad over towel; kept in place for desired duration. ___ ___ ___ _____

l. Changed warm compress using sterile technique as ordered if pad or heat pack was not used. ___ ___ ___ _____

m. Applied clean gloves; removed pad, towel, and compress; reassessed wound and condition of skin; replaced dry sterile dressing. ___ ___ ___ _____

n. Helped patient to preferred comfortable position. ___ ___ ___ _____

o. Disposed of equipment and soiled compress, performed hand hygiene. ___ ___ ___ _____

Copyright © 2018 by Elsevier Inc. All rights reserved.

	S	U	NP	Comments

6. Sitz bath or warm soak to intact skin or wound:

   a. Performed hand hygiene, applied clean gloves, removed any existing dressing covering wound, disposed of gloves and dressings, performed hand hygiene. ___ ___ ___ _____

   b. Inspected condition of wound and skin, paid attention to suture line. ___ ___ ___ _____

   c. Applied gloves and cleansed intact skin around open area when exudate was present, disposed of gloves, performed hand hygiene. ___ ___ ___ _____

   d. Filled bath with warmed solution, checked temperature. ___ ___ ___ _____

   e. Assisted patient to bathroom, immersed body part in bath, covered patient with bath blanket or towel as needed. ___ ___ ___ _____

   f. Assessed heart rate, ensured that patient was not lightheaded and that call light was within reach. ___ ___ ___ _____

   g. Removed patient from soak, dried body throughout. ___ ___ ___ _____

   h. Drained solution from basin or tub, cleaned and placed in proper storage area, disposed of soiled linen and gloves, performed hand hygiene. ___ ___ ___ _____

EVALUATION

1. Inspected condition of body part or wound for evidence of healing, observed skin color, temperature, edema, and sensitivity to touch. ___ ___ ___ _____

2. Asked patient to describe level of comfort, asked about any sensation of burning following treatment. ___ ___ ___ _____

3. Obtained vital signs, compared with baseline. ___ ___ ___ _____

4. Asked patient to demonstrate how to apply compress at home. ___ ___ ___ _____

5. Identified unexpected outcomes. ___ ___ ___ _____

RECORDING AND REPORTING

1. Recorded and reported all pertinent information of procedure. ___ ___ ___ _____

2. Recorded preprocedure and postprocedure vital signs. ___ ___ ___ _____

3. Documented evaluation of patient or caregiver learning. ___ ___ ___ _____

Copyright © 2018 by Elsevier Inc. All rights reserved.

Student _____ Date _____

Instructor _____ Date _____

PERFORMANCE CHECKLIST SKILL 42.2 **APPLYING AQUATHERMIA AND DRY HEAT**

	S	U	NP	Comments

ASSESSMENT

1. Identified patient using at least two identifiers.

2. Referred to health care provider's order for location of application and duration of therapy.

3. Performed hand hygiene; assessed condition of skin and underlying tissue area where applying pad for skin integrity, color, temperature, sensitivity to touch, blistering, and excessive dryness.

4. Asked patient to describe level of comfort, assessed ROM if necessary.

5. Checked electrical plugs and cords for fraying or cracking.

6. Determined patient's or caregiver's knowledge of procedure.

PLANNING

1. Identified expected outcomes.

2. Prepared equipment and supplies.

3. Explained procedure and precautions.

IMPLEMENTATION

1. Provided privacy.

2. Performed hand hygiene, positioned patient to expose area being treated.

3. Applied heat therapy:

   a. Applied aquathermia heating pad.

      (1) Covered or wrapped area to be treated with towel or enclosed pad with pillowcase.

      (2) Placed pad over affected area, secured with tape, tie, or gauze.

      (3) Turned on aquathermia unit, checked temperature setting.

   b. Applied commercially prepared heat pack properly.

Copyright © 2018 by Elsevier Inc. All rights reserved.

	S	U	NP	Comments

4. Monitored condition of skin over site at appropriate intervals, asked patient about sensation of burning. ____ ____ ____ _____

5. Performed hand hygiene, applied clean gloves, removed pad at appropriate time and stored. ____ ____ ____ _____

6. Helped patient return to preferred comfortable position, disposed of soiled linen, performed hand hygiene. ____ ____ ____ _____

EVALUATION

1. Inspected condition of skin for response to heat exposure, evaluated at appropriate interval. ____ ____ ____ _____

2. Assessed ROM, asked patient to rate pain. ____ ____ ____ _____

3. Asked patient to explain why keeping a layer of cloth between skin and heating pad is important. ____ ____ ____ _____

4. Identified unexpected outcomes. ____ ____ ____ _____

RECORDING AND REPORTING

1. Recorded type of application, temperature, duration of therapy, and patient's response in the appropriate log. ____ ____ ____ _____

2. Documented evaluation of patient or caregiver learning. ____ ____ ____ _____

3. Reported pain level, ROM of body part, skin integrity, color, temperature, sensitivity to touch, blistering, and dryness. ____ ____ ____ _____

Copyright © 2018 by Elsevier Inc. All rights reserved.

Student _____ Date _____

Instructor _____ Date _____

PERFORMANCE CHECKLIST SKILL 42.3 **APPLICATION OF COLD**

	S	U	NP	Comments
ASSESSMENT				
1. Identified patient using at least two identifiers.	___	___	___	_____
2. Referred to health care provider's order for type, location, and duration of application.	___	___	___	_____
3. Performed hand hygiene, inspected condition or affected part, palpated area for edema.	___	___	___	_____
4. Considered time elapsed since injury occurred.	___	___	___	_____
5. Asked patient to describe severity and character of pain.	___	___	___	_____
6. Performed neurovascular check, inspected surrounding skin for integrity, circulation, color, temperature, and sensitivity to touch.	___	___	___	_____
7. Reviewed medical history for conditions that contraindicate use of cold therapy.	___	___	___	_____
8. Assessed patient's LOC and responsiveness.	___	___	___	_____
9. Assessed patient's understanding and awareness of procedure.	___	___	___	_____
PLANNING				
1. Identified expected outcomes.	___	___	___	_____
2. Prepared equipment and supplies.	___	___	___	_____
3. Explained procedure and precautions.	___	___	___	_____
IMPLEMENTATION				
1. Provided privacy, performed hand hygiene, applied clean gloves.	___	___	___	_____
2. Positioned patient properly, exposed area to be treated, draped patient with blankets.	___	___	___	_____
3. Placed towel or pad under area to be treated.	___	___	___	_____
4. Applied cold compress:				
a. Placed ice water in basin, tested temperature.	___	___	___	_____
b. Submerged gauze into basin, wrung out excess moisture.	___	___	___	_____
c. Applied compress to affected area, molded over site.	___	___	___	_____
d. Removed, remoistened, and reapplied to maintain temperature as needed.	___	___	___	_____

Copyright © 2018 by Elsevier Inc. All rights reserved.

	S	U	NP	Comments

5. Applied ice pack or bag:

   a. Filled bag with water, secured cap, inverted bag.   ____ ____ ____ _____

   b. Emptied water, filled bag properly with ice chips and water.   ____ ____ ____ _____

   c. Expressed excess air from bag, secured bag closure, wiped bag dry.   ____ ____ ____ _____

   d. Squeezed or kneaded commercial ice pack.   ____ ____ ____ _____

   e. Wrapped pack or bag with towel, applied over injury, secured with tape as needed.   ____ ____ ____ _____

6. Applied commercial gel pack:

   a. Removed from freezer.   ____ ____ ____ _____

   b. Wrapped in towel, applied over injury.   ____ ____ ____ _____

   c. Secured with tape or gauze as needed.   ____ ____ ____ _____

7. Applied electrically controlled cooling device:

   a. Prepared device appropriately.   ____ ____ ____ _____

   b. Ensured all connections are intact and temperature is set.   ____ ____ ____ _____

   c. Wrapped cool-water flow pad in towel or pillowcase.   ____ ____ ____ _____

   d. Wrapped cool pad around body part.   ____ ____ ____ _____

   e. Turned device on and set correct temperature.   ____ ____ ____ _____

   f. Secured with elastic wrap bandage, gauze roll, or ties.   ____ ____ ____ _____

8. Removed gloves, disposed of properly, performed hand hygiene.   ____ ____ ____ _____

9. Checked condition of skin at appropriate intervals:

   a. Used extra caution if area was edematous, assessed site more often.   ____ ____ ____ _____

   b. Stopped if patient complained of burning sensation or skin began to feel numb.   ____ ____ ____ _____

10. Applied clean gloves, removed compress or pad at appropriate time, dried any moisture.   ____ ____ ____ _____

11. Helped patient to comfortable position.   ____ ____ ____ _____

12. Removed and disposed of supplies, emptied basin and dried, disposed of soiled linens and gloves, performed hand hygiene.   ____ ____ ____ _____

Copyright © 2018 by Elsevier Inc. All rights reserved.

	S	U	NP	Comments

EVALUATION

1. Inspected affected area for integrity, color, temperature, and sensitivity to touch; reevaluated at appropriate interval. ___ ___ ___ _____

2. Palpated affected area for edema, bruising, and bleeding. ___ ___ ___ _____

3. Asked patient to report pain level. ___ ___ ___ _____

4. Asked patient to demonstrate how to apply ice pack. ___ ___ ___ _____

5. Identified unexpected outcomes. ___ ___ ___ _____

RECORDING AND REPORTING

1. Recorded procedure and patient's response in the appropriate log. ___ ___ ___ _____

2. Documented evaluation of patient or caregiver learning. ___ ___ ___ _____

3. Reported any sensations of burning, numbness, or unrelieved skin color changes to health care provider. ___ ___ ___ _____

Copyright © 2018 by Elsevier Inc. All rights reserved.

Student _____   Date _____

Instructor _____   Date _____

PERFORMANCE CHECKLIST SKILL 42.4 **CARING FOR PATIENTS REQUIRING HYPOTHERMIA OR HYPERTHERMIA BLANKETS**

	S	U	NP	Comments
ASSESSMENT				
1. Identified patient using at least two identifiers.	___	___	___	_____
2. Referred to health care provider's order, checked that patient's current body temperature indicated use of blanket.	___	___	___	_____
3. Assessed vital signs, neurologic status, mental status, and peripheral circulation.	___	___	___	_____
4. Verified that less intensive measures cannot return patient's body temperature to normal.	___	___	___	_____
5. Performed hand hygiene, assessed patient's skin on chest and extremities, paid attention to bony prominences.	___	___	___	_____
PLANNING				
1. Identified expected outcomes.	___	___	___	_____
2. Explained procedure to patient.	___	___	___	_____
3. Positioned patient comfortably.	___	___	___	_____
4. Prepared blanket according to policy and instructions.	___	___	___	_____
IMPLEMENTATION				
1. Performed hand hygiene, applied clean gloves.	___	___	___	_____
2. Turned on blanket, observed that light was on, set pad temperature as desired.	___	___	___	_____
3. Verified that pad temperature limits were set safely.	___	___	___	_____
4. Covered blanket with thin sheet or bath blanket.	___	___	___	_____
5. Positioned blanket on top of patient properly, wrapped body parts as necessary.	___	___	___	_____
6. Lubricated rectal probe and inserted in patient's rectum.	___	___	___	_____
7. Positioned patient to protect from pressure injury development and impaired body alignment, kept linens free of perspiration and condensation.	___	___	___	_____
8. Double-checked fluid thermometer on control panel before leaving.	___	___	___	_____
9. Removed gloves, performed hand hygiene.	___	___	___	_____

Copyright © 2018 by Elsevier Inc. All rights reserved.

	S	U	NP	Comments

EVALUATION

1. Monitored patient's temperature and vital signs at appropriate intervals. ____ ____ ____ _____

2. Evaluated automatic temperature control properly and at appropriate intervals. ____ ____ ____ _____

3. Observed skin for burns, changes in color, and other signs of injury. ____ ____ ____ _____

4. Observed patient for signs of shivering. ____ ____ ____ _____

5. Determined patient's level of comfort. ____ ____ ____ _____

6. Asked patient to explain why blanket is in use. ____ ____ ____ _____

7. Identified unexpected outcomes. ____ ____ ____ _____

RECORDING AND REPORTING

1. Recorded baseline data. ____ ____ ____ _____

2. Charted on temperature graphic repeated measurements of vital signs. ____ ____ ____ _____

3. Documented your evaluation of family caregiver learning. ____ ____ ____ _____

4. Reported any unexpected outcome to health care provider. ____ ____ ____ _____

Copyright © 2018 by Elsevier Inc. All rights reserved.

Student _____ Date _____

Instructor _____ Date _____

PERFORMANCE CHECKLIST SKILL 43.1   **HOME ENVIRONMENT ASSESSMENT AND SAFETY**

	S	U	NP	Comments
ASSESSMENT				
1. Reviewed risk factors that predispose patient to accidents in the home.	——	——	——	_____
2. Determined if patient had history of falls or other home injuries, used mnemonic SPLATT.	——	——	——	_____
3. Had patient who had a near fall or an actual fall maintain a fall diary.	——	——	——	_____
4. Conducted a TUG test properly.	——	——	——	_____
5. Determined if patient had fear of falling.	——	——	——	_____
6. Partnered with patient and family caregivers to conduct home safety assessment:				
a. Assessed front and back entrances.	——	——	——	_____
b. Assessed kitchen.	——	——	——	_____
c. Assessed bathroom.	——	——	——	_____
d. Assessed bedroom.	——	——	——	_____
e. Assessed living room/family room.	——	——	——	_____
f. Assessed other general house areas.	——	——	——	_____
g. Assessed general fire safety.	——	——	——	_____
h. Assessed general electric safety.	——	——	——	_____
i. Assessed carbon monoxide prevention.	——	——	——	_____
7. Assessed patient's financial resources, determined monthly income used for expenses.	——	——	——	_____
8. Assessed patient's and family caregiver's willingness to make changes, determined importance of functional independence for patient.	——	——	——	_____
PLANNING				
1. Identified expected outcomes.	——	——	——	_____
2. Prioritized environmental barriers that pose greatest risk.	——	——	——	_____
3. Recommended calling in reliable contractor if repairs were necessary.	——	——	——	_____

Copyright © 2018 by Elsevier Inc. All rights reserved.

	S	U	NP	Comments

IMPLEMENTATION

1. General home safety:

   a. Provided direct light source in places where patient works.

   b. Considered nonglossy finishes, had curtains or adjustable shades in other living areas.

   c. Color coded controls of appliances.

   d. Considered installing lazy Susans, pull-out drawers, or C-rings if necessary.

   e. Installed automatic door openers, level door-knob handles, and hook-and-chain locks.

2. Fall prevention steps:

   a. Painted edges of concrete stairs.

   b. Installed treads on steps.

   c. Rearranged furniture to open space.

   d. Reduced clutter in living areas.

   e. Secured all carpet, mats, and tiles; placed backing under rugs; removed rugs in dry areas.

   f. Padded floor, used specialized tile that absorbs impact.

   g. Used low-rise bed or mattress on the ground.

   h. Installed extra electrical outlets, secured electrical cords against baseboards.

   i. Installed nonskid surface in tub or shower, ensured floor was clean and dry.

   j. Had grab bars installed in bathroom, allowed patient to select placement, ensured bar was different color from wall.

   k. Had handrails installed along stairways, ensured stairways were well lit with switches at top and bottom of steps.

   l. Installed appropriate lighting for outside walkways.

   m. Kept a lighted phone accessible.

   n. Installed motion sensor exterior lighting for walks/driveways.

   o. Had patient use padding or clothing to cushion bony prominences.

Copyright © 2018 by Elsevier Inc. All rights reserved.

	S	U	NP	Comments

3. Prevented spread of infection:

   a. Instructed patient and caregiver in cleaning practices.

   b. Instructed patient not to share utensils.

   c. Instructed patient to clean appliances and surfaces daily.

   d. Instructed patient in safe food preparation and storage.

4. Burn safety:

   a. Adjusted setting on hot water heater appropriately.

   b. Instructed patient to always turn cold water on first.

   c. Installed touch pads on lamps.

   d. Used color codes on faucets.

5. Carbon monoxide safety:

   a. Had condition of furnace venting checked annually.

   b. Cautioned patients against using gas stove or barbecue grill for heating inside.

   c. Had battery-operated carbon monoxide detector installed in home, checked batteries at appropriate times.

6. Firearm safety:

   a. Taught patient about dangers of guns in the home.

   b. Taught patient to install trigger locks, store guns in a locked cabinet, store ammunition separately, and store keys in a place inaccessible to children.

EVALUATION

1. Had patient and caregiver identify safety risks revealed in home assessment.

2. Asked patient to discuss modification plans during follow-up, observed what changes had been implemented.

3. Asked if patient had experienced falls or other injuries in the home.

4. Reassessed for progression of dementia.

5. Asked patient to explain why home modifications are important.

6. Identified unexpected outcomes.

Copyright © 2018 by Elsevier Inc. All rights reserved.

	S	U	NP	Comments

RECORDING AND REPORTING

1. Retained copy of home safety assessment in patient's home care record.   ____ ____ ____ _____

2. Recorded any instruction provided, patient response, and changes made within environment in progress notes.   ____ ____ ____ _____

Copyright © 2018 by Elsevier Inc. All rights reserved.

Student _____ Date _____

Instructor _____ Date _____

PERFORMANCE CHECKLIST SKILL 43.2   **ADAPTING THE HOME SETTING FOR PATIENTS WITH COGNITIVE DEFICITS**

	S	U	NP	Comments

ASSESSMENT

1. Assessed patient over a short period of time, was sensitive to any sensory disability.

2. Ensured room was well lit with minimal noise or interruption, spoke clearly and in a normal tone.

3. Asked patient to describe own level of health and ability to perform self-care skills.

4. Asked how patient was doing with home management responsibilities.

5. Assessed patient's adherence to taking medications, reviewed numbers and types of medications and patient's understanding of purpose, time, and dosage.

6. Assessed where patient stores medications, had patient or caregiver keep medication list.

7. Determined if patient had family caregiver who assisted with self-care or home management, assessed relationship and support given.

8. Observed patient's dress, nonverbal expressions, appearance, and cleanliness.

9. Observed immediate home environment.

10. Completed Folstein's examination or SGDS if cognitive or mental status change was suspected.

11. Observed for potentially hazardous behaviors if patient was suspected to be at risk for wandering.

12. Assessed which current environmental strategies caregivers were using to deal with wandering.

13. Assessed caregiver for signs of stress.

PLANNING

1. Identified expected outcomes.

2. Referred family to occupational therapy, homemaker services, or respite care if patient had difficulty with self-care or fine motor skills.

Copyright © 2018 by Elsevier Inc. All rights reserved.

	S	U	NP	Comments

3. Considered patient's level of cognitive impairment when making changes to patient's living environment. ____ ____ ____ _____

4. Determined best time of day for approaches that result in desired response. ____ ____ ____ _____

IMPLEMENTATION

1. Helped create a list or posted reminder notes if patient had difficulty remembering when to perform tasks. ____ ____ ____ _____

2. Provided organized medication, recommended a wristwatch with an alarm or scheduled text messages if patient has difficulty remembering when to take medications. ____ ____ ____ _____

3. Reduced steps it takes to complete tasks such as paying bills or bringing in groceries. ____ ____ ____ _____

4. Offered assistive devices if patient has difficulty bathing, dressing, writing, and feeding. ____ ____ ____ _____

5. Helped patient and caregiver determine routine schedule for ADLs, posted a large calendar conspicuously. ____ ____ ____ _____

6. Instructed caregiver to focus on patient's abilities rather than disabilities in modifying approaches. ____ ____ ____ _____

7. Had caregiver assist in setting up activities so patient could complete tasks. ____ ____ ____ _____

8. Discussed with patient, caregiver, pharmacist, and health care provider options for scheduling multiple medications. ____ ____ ____ _____

9. Instructed caregiver in how to use simple and direct communication. ____ ____ ____ _____

10. Placed clocks, calendars, and personal mementos throughout the home; enhanced the environment as necessary. ____ ____ ____ _____

11. Had caregiver routinely orient patient to caregiver and activities. ____ ____ ____ _____

12. Ensured patient had regular naps or rest. ____ ____ ____ _____

13. Had caregiver support visits by family and friends, instructed caregiver in how to promote social interaction. ____ ____ ____ _____

14. Provided safe place for a person to wander. ____ ____ ____ _____

15. Recommended family install door locks or guards. ____ ____ ____ _____

16. Created calm, safe setting for patient's abilities. ____ ____ ____ _____

17. Monitored patient for personal comfort. ____ ____ ____ _____

Copyright © 2018 by Elsevier Inc. All rights reserved.

	S	U	NP	Comments

18. Kept a list of places to which patient may wander.

19. Considered having patient wear GPS device to help manage location, installed motion detector near exit.

20. Considered need for full-time care.

EVALUATION

1. Asked patient to review activities completed recently during follow-up visits.

2. Reviewed revised schedule for medication administration with patient and caregiver.

3. Checked pill counts maintained by patient/family for a week.

4. Asked caregiver to describe ways that would increase patient's success in completing tasks.

5. Had caregiver show schedules of daily routines and review approaches used, observed environment for presence of reality-oriented cues.

6. Had family caregivers describe options for minimizing wandering.

7. Had family caregivers report number of occurrences of wandering.

8. Asked caregiver to explain how to help minimize patient's wandering.

9. Identified unexpected outcomes.

RECORDING AND REPORTING

1. Recorded assessment of patient's cognitive and mental status, recommended interventions, and patient's and caregiver's response in the appropriate log.

2. Reported any change in patient's behavior that reflects a decline in cognitive or mental status to health care provider.

Copyright © 2018 by Elsevier Inc. All rights reserved.

Student _____ Date _____

Instructor _____ Date _____

PERFORMANCE CHECKLIST SKILL 43.3 **MEDICATION AND MEDICAL DEVICE SAFETY**

	S	U	NP	Comments

ASSESSMENT

1. Assessed patient's sensory, musculoskeletal, and neurologic function.

2. Assessed caregiver's concerns about providing care for patient.

3. Assessed patient's medication regimen and length of time patient had been receiving each drug, asked patient and caregiver to describe doses taken daily.

4. Assessed patient's and caregiver's health literacy level.

5. Asked patient to show you where medications were stored, looked at each container.

6. Assessed temperature of storage area.

7. Assessed patient's daily schedule for drug administration, asked patient to describe schedule and problems following it.

8. Asked to see where patient stores injection supplies and disposed of needles if necessary.

9. Asked to see where glucose monitor, lancets, and strips were stored and how lancets were disposed of if necessary.

PLANNING

1. Identified expected outcomes.

IMPLEMENTATION

1. Educated patient and caregiver in principles to ensure medications were safe to use:

   a. Ensure medication was taken by patient for whom it was prescribed.

   b. Did not take medication more than 1 year old or past expiration.

   c. Did not place different medications in the same containers.

   d. Did not place medications in containers other than their original ones.

   e. Finished prescribed medication.

Copyright © 2018 by Elsevier Inc. All rights reserved.

	S	U	NP	Comments

f. Washed hands before and after administering medication. ____ ____ ____ _____

2. Recommended approaches for preparation of medications if necessary:

   a. Placed medications in screw-top container. ____ ____ ____ _____

   b. Had pharmacy-type larger labels on medication containers. ____ ____ ____ _____

   c. Had Braille labels placed on medication containers, if necessary. ____ ____ ____ _____

   d. Introduced a color-coding system. ____ ____ ____ _____

   e. Provided syringes with large numerals or a syringe magnifier. ____ ____ ____ _____

   f. Offered spring-loaded needle insertion aid. ____ ____ ____ _____

   g. Instructed caregivers in how to draw medication into syringe. ____ ____ ____ _____

3. Recommended approaches for medication and supply storage:

   a. Stored medications in a safe place. ____ ____ ____ _____

   b. Kept liquid medications and parenteral drugs in a cool place. ____ ____ ____ _____

   c. Kept medical supplies in airtight containers and in a cool place. ____ ____ ____ _____

   d. Instructed patient and caregiver to use a new needle with each medication administration. ____ ____ ____ _____

4. Reviewed proper techniques for disposal of medications, "sharps," and other supplies:

   a. Discarded unused or outdated drugs in a bag containing coffee grounds or kitty litter. ____ ____ ____ _____

   b. Obtained sharps container. ____ ____ ____ _____

   c. Cautioned against overfilling sharps container. ____ ____ ____ _____

   d. Stored container in an area inaccessible to children. ____ ____ ____ _____

   e. Disposed of soiled supplies in a separate, sealed, plastic bag; placed in second bag; discarded appropriately. ____ ____ ____ _____

   f. Consulted local public health department or community regarding proper waste disposal. ____ ____ ____ _____

EVALUATION

1. Had patient/caregiver describe steps to ensuring safe medication. ____ ____ ____ _____

2. Observed patient/caregiver prepared and administered medication. ____ ____ ____ _____

Copyright © 2018 by Elsevier Inc. All rights reserved.

	S	U	NP	Comments
3. Observed home setting for location of medication and supplies.	——	——	——	———————
4. Had patient describe how sharps and equipment were discarded.	——	——	——	———————
5. Did pill counts at appropriate intervals.	——	——	——	———————
6. Asked patient to describe how sharps are disposed of and why proper disposal is important.	——	——	——	———————
7. Identified unexpected outcomes.	——	——	——	———————

RECORDING AND REPORTING

	S	U	NP	Comments
1. Recorded instructions and recommendations in the appropriate log, notified health care provider of unsafe situations.	——	——	——	———————
2. Reported unsafe situation to health care provider.	——	——	——	———————

Copyright © 2018 by Elsevier Inc. All rights reserved.

Student _____   Date _____

Instructor _____   Date _____

PERFORMANCE CHECKLIST SKILL 44.1   **TEACHING CLIENTS TO MEASURE BODY TEMPERATURE**

	S	U	NP	Comments
ASSESSMENT				
1. Identified client using at least two identifiers during first visit.	____	____	____	_____
2. Assessed client's/caregiver's ability to manipulate and read thermometer, had client put on glasses if necessary.	____	____	____	_____
3. Assessed client's knowledge of normal temperature ranges, symptoms of fever and hypothermia, and client's risk for body temperature alterations.	____	____	____	_____
4. Assessed client's ability to determine appropriate type of thermometer to use.	____	____	____	_____
5. Assessed client's learning readiness and ability to concentrate.	____	____	____	_____
6. Assessed client's/caregiver's previous knowledge and experience in measuring temperature and maintaining thermometer, had client or caregiver perform demonstration if necessary.	____	____	____	_____
PLANNING				
1. Identified expected outcomes.	____	____	____	_____
2. Selected setting in home where client was most likely to measure temperature.	____	____	____	_____
3. Selected good location for teaching session:				
a. Selected room that is well lit with comfortable seating.	____	____	____	_____
b. Ensured client can see nurse clearly.	____	____	____	_____
c. Controlled sources of noise and distractions.	____	____	____	_____
4. Discussed and demonstrated normal temperature ranges, instructed caregiver to remain with patient if necessary.	____	____	____	_____

512

Copyright © 2018 by Elsevier Inc. All rights reserved.

	S	U	NP	Comments

IMPLEMENTATION

1. Demonstrated steps of thermometer preparation, insertion, and reading; provided rationale for steps:

   a. Instructed client to take oral temperature at appropriate times and when to select a different temperature site. ____ ____ ____ _____

   b. Performed hand hygiene, instructed caregiver to wear clean, disposable gloves. ____ ____ ____ _____

   c. Taught client or caregiver proper positioning for temperature measurement. ____ ____ ____ _____

   d. Demonstrate temperature measurement technique, had client or caregiver perform each step. ____ ____ ____ _____

   e. Explained any special precautions in using thermometers. ____ ____ ____ _____

   f. Discussed typical time frame for each type of temperature to register and how to take reading. ____ ____ ____ _____

   g. Taught proper method for removing, cleaning, and storing thermometer, selected suitable storage location. ____ ____ ____ _____

2. Discussed common symptoms of fever. ____ ____ ____ _____

3. Discussed common signs and symptoms of hypothermia, explained risk factors. ____ ____ ____ _____

4. Discussed importance of notifying health care provider when temperature elevations occur, reviewed common therapies for temperature reduction that are safe to perform at home. ____ ____ ____ _____

5. Provided written guidelines for client's reference at appropriate level of health literacy. ____ ____ ____ _____

6. Gave client/caregiver logbook to record temperature and time, instructed client to use record to report temperature to health care provider. ____ ____ ____ _____

Copyright © 2018 by Elsevier Inc. All rights reserved.

	S	U	NP	Comments

EVALUATION

1. Had client/caregiver demonstrate technique for temperature measurement.

2. Asked client/caregiver to identify normal temperature range and influences on readings, discussed safety implications.

3. Had client/caregiver describe common signs of fever and hypothermia and method for control.

4. Watched client/caregiver clean and store equipment.

5. Watched client/caregiver record values and times, reviewed logbook periodically to ensure correctness.

6. Asked patient to explain importance of knowing how to take own temperature.

7. Identified unexpected outcomes.

RECORDING AND REPORTING

1. Recorded information taught and client's demonstration in home care record.

2. Recorded temperature in appropriate logs.

3. Reported high and low temperatures to health care provider.

Copyright © 2018 by Elsevier Inc. All rights reserved.

Student _____ Date _____

Instructor _____ Date _____

PERFORMANCE CHECKLIST SKILL 44.2 **TEACHING BLOOD PRESSURE AND PULSE MEASUREMENT**

	S	U	NP	Comments
ASSESSMENT				
1. Identified client using at least two identifiers during first visit.	___	___	___	_____
2. Assessed client's or caregiver's psychomotor function.	___	___	___	_____
3. Assessed client's/caregiver's knowledge of normal BP, pulse ranges, and symptoms and causes of high or low readings.	___	___	___	_____
4. Assessed client's/caregiver's knowledge of BP and pulse measure, medical issues that affect them, why awareness was important to client health.	___	___	___	_____
5. Assessed client's/caregiver's previous knowledge and experience in measuring blood pressure, had client or caregiver perform demonstration if appropriate.	___	___	___	_____
6. Assessed client's learning readiness and ability to concentrate, considered presence of pain, nausea, or fatigue and client interest in instruction.	___	___	___	_____
7. Assessed home environment for favorable place to measure BP and pulse.	___	___	___	_____
PLANNING				
1. Identified expected outcomes.	___	___	___	_____
2. Encouraged client or caregiver to perform measurements on routine schedule for long-term monitoring plan.	___	___	___	_____
3. Encouraged client to avoid exercise, caffeine, and smoking for 30 minutes before assessment.	___	___	___	_____
4. Had client or caregiver perform measurement in comfortable, correct position and in warm, quiet environment.	___	___	___	_____

Copyright © 2018 by Elsevier Inc. All rights reserved.

	S	U	NP	Comments

IMPLEMENTATION

1. Blood pressure measurement:

   a. Explained importance of client sitting quietly before measurement. ___ ___ ___ _____

   b. Discussed best sites for assessing BP, explained when not to apply cuff. ___ ___ ___ _____

   c. Demonstrated steps for measuring BP.

      (1) Use of sphygmomanometer and stethoscope.

         (a) Taught palpation of artery, positioning and wrapping of cuff, placement of stethoscope, inflation and release of cuff, and listening for Korotkoff sounds. ___ ___ ___ _____

         (b) Described sounds of measurement and relationship to observation of gauge during reading, cautioned client about level and time appropriate for cuff inflation. ___ ___ ___ _____

         (c) Taught client or caregiver to routinely clean stethoscope properly. ___ ___ ___ _____

      (2) Use of electronic BP monitor.

         (a) Taught correct placement of cuff and used to electronic inflation. ___ ___ ___ _____

2. Pulse measurement:

   a. Discussed with client/caregiver best sites for assessing pulse. ___ ___ ___ _____

   b. Demonstrated steps for palpating pulse properly.

      (1) Instructed in use of gentle pressure. ___ ___ ___ _____

      (2) Instructed in use of clock with second hand. ___ ___ ___ _____

      (3) Instructed to count for full 60 seconds, started with second hand at 12:00 o'clock position. ___ ___ ___ _____

Copyright © 2018 by Elsevier Inc. All rights reserved.

	S	U	NP	Comments

3. Educated client about desired BP and pulse ranges, purposes for monitoring, and when to take measurements. _____ _____ _____ _____

4. Described symptoms that indicated need to perform BP and/or pulse measurement. _____ _____ _____ _____

5. Had client/caregiver attempt each skill on you or family member. _____ _____ _____ _____

6. Observed client demonstrate techniques on self, did not allow multiple repetitive BP attempts on any one limb. _____ _____ _____ _____

7. Taught client or caregiver to monitor BP and pulse even if they remain in normal range. _____ _____ _____ _____

8. Provided client or caregiver with printed instructions with guide or video demonstration of procedure if possible. _____ _____ _____ _____

9. Gave client log to record BP and pulse and time taken, instructed client to record whether medications that affect BP or pulse were taken, instructed client to use written record to report readings to health care provider. _____ _____ _____ _____

10. Instructed client or caregiver in proper care of equipment. _____ _____ _____ _____

EVALUATION

1. Observed client or caregiver demonstrate technique for BP/pulse measurement on three different occasions, verified client adds information to log correctly. _____ _____ _____ _____

2. Asked client if readings were within range and when to report abnormal readings to health care provider. _____ _____ _____ _____

3. Asked client or caregiver to describe reason for BP or pulse monitoring and any related medications or treatment. _____ _____ _____ _____

4. Had client or caregiver demonstrate proper care of equipment. _____ _____ _____ _____

5. Asked client to explain how medications can affect BP readings. _____ _____ _____ _____

6. Identified unexpected outcomes. _____ _____ _____ _____

Copyright © 2018 by Elsevier Inc. All rights reserved.

	S	U	NP	Comments
RECORDING AND REPORTING				
1. Recorded teaching, client responses, and demonstration in the appropriate log.	____	____	____	_____
2. Recorded BP and pulse in home care record and logbook.	____	____	____	_____
3. Reported changes in readings of BP/pulse.	____	____	____	_____

Copyright © 2018 by Elsevier Inc. All rights reserved.

Student _____ Date _____

Instructor _____ Date _____

PERFORMANCE CHECKLIST SKILL 44.3   **TEACHING INTERMITTENT SELF-CATHETERIZATION**

	S	U	NP	Comments
ASSESSMENT				
1. Identified client using at least two identifiers during first visit.	——	——	——	_____
2. Reviewed client's medical record; gathered information about voiding history, medical and surgical history, client's fluid intake, postvoid residual amount, and daily voiding routine.	——	——	——	_____
3. Assessed client's ability to perform CISC.	——	——	——	_____
4. Assessed client's/caregiver's knowledge about CISC, observed performance of CISC.	——	——	——	_____
PLANNING				
1. Identified expected outcomes.	——	——	——	_____
2. Selected setting that client/caregiver would most likely use when performing CISC.	——	——	——	_____
3. Helped client/caregiver select proper catheter.	——	——	——	_____
IMPLEMENTATION				
1. Taught client/caregiver how to perform appropriate hand hygiene using soap and water, had involved caregiver apply clean gloves.	——	——	——	_____
2. Performed hand hygiene, helped client get comfortable in a place with adequate lighting.	——	——	——	_____
3. Taught client how to properly clean urethral meatus.	——	——	——	_____
4. Taught female client how to insert catheter:				
a. Selected appropriate catheter.	——	——	——	_____
b. Helped client locate meatus.	——	——	——	_____
c. Placed outflow end of catheter in urine collection container or toilet, inserted catheter tip into meatus until urine began to flow.	——	——	——	_____

Copyright © 2018 by Elsevier Inc. All rights reserved.

	S	U	NP	Comments

5. Taught male client how to insert catheter:

   a. Selected appropriate catheter. ___ ___ ___ _____

   b. Lubricated tip of catheter with water-soluble jelly, rotated tip. ___ ___ ___ _____

   c. Placed outflow end of catheter into urine collection container or toilet bowl, inserted catheter into meatus until urine began to flow. ___ ___ ___ _____

6. Instructed client to hold catheter in place while urine flowed. ___ ___ ___ _____

7. Taught client to remove catheter when urine flow stopped and to perform hand hygiene. ___ ___ ___ _____

8. Gave client logbook to record amount of urine if needed. ___ ___ ___ _____

9. Instructed client to clean reusable catheter with soap and water immediately; rinsed catheter, allowed it to air dry, and stored it in dry towel or paper bag. ___ ___ ___ _____

10. Taught client to replace catheter at appropriate time. ___ ___ ___ _____

EVALUATION

1. Observed client/caregiver independently demonstrate technique for CISC. ___ ___ ___ _____

2. Asked client to identify plan for timing of CISC and steps to take when problems arise. ___ ___ ___ _____

3. Reviewed client's logbook, observed as client entered information. ___ ___ ___ _____

4. Asked patient to explain how to clean and store reusable catheter. ___ ___ ___ _____

5. Identified unexpected outcomes. ___ ___ ___ _____

RECORDING AND REPORTING

1. Recorded the information taught, client's response, and demonstration in home care record. ___ ___ ___ _____

2. Recorded urine output in home care record and logbook. ___ ___ ___ _____

3. Reported signs and symptoms of UTIs and difficulty performing CISC. ___ ___ ___ _____

Copyright © 2018 by Elsevier Inc. All rights reserved.

Student _____   Date _____

Instructor _____   Date _____

PERFORMANCE CHECKLIST SKILL 44.4   **USING HOME OXYGEN EQUIPMENT**

	S	U	NP	Comments
ASSESSMENT				
1. Identified client using at least two identifiers at hospital during first home visit.	___	___	___	_____
2. Determined client's or caregiver's ability to use oxygen equipment correctly while in hospital, assessed for appropriate use of equipment in home setting.	___	___	___	_____
3. Determined appropriate resource in community for equipment and assistance.	___	___	___	_____
4. Determined appropriate backup system in event of power failure, had space oxygen tank available.	___	___	___	_____
5. Assessed client's learning readiness and ability to concentrate, considered presence of pain, nausea, or fatigue and client interest in instruction.	___	___	___	_____
PLANNING				
1. Identified expected outcomes.	___	___	___	_____
2. Selected setting in home where client is most likely to use oxygen equipment, ensured client can see nurse clearly, controlled noise and distractions.	___	___	___	_____
IMPLEMENTATION				
1. Taught client/caregiver how to perform hand hygiene.	___	___	___	_____
2. Placed oxygen delivery system in appropriate environment.	___	___	___	_____
3. Demonstrated steps for preparation and maintenance of oxygen therapy:				
a. Compressed oxygen system.				
(1) Turned cylinder valve properly with wrench.	___	___	___	_____
(2) Checked pressure gauge on cylinder.	___	___	___	_____
(3) Stored wrench with oxygen tank.	___	___	___	_____
b. Oxygen concentrator system.				
(1) Plugged concentrator into appropriate outlet.	___	___	___	_____

Copyright © 2018 by Elsevier Inc. All rights reserved.

	S	U	NP	Comments

(2) Turned on power switch.

c. Liquid oxygen system.

   (1) Checked liquid system by reading dial on reservoir or tank.

   (2) Collaborated with DME provider to provide instruction in refilling ambulatory tank.

   (3) Taught to refill liquid oxygen tank.

     (a) Wiped both filling connectors clean.

     (b) Turned off flow selector of ambulatory unit.

     (c) Attached ambulatory unit to stationary reservoir properly.

     (d) Opened fill valve on ambulatory tank, applied pressure to top of stationary reservoir, stayed with unit while it filled.

     (e) Disconnected ambulatory unit from stationary reservoir when hissing changed and vapor cloud began to form.

     (f) Wiped both filling connectors clean.

4. Connected oxygen delivery device to oxygen delivery system.

5. Adjusted oxygen flow rate.

6. Had client/caregiver apply oxygen delivery device correctly, ensured client had two sets of delivery devices and tubing.

7. Instructed client not to change oxygen flow rate.

8. Had client/caregiver perform each step, provided written material for reinforcement or review.

9. Instructed client/caregiver to notify health care provider if signs of hypoxia or respiratory tract infection occurred.

10. Discussed emergency plans, had caregiver/client call 911 and notify health care provider and home care agency.

11. Instructed client in safe home oxygen practices.

EVALUATION

1. Monitored rate at which oxygen is being delivered.

2. Asked client/caregiver about ease or problems associated with home oxygen.

Copyright © 2018 by Elsevier Inc. All rights reserved.

	S	U	NP	Comments

3. Asked client/caregiver to state safety guidelines, emergency precautions, and emergency plan.   ___ ___ ___ _____

4. Asked client/caregiver to describe why oxygen is needed and signs of hypoxia.   ___ ___ ___ _____

5. Identified unexpected outcomes.   ___ ___ ___ _____

RECORDING AND REPORTING

1. Recorded teaching plan and information provided in home care record.   ___ ___ ___ _____

2. Communicated client's/caregiver's learning progress to other health care providers.   ___ ___ ___ _____

3. Recorded oxygen delivery system, related supplies, and prescribed oxygen flow rate in home care record.   ___ ___ ___ _____

4. Reported respiratory complications/concerns to health care provider.   ___ ___ ___ _____

Copyright © 2018 by Elsevier Inc. All rights reserved.

Student _____ Date _____

Instructor _____ Date _____

PERFORMANCE CHECKLIST SKILL 44.5 **TEACHING HOME TRACHEOSTOMY CARE AND SUCTIONING**

	S	U	NP	Comments

ASSESSMENT

1. Identified client using at least two identifiers during home visit.

2. Assessed client's/caregiver's ability to perform tracheostomy care and suctioning properly, assessed client's LOC and ability to problem solve.

3. Assessed client's/caregiver's knowledge of need to perform tracheostomy care and suctioning.

4. Assessed client's/caregiver's ability to assess pulse rate and respirations.

5. Assessed client's learning readiness and ability to concentrate; considered presence of pain, nausea, or fatigue and client interest in instruction.

6. Observed client/caregiver performing complete tracheostomy tube care and suctioning.

PLANNING

1. Identified expected outcomes.

2. Selected setting in home that was most likely to be used when completing tube care, ensured patient can see nurse clearly, controlled noise and distractions.

3. Discussed and demonstrated proper position for procedure.

IMPLEMENTATION

1. Suctioning:

   a. Verified health care provider's orders for suctioning, ensured client and caregiver understand suctioning order.

   b. Instructed client/caregiver on techniques for hand hygiene and application of clean gloves.

   c. Taught and demonstrated preparation and completion of tube suctioning.

   d. Taught client/caregiver to suction nasal and oral pharynx and perform mouth care, encouraged client/caregiver to brush teeth and use mouth and lip moisturizer at appropriate intervals.

   e. Had client take deep breaths at end of procedure to reassess lungs.

Copyright © 2018 by Elsevier Inc. All rights reserved.

	S	U	NP	Comments

f. Disconnected suction catheter, discarded catheter appropriately or set aside to be disinfected, removed and disposed of gloves properly, performed hand hygiene. _____ _____ _____ _____

2. Tracheostomy care:

 a. Had client sit at table with mirror, instructed client or caregiver how to perform hand hygiene and apply clean gloves, taught skills of tracheostomy care. _____ _____ _____ _____

 b. Had client/caregiver remove and discard gloves, performed hand hygiene. _____ _____ _____ _____

 c. Instructed client or caregiver to apply clean gloves, demonstrated technique for cleaning reusable supplies, rinsed and dried, stored supplies in labeled bag. _____ _____ _____ _____

 d. Had client or caregiver remove and discard gloves, performed hand hygiene. _____ _____ _____ _____

3. Explained procedure for disinfecting reusable supplies by boiling or soaking. _____ _____ _____ _____

4. Had client/caregiver perform each step with guidance. _____ _____ _____ _____

5. Taught client/caregiver signs of stoma infection, respiratory tract infection, and transesophageal fistula. _____ _____ _____ _____

EVALUATION

1. Observed client or caregiver demonstrate technique for tracheostomy tube care and suctioning. _____ _____ _____ _____

2. Asked client or caregiver to describe signs indicating need for tracheostomy care and suctioning and factors influencing tracheostomy airway functioning. _____ _____ _____ _____

3. Had client and caregiver explain problems that need to be reported to their health care provider. _____ _____ _____ _____

4. Asked client to describe signs for need to suction tracheostomy. _____ _____ _____ _____

5. Identified unexpected outcomes. _____ _____ _____ _____

RECORDING AND REPORTING

1. Recorded client instruction and accuracy of care demonstrated by client/caregiver. _____ _____ _____ _____

2. Developed system of recording home care for client/caregiver. _____ _____ _____ _____

Copyright © 2018 by Elsevier Inc. All rights reserved.

Student _____ Date _____

Instructor _____ Date _____

PERFORMANCE CHECKLIST SKILL 44.6 **TEACHING MEDICATION SELF-ADMINISTRATION**

	S	U	NP	Comments
ASSESSMENT				
1. Identified client using at least two identifiers during first home visit.	___	___	___	_____
2. Assessed client's cognitive, sensory, and motor function.	___	___	___	_____
3. Assessed resources client has to obtain medications.	___	___	___	_____
4. Assessed client's learning readiness and ability to concentrate.	___	___	___	_____
5. Assessed client's and caregiver's knowledge regarding medication therapy.	___	___	___	_____
6. Assessed client's belief in need for medication therapy.	___	___	___	_____
7. Assessed client's prescribed and OTC medications, included herbal supplements.	___	___	___	_____
8. Ensured caregiver knew client's drug allergies.	___	___	___	_____
9. Consulted with health care provider to review medications and simplify medications if possible.	___	___	___	_____
PLANNING				
1. Identified expected outcomes.	___	___	___	_____
2. Prepared environment for teaching session properly.	___	___	___	_____
3. Prepared proper teaching materials.	___	___	___	_____
4. Ensured client was wearing glasses or hearing aids if needed.	___	___	___	_____
5. Arranged teaching time to allow participation of family members.	___	___	___	_____
IMPLEMENTATION				
1. Instructed client/caregiver in importance of performing hand hygiene before medication administration.	___	___	___	_____
2. Presented information clearly and concisely.	___	___	___	_____

Copyright © 2018 by Elsevier Inc. All rights reserved.

	S	U	NP	Comments

3. Provided frequent pauses so client/caregiver could ask questions and express understanding.

4. Instructed client/caregiver on purpose of medications and desired effects, how medication works, schedules and rationale, side effects and relief from them, what to do if dose is missed, when to call health care provider, medication safety guidelines, and implications of not taking medication.

5. Instructed client in appropriate route of medication delivery.

6. Provided teaching sessions, planned several sessions if necessary.

7. Provided teaching about OTC medications and herbal supplements.

8. Provided client with written instructions for review, including charts, diagrams, learning aids, written information, and Internet resources.

9. Offered assistance as client practiced preparing medication.

10. Had pharmacy provide clear, large-print labels and teaching handouts if appropriate.

11. Had pharmacy provide containers client can open independently.

12. Facilitated arrangements for pharmacy to receive written prescriptions in a timely fashion, arranged for pharmacy to deliver medications to the home if necessary.

13. Discussed with client or caregiver how to dispose of discontinued or expired medications.

EVALUATION

1. Asked client/caregiver to explain information about each drug.

2. Asked client to describe when to call health care provider or refer to printed information for resources.

Copyright © 2018 by Elsevier Inc. All rights reserved.

	S	U	NP	Comments
3. Had client/caregiver prepare doses for all prescribed medication.	___	___	___	_____
4. Asked client to describe correct way to dispose of tablets at home.	___	___	___	_____
5. Identified unexpected outcomes.	___	___	___	_____

RECORDING AND REPORTING

	S	U	NP	Comments
1. Documented instruction provided and learning outcomes achieved by client in home record.	___	___	___	_____
2. Developed client/caregiver recording system for dosage schedules and self-monitoring of regimen.	___	___	___	_____
3. Left phone number and directions about how to reach home care nurse if needed.	___	___	___	_____

Copyright © 2018 by Elsevier Inc. All rights reserved.

Student _____ Date _____

Instructor _____ Date _____

PERFORMANCE CHECKLIST SKILL 44.7   **MANAGING FEEDING TUBES IN THE HOME**

	S	U	NP	Comments

ASSESSMENT

1. Identified client using at least two identifiers during first home visit.

2. Assessed client's health status and tolerance to enteral feedings.

3. Assessed client's/caregiver's physical, emotional, financial, and community resources.

4. Assessed environmental conditions of home.

5. Assessed client's/caregiver's understanding of purpose of enteral feedings and positive expected outcomes.

6. Assessed client's/caregiver's understanding of storage and management of equipment and supplies, as well as where and how to obtain supplies.

7. Assessed client's learning readiness, ability to concentrate, and learning style preference.

8. Assessed client's/caregiver's ability to manipulate feeding equipment.

PLANNING

1. Identified expected outcomes.

2. Prepared environment appropriately for teaching session.

IMPLEMENTATION

1. Had client/caregiver perform hand hygiene.

2. Discussed purpose of enteral feeding and enhanced nutritional health.

3. Assisted client/caregiver in determining feeding schedule that will maintain nutritional requirements and fit within client's or family's schedule.

4. Had client/caregiver apply clean gloves, demonstrated how to identify placement of feeding tube.

5. Observed client/caregiver in determining placement of nasally placed tube.

Copyright © 2018 by Elsevier Inc. All rights reserved.

	S	U	NP	Comments

6. Observed client/caregiver check for gastric residual volume, instructed to return aspirated contents to stomach if appropriate.

7. Discussed use of medical asepsis in setting up and changing administration sets, mixing and refrigerating formula, limiting formula "hung," and maintaining and caring for bag.

8. Instructed client/caregiver in how to position client properly for feeding or medications.

9. Observed client/caregiver mixing, administering, and storing formulas; discussed flushing of tube.

10. Observed client/caregiver change administration sets and clean bags, had him or her dispose of supplies, remove gloves, and perform hand hygiene.

11. Observed client/caregiver administering medications and flushing tube.

12. Discussed and observed use of infusion pump if necessary.

13. Discussed measures to stabilize feeding tube in clients.

14. Provided contact information for ordering equipment and supplies or who to call in case of equipment failure.

15. Discussed emergency plan and actions to take for signs and symptoms of aspiration.

16. Discussed who to contact and when for signs of diarrhea, constipation, or weight loss.

EVALUATION

1. Asked client or caregiver to state purpose of home enteral nutrition therapy.

2. Observed client/caregiver performing medical asepsis techniques, checking tube placement, aspirating residuals, administering medications and feedings, and using equipment.

3. Asked client/caregiver to state measures used to prevent complications.

4. Asked client/caregiver how to care for open formula cans.

5. Asked patient to describe how to manage nausea, stomach fullness or distention, and diarrhea.

6. Identified unexpected outcomes.

Copyright © 2018 by Elsevier Inc. All rights reserved.

	S	U	NP	Comments

RECORDING AND REPORTING

1. Recorded instructions given to client/caregiver and response in home care record.   ___ ___ ___ _____

2. Recorded specifics of enteral feeding plan.   ___ ___ ___ _____

3. Instructed client/caregiver in documentation needed.   ___ ___ ___ _____

Copyright © 2018 by Elsevier Inc. All rights reserved.

Student _____ Date _____

Instructor _____ Date _____

PERFORMANCE CHECKLIST SKILL 44.8 **MANAGING PARENTERAL NUTRITION IN THE HOME**

	S	U	NP	Comments

ASSESSMENT

1. Identified client using at least two identifiers during first home visit.   ___ ___ ___ _____

2. Assessed client's nutritional status and risk for malnutrition, identified signs of malnutrition, included measurement of vital signs.   ___ ___ ___ _____

3. Assessed client's fluid and electrolyte levels, serum albumin, total protein, transferrin, prealbumin, triglycerides, and glucose levels.   ___ ___ ___ _____

4. Assessed client's venous access device for edema, drainage, tenderness, and signs of inflammation; measured circumference and marked arm if necessary.   ___ ___ ___ _____

5. Verified health care provider's order for PN.   ___ ___ ___ _____

6. Assessed client's learning readiness, anxiety and ability to concentrate, and learning style preference.   ___ ___ ___ _____

7. Assessed client's/caregiver's previous knowledge and experience in managing PN in the home, had client/caregiver perform return demonstration if able.   ___ ___ ___ _____

PLANNING

1. Identified expected outcomes.   ___ ___ ___ _____

2. Selected setting in home where client was most likely to administer PN and is conducive to teaching session.   ___ ___ ___ _____

IMPLEMENTATION

1. Provided name and phone number of resources available if problems arise.   ___ ___ ___ _____

2. Explained type of infusion, volume and infusion rate, expected outcomes, and components of PN; explained that PN needs to be stored in refrigerator.   ___ ___ ___ _____

3. Had client/caregiver perform each step with guidance, did not rush client.   ___ ___ ___ _____

4. Instructed client/caregiver to inspect label of bag, ensured bag was not expired or leaking.   ___ ___ ___ _____

Copyright © 2018 by Elsevier Inc. All rights reserved.

	S	U	NP	Comments

5. Suggested taking PN solution out of refrigerator 30 to 60 minutes before scheduled infusion time. ___ ___ ___ _____

6. Explained need to inspect fluid in bag for color and precipitates. ___ ___ ___ _____

7. Had client/caregiver perform hand hygiene and apply gloves; demonstrated how to attach IV tubing and filter, how to prime tubing, and how to load tubing into electronic infusion pump. ___ ___ ___ _____

8. Wiped CVC port with alcohol, showed how to flush CVC and connect tubing to port, used needleless system whenever possible. ___ ___ ___ _____

9. Explained how to determine appropriate rate of infusion and program infusion pump. ___ ___ ___ _____

10. Had client/caregiver remove and dispose of gloves and perform hand hygiene. ___ ___ ___ _____

11. Explained how to disconnect tubing and flush CVC, ensured client/caregiver performed hand hygiene. ___ ___ ___ _____

12. Described appropriate use and storage of infusion pump and supplies, explained tubing replacement schedules. ___ ___ ___ _____

13. Helped in developing plan for appropriate disposal of supplies. ___ ___ ___ _____

14. Demonstrated appropriate care of CVC site, discussed dressing changes and signs of infection. ___ ___ ___ _____

15. Taught client/caregiver about signs and symptoms indicating complications from PN therapy and when to call for help. ___ ___ ___ _____

16. Demonstrated use of self–blood glucose monitor; explained frequency of testing, normal glucose values, and what to do if values fall outside expected range. ___ ___ ___ _____

17. Provided client with logbook to record administration of PN, weights, I&O, and blood glucose levels. ___ ___ ___ _____

18. Helped client develop a plan to reorder supplies, an emergency plan, and a home safety plan. ___ ___ ___ _____

EVALUATION

1. Had client/caregiver independently demonstrate initiation, infusion, and discontinuation of PN infusion, as well as CVC site care. ___ ___ ___ _____

2. Watched client clean and store PN, equipment, and supplies. ___ ___ ___ _____

Copyright © 2018 by Elsevier Inc. All rights reserved.

	S	U	NP	Comments

3. Asked client/caregiver to identify expected outcomes.

4. Had client or caregiver independently demonstrate blood glucose monitoring and recording.

5. Watched client record information in logbook, reviewed book periodically.

6. Asked client to describe signs and symptoms of infection.

7. Identified unexpected outcomes.

RECORDING AND REPORTING

1. Recorded information taught, client's response, and outcomes of PN therapy in home care record.

2. Recorded appearance of CVC site, infusions, glucose monitoring results, and client's weight in home logbook.

Copyright © 2018 by Elsevier Inc. All rights reserved.